EATING YOUR WAY TO HEALTH

RUTH KUNZ-BIRCHER is the daughter of
Dr. M. O. Bircher-Benner, founder of the
celebrated Bircher-Benner Clinic in Switzerland. She was born in Zurich in 1902.
Abandoning a successful career as a con-
cert violinist, she assumed direction of the
clinic in 1944 and continues to guide it
today. Her husband, Dr. Alfred Kunz-
Bircher, is head of the clinic's chemical
and diagnostic department. Dr. Ralph
Bircher, Ruth Kunz-Bircher's brother, is a
graduate of Zurich University and the
author of numerous studies on the history
and geography of nutrition. In 1952, he
founded the Bircher-Benner Verlag, pub-
lisher of books on food and health. Dr.
Dagmar Liechti-von Brasch is the niece of
Dr. M. O. Bircher-Benner. After her gradu-
ation from medical school, she studied
with him and, since 1947, has served as
the clinic's medical director.

RUTH KUNZ-BIRCHER

DAGMAR LIECHTI-VON BRASCH

RALPH BIRCHER

ALFRED KUNZ-BIRCHER

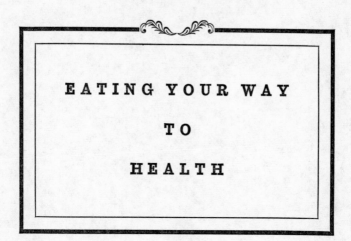

EATING YOUR WAY

TO

HEALTH

PENGUIN BOOKS INC.

BALTIMORE • MARYLAND

Penguin Books Inc
7110 Ambassador Road
Baltimore, Maryland 21207, U.S.A.

Original English translation and edition
© Ruth Bircher and Claire Loewenfeld, 1961

This American version © Penguin Books, 1972

Published in Penguin Books 1972

Library of Congress Catalogue Card Number 70–172530

Printed in the United States of America
by Kingsport Press, Inc., Kingsport, Tennessee

Set in Linotype Primer

Typography by Martin Connell

IMPORTANT

★

The recipes marked D are suitable for Diet Menus
(see *Low-Fat Diet*, p. 308).
Where necessary, a modification is clearly given.

★

CONTENTS

PART III

SPECIAL DIET SUGGESTIONS

Dr. M. O. Bircher-Benner (1867–1939) has long been accepted as one of the great pioneers of the science of dietetics. His Clinic, founded in 1897, situated on a hill overlooking the lake and town of Zurich, has gradually become a Mecca for sick people and dieticians of all nationalities.

On what is this reputation based? At the start of his career in 1891, Dr. Bircher himself certainly had no idea of the direction in which his work would develop. For a few years he ran his flourishing medical practice in the orthodox manner, until one day a woman came to him suffering from a gastric disorder. No treatment had been able to help her; she had gradually become worse and worse until finally she was able to digest scarcely any food. A friend suggested a diet of raw vegetables and fruit, and to everyone's amazement she recovered completely.

It was only five years later that Bircher, after having studied the question from every angle, even taking lessons from leading scientists, found an explanation for this first of many amazing cures. He came to the conclusion that it was the high quality of food energy obtained from the very freshest food, in a state as near as possible to the living state, that was of vital importance. The deterioration of foodstuffs, generally taking place during cooking and other processing, was at the root of many evils.

His ideas were at first contemptuously dismissed by his colleagues. But, unperturbed by such criticism, Bircher continued to treat his patients in his expanding Clinic, where he was putting his own ideas into practice by keeping patients and every item of their diet under constant observation and demanding of them that they give up their old eating habits and 'return to nature' in the truest sense of the word.

Many of the things for which Bircher fought have become a matter of course for us today, for like many great men he was in advance of his time. Long before his contemporaries he recognized the value of vitamins, the vital influence of nutrition on health, and the supreme importance of fresh foods of all kinds. His ideas continued to expand and to find a hearing even after his death in 1939, for they are not founded on any fashionable craze, but are based on fundamental principles.

With this new diet and cookery book we want to help patients who have frequently expressed the wish to be initiated into the present-day secrets of the cuisine of the Bircher-Benner Clinic, in order to use at home a knowledge and experience obtained during their time at Zurich. This is the third diet cook book to be published containing recipes and menus of the Bircher-Benner school. The first was in 1907 (4 editions), the second in 1926 (32 editions)—the English edition was published by Arnold under the title *Health-giving Dishes* —and now it has become imperative to adapt these recipes to the changed conditions of today. The endeavors of both the medical staff and management in constant co-operation to improve on the combination of dietetic and culinary values in the preparation of menus, have created a new situation. All recipes and menus have been changed since the last book, *Health-giving Dishes,* was published. Recipes have been added, others omitted, while menus of a festive as well as of an austere character have also been added. A new paragraph on the feeding of children and detailed directions on diets for certain chronic conditions widen the scope of the book considerably. Since Dr. Bircher's death in 1939, dietetics has gone through many a change and many a development but we who have been able to study his ideas from the beginning are constantly surprised and impressed to find how they are confirmed time after time by the general scientific development and the experience of doctors and former patients.

My thanks are due to my sister, Mrs. Betty Favaretto-Bircher; my cousin, Dr. Dagmar Liechti-von Brasch; my brother, Dr. Ralph Bircher; and my husband, Dr. Alfred Kunz, for their valuable co-operation; and to Miss Bosshard, housekeeper at our Clinic, and Miss Keller, head cook, who were of great assistance to me in compiling the menus and working out the recipes.

RUTH KUNZ-BIRCHER

Zurich, Switzerland,
Spring, 1954

A great deal of interest seems to have been caused by the previous editions of this book. Many letters reached us reporting on an improvement in health gained through a change of diet carried out with the help offered in this book. They expressed satisfaction about the feeling of confidence which grew steadily when following the directions. We have also received valuable suggestions which have been incorporated in this new edition. For all this I would like to express my gratitude.

I should also like to point out the purpose of this book. It is, firstly, intended to introduce our contemporaries to a still unknown culinary art and guide them into a new realm of enjoyable meals. It is intended to familiarize them with how one can best preserve the natural properties of food as one goes about its daily preparation. It is also intended to guide people out of the danger zone of ill health, stress and strain, disease and possible breakdown by renewing the physical basis of personality and thus providing new strength and fresh resources with which to tackle their lives.

Today it is of vital import that people with insight realize and practice this health-giving change in food habits for themselves, for their families, in the hotels they run for other people, and in their hospitals. In recent times there has been a marked increase in warnings against the exhaustion of one's vital force. They confirm the warnings which my father gave more than sixty years ago. His suggestions for averting this danger, expressed in the introduction of this book in a more contemporary way, have found new confirmation. They have also been demonstrated at the exhibition of Modern Food and Diet in the HOSPES 1954 (International Cookery Exhibition in Berne, Switzerland). They aroused much interest, and the technique taught in this book was awarded a gold medal.

The resolutions of the Scientific Council of the International Society for Research into Vital Substances and Nutrition, meeting in the years 1955–6–7–8, were influenced by the theories on which the book is based.

During one of the first Conferences of this Society I was

surprised and very delighted to learn that a Bircher-Benner medal had been created as an appreciation of my father's lifelong pioneer work in the field of nutrition. The first medal was presented to Dr. W. Kollath for his services in bringing about changes in general nutrition. Dr. Kollath, in a broadcast on 19 January 1958, gave a serious warning of the danger in which Western humanity will find itself if people continue with their present methods of feeding. If they will not, with speed and energy, change over to a healthier, more balanced diet, they will find themselves confronted with the greater strength and vitality of the Eastern people. Does it help us when the many new discoveries in medicine extend life a few years, if these years gained are spent in a weakened condition, a twilight zone of health, and in fear before the increasing number of chronic illnesses of our time? We should not forget also that in a healthy virile body, the mind can develop more fully.

A decisive change of attitude is urgently needed and as a practical guide to this, it might be said there is, perhaps, none better than this book. It is in this hope that a more detailed theoretical introduction than is usual with cookbooks, has been given here before the actual recipes. Those already convinced of the book's basic principles will tend to start immediately on the practical sections and perhaps rarely refer to the theory. However, even those long familiar with these matters may be interested to read that modern knowledge is already beginning to provide a basis for and explanation of our theory. Then there are those who have until now only known the orthodox feeding methods, and those who are already bewildered by the contradictions of the varying unorthodox schools of thought and would like to know once and for all what to do. Both should first carefully study the introductory chapters.

It has not, of course, been possible within the scope of this book to discuss everything in detail, but perhaps the reader can feel that there is behind each statement many years' experience in the crusade for healthier food and the re-education of the palate to enjoy natural foods; this experience is backed by our continuous contact with the medical and dietetic research of many countries and a long experience in teaching these methods. The study of physiological and clinical results in the field of nutrition in many countries has been pursued in order to compare them with our results and our approach and there has always been unbiased study of different, even controversial, teaching to examine and learn from this. All this has been done for more than sixty years and at present it is carried out through the co-operation of doctors, biochemists, an economist and last, but not least, cookery experts in the kitchen. Though some of the principles are given without cumbersome detail the reader should know that these have all been carefully examined and evaluated and that we are always ready to provide more information if required.

We hope the fact that French, Italian, Dutch, Portuguese and English editions have been published, and that this American edition has now appeared, proves that the book has been useful to people in different countries.

And now, dear reader, will you help in the great undertaking of rebuilding health for yourself, your family and your nation?

RUTH KUNZ-BIRCHER

NOTE

The increasing recognition for the Bircher-Benner school of thought in dietetics is shown by official awards during the last years:

Golden Medal of the Department 'Modern Nutrition and Diet', of the International Cooking Exhibition 'Hospes' 1954 in Berne, Switzerland.

Golden Bircher-Benner Medal created by the 'International Society for Research into Vital Substances and Nutrition' in 1956; this medal was awarded in 1958 to Dr. W. Kollath, in 1961 to Dr. Clive McCay (Cornell University), in 1964 to Dr. Fritz Eichholtz (University of Heidelberg) and in 1967 to Dr. Silverio Palafox (University of Madrid).

GENERAL INTRODUCTION

by DR. RALPH BIRCHER

The Bircher-Benner Clinic in Zurich, Switzerland, birthplace of this book, is the center from which (to quote a recent official handbook) fresh stimuli, important for the development of dietetics, have emerged time and again during the past fifty years.

There are, of course, already a number of cookery books dealing with the Bircher and similar 'cuisines', with or without additions and omissions. They are all based on ideas which came originally from this Clinic and we are indebted to them for their work as they have, no doubt, helped to spread the idea of wholesome foods and their preparation. We hope that this new book will provide fresh ideas: the results of medical experience and research in the Clinic combined with new cookery possibilities offered by improved kitchen methods and new ways of marketing. The physician's task is to maintain the vital, curative and regenerative quality of nutrition; that of the kitchen—by contrast—to provide tempting food of a quality acceptable to the gourmets of many countries who may have to be asked to renounce cherished habits. The authors of this book—standing midway between these two viewpoints—have had the difficult task of combining both aims, while doing justice to each of them. The pages of recipes will show how this has been carried out.

It should be a simple matter to eat in such a way that the greatest possible health of body and spirit results. Consider, for instance, the Hunza people, whose food was plain and wholesome until recently, and who enjoyed magnificent health. Alternatively, if one could return to the frugal eating habits of the early Greeks and Romans, or to those of the ancient Swiss at the time the Federation was founded (in many respects similar to the principles on which this book is based), one would soon feel the resurgence of vitality, resulting in new powers of resistance and energy.

1

We are, however, living in the twentieth century. We cannot go back, we must go forward. Compared with the ancient Swiss, with the early Greeks and Romans or with the Hunzas, we are not only pampered but are more dependent on civilization: we live in a world full of social and business obligations. It is essential, therefore, that the new nutrition, despite its simplicity and closeness to nature, be more discriminating and attractive than even the best 'cuisine' of the 'old school', otherwise conversion will never be complete.

This book will, we believe, make it easy to solve this apparent paradox. 'This way it's certainly not hard to accept the new ideas. It is not difficult to give up sweet things, spirits, coffee and even meat. I have practically no craving for them as long as I am given such food as I find here.' Similar remarks are constantly made to me. Our patients find that their palate is satisfied in a novel, pleasing manner and that they have an agreeable feeling of satiety without the sensation of heaviness so commonly associated with it.

Invalid diet as laid down by Dr. Bircher-Benner has now been introduced into many clinics and hospitals and used by many physicians. Even greater use would be made of it, however, if its introduction were easier and did not depend to such an extent on the goodwill and understanding of those responsible for carrying it out. A diet cannot be prescribed in the same manner as a drug. We have repeatedly found that clinics and hospitals farsighted enough to send someone competent to us for training beforehand, someone able to study at first hand for an adequate period the application of this system, subsequently obtained excellent results that confirmed our own experience. In cases where its introduction was attempted without such thorough personal training, it was usually unsuccessful or the results inconclusive. This book cannot, of course, wholly serve as a substitute for such personal contact, but should prove a valuable aid.

Nevertheless, this is not intended as a book for invalid diet but as a textbook for the teaching of a *natural, whole-food diet* which can help the healthy as well as the convalescent and those of indifferent health. This diet can prevent illness by increasing resistance and can help one withstand the diseases of old age. It can also be immensely useful to the average person who is concerned about the current devitalization of over-packaged, chemically preserved food and is trying to discover a healthier way to eat (and thus live).

This basic *normal diet* has been adapted in this book, for the first time, to meet various circumstances and requirements— for everyday life; for festive occasions; for the smallest of

purses; for busy housewives; for the most elaborate and so-
phisticated cooking; for brain and manual workers; for children and adults and (what is fundamentally new), for certain
types of people with delicate, susceptible or weakened constitutions and decreased organic functions. It thus serves as a long-
term guide to carrying out conscientiously medical diet prescriptions.

It is sometimes stated that such a 'normal diet' may well suit
women and those with a sedentary occupation, but that men,
particularly athletes and manual workers, require more concentrated and sustaining food, by which is generally meant
meat, fish, eggs and so on. This is a great mistake. Their efficiency usually does not suffer in the least; on the contrary,
after a period of transition it is even increased if they follow
the precepts laid down in this book. This has been proved by
exhaustive scientific tests. Even laborers, who carry heavy
loads every day, can benefit from this diet.

It is probable that anyone embarking on so great a change
will meet many difficulties—the prejudices of his family, his
own many cherished habits and, very often, temporary reactions to the eliminating processes which he is likely at first to
misinterpret.

So many of us have unconscious cravings and an eternal
greed typical of the 'hunger pangs' of mankind. Yet at the same
time there is a latent but powerful desire for fresh vitality.
These problems may be helped by a careful study of the following summary and the book should be of service to those who
follow its teaching intelligently.

THE INFLUENCE OF NUTRITION ON HEALTH

Health and disease depend on a number of factors—climate,
hygiene, exercise, disposition, nutrition, heredity, etc., and not
least on psychological influences. Each of them has its own in-
trinsic importance which may predominate. However, on the
whole nutrition often has the greatest and most decisive influence. In a damp unhygienic home devoid of light, health and
powers of resistance can be built up with suitable nutrition;
whilst in the sunniest home, in spite of meticulous cleanliness
and abundant exercise, health can be undermined and ruined
by incorrect food. We can see for ourselves, looking around us,
the truth of this statement and find it confirmed again and
again in investigations. It is therefore worth making every en-
deavor to restore health by means of nutrition.

Constant Friction will wear away a Stone

It is those seemingly unimportant eating habits, regularly repeated, which decisively influence health, not the occasional lapses. The regular consumption of devitalized food which has been overprocessed (and is thus far from its natural state) and too rich food, may impair health: partly by over-stimulating the nervous system with the help of toxins (tea, coffee, cocoa, hot chocolate, soft drinks, alcohol, tobacco and uric acid) and partly by supplying a one-sided food, that is, one which is too highly concentrated and is devoid of essential nutrients and important active principles (pastries, cakes, candies—in fact, any 'food' with excess sugar. 200 grams of sugar raise the adrenalin level by 30 to 120 per cent within 5 to 20 minutes. Excess protein, too, as found in meat and fish, can be harmful). A healthy organism can deal with these foods as an occasional exception, but not if they become a daily habit. In the case of invalid diet, however, no compromises or exceptions should be made: for the healthy, the art of cooking should facilitate the necessary change in eating habits.

Civilization and Nutrition

The consumption of food is not of a merely animal nature, but an act that requires all our attention. Correct and careful nutrition may greatly influence our thoughts and emotions, a fact known to the wise men of all ages. A different attitude towards nutrition may lead to a more mature personality with a change in spiritual outlook. At the end of his life Dr. Bircher-Benner wrote from his insight and experience these words: 'To concern oneself about one's body or one's nutrition is of no avail unless a new awakening, a new awareness of one's inner forces results. The wonders of the spirit remain a closed book to those who constantly disregard the laws of nutrition. The force and depth of inner experience depend on nutrition to an inconceivable extent.'

What is Meant by 'Raw Foods'?

Fresh, unspoiled plant food from healthy soil has unequalled health-promoting powers. This is a fact which has been proved by prolonged clinical experience and in the most painstaking tests. It may be because such nutrition is the ancient and original food of man, for the absorption of which our organism was primarily constructed. Fresh, vital raw foods restore the conditions essential to life, and will relieve and regenerate the regulative systems and that of the endocrine glands. This nutrition at the source, where as yet no contamination or devitalization can have taken place, preserves the natural wholeness of foods and their rare qualities. The treatment of many a disease demands, according to our experience, an almost complete return to such primary nutrition for a short time. This is something which must be done under a doctor's supervision and generally for a brief period only. For the regeneration of vitality in the healthy, however, a milder régime is sufficient. For such a daily diet *it is enough if half of the daily intake should consist of raw foods*.

WHY RAW FOOD AT THE START OF EVERY MEAL?

What is it that gives uncooked foods their particular health value as compared with heated or cooked foods? What distinguishes the fresh apple from the cooked, fresh milk from pasteurized or boiled milk? Though the results of our clinical experience answer these questions daily for us, the theoretical answers cannot yet be stated in short, simple terms. Too much of the total picture is still unknown but a number of individual factors have already come to light and are presented here for those who are really interested in the reasons.

A large number of chemical and physical properties, the significance of which has as yet not been properly investigated, are altered by heat, and some important vitamins are lost (Vitamin C, P, folic acid, and in part Vitamin A), vitamins that are important for the healthy functioning of the endocrine glands, the mucous membranes, the blood vessels, the cell walls and the formation of blood. Food that has to be cooked before being eaten should be steamed, since many minerals and trace elements (for example, iodine, larger quantities of which are necessary for the development of the intellect than for the prevention of goiter) are lost in the water in which the food has been boiled.

However, all the foregoing provides only a partial explanation of the curative effect of raw foods. Chemical analysis throws little light on the subject and calculation of the calories none whatever. Furthermore, heating also destroys the numerous enzymes present in the plant cells. As has recently been found, these enzymes perform two functions that offer a further explanation for the curative effect of raw foods. To start with, they produce, as it were, a self-digestion of the raw food within the intestinal tract, thus relieving the digestive glands. Previously it was doubted whether the enzymes reached the colon in an efficient state, it has now been shown that 60–80 per cent of them arrive there unimpaired and—by oxygen fixation—establish anaerobic conditions in the intestinal tract, the medium in which the beneficial coli bacteria grow and multiply, and thus drive away the pathogenic ones. Both these factors are of tremendous importance for health and would in themselves be sufficient to merit raw foods having a special place of honor. But this is not all. Special aromatic substances in uncooked foods appear to be responsible for preventing the 'digestive leucocytosis', unavoidable when cooked food is consumed. Leucocytosis is a mobilization of white blood corpuscles and their concentration in the walls of the intestines. Even if cooked food is eaten afterwards this leucocytosis fails to materialize, provided a sufficient portion of raw food was eaten at the beginning of the meal. The absence of leucocytosis frees the white blood corpuscles for other tasks, saves the body the effort of a defensive action and therefore strengthens the powers of resistance to disease. Hence the Bircher-Benner maxim: *Begin each meal with raw food. Raw food before, not after, the cooked food.*

THE ACTION OF RAW FOODS ON CELL TISSUES

All the foregoing phenomena, the loss of vitamins sensitive to heat and of mineral substances, the importance of the specific enzymes for the intestinal bacteria and the aromatic substance for preventing digestive leucocytosis, are nevertheless insufficient to explain what is actually the chief effect of raw foods, the increase of micro-electric tension in the cell tissue of the whole body, discovered by the Viennese school investigating permeability. Raw plant nutrition alone is capable of producing this. With the increase of micro-electric tension, cell respiration improves, cell metabolism is stimulated, the powers of resistance and cell renewal increase, metabolism as a whole proceeds more economically, and all natural healing processes are intensified. The most recent Japanese researches at the University of Kyushu have shown that raw plant foods prevent even hunger edema and hunger anemia, and that they strengthen the powers of resistance in the blood in its fight against disease-producing agents.

ANOTHER MAXIM—GREEN LEAVES DAILY

We maintain that green vegetables, and in particular leafy green vegetables, benefit health to a greater extent than any other food. Chlorophyll, the green coloring matter of plants, is becoming an object of ever-increasing interest to doctors on ac-

count of its apparently inexhaustible fund of curative properties. It promotes the formation of red blood cells better than
iron therapy, stimulates respiration and nitrogen metabolism
of the cell tissues, improves utilization of protein, normalizes
blood-pressure, reduces insulin requirements, improves circulation, increases the healing tendency in tuberculosis, causes
unpleasant body odor to disappear, heals wounds and improves
thyroid activity. The green leaf restores a favorable acid-
alkaline balance of the ashes after combustion of foods more
rapidly and effectively than anything else could do. It supplies
a protein of extremely high biological value which supplements, even in minute quantities, that of cereal food, also a
great variety of vitamins in correct proportions, particularly
Vitamins A, C and the folic acids. At a time when the green
leaf was universally despised, Dr. Bircher-Benner recognized
its significance and recommended that it be given a place of
honor in the daily menu, particularly in its fresh form as raw
vegetable salad. Since he was aware of its importance and wit-
nessed how it was despised by his contemporaries, he searched
for methods of preparation to make it palatable and attractive.
The results will be found in this book. *Whenever and however
possible: No day without green leaves.*

BREAD AND OTHER CEREAL FOODS

Whole-grain nutrition is also of decisive value for health.
Cereals are indeed one of the principal foods in our daily diet.
Many particularly healthy and resilient races have lived mainly
on bread or a dish of whole groats and grain, like porridge or
frumenty. Foods made of finely milled flour are also known to
them but are given their proper place, that is, used for special
occasions. The introduction and subsequently all too plentiful
use in everyday life of these festive and refined forms of cereal
food began some fifty or a hundred years ago. They have con-
tributed more than anything else to the degeneration of the
constitution, and especially of the teeth. Thus return to whole-
grain foods as part of the daily menu would inestimably benefit
general health. Separation of bran from the grain reduces its
content of the entire Vitamin B group and Vitamin E to such
an extent that it is very difficult to restore the original balance.
Only whole-grain foods can supply this. They help to preserve
youthful freshness in old age and the healthy balance of the
intestinal bacterial flora. The germ of the grain is of prime
importance: anyone buying whole-grain products should make
sure that it is present. It is the germ which gives the delicate,
nutty flavor and it is this flavor which makes it easier to give

up white flour products. Many recipes for whole-grain dishes will be found in this book.

SEASONING

In this book seasoning is suggested in a different manner from what is usual in present-day 'homely' fare, or still more in hotel cooking. Cooking salt, strong condiments, or a heap of sugar disguise the natural taste of food, blunt the palate and distort the normal appetite by titillating the palate to an even greater consumption of food and drink. Continued excess can lead to ill health, which in turn can suddenly cause disease. Skilful additions of aromatic herbs, a little sea salt and practically no ordinary salt, on the other hand, emphasize and enrich the natural taste.

Not more than a bare level teaspoonful of salt—and this preferably in the form of sea salt—should be taken and not more than 1 level tablespoonful of refined sugar per day, unless brown sugar or honey can be used for sweetening. Raw salad foods should be prepared without any salt at all. Pungent spices, such as pepper, mustard, ginger, curry or paprika, should be used as an exception, if at all, and then only in the most minute quantity. In their stead, use is made of natural herbs, sea salt and valuable yeast flavorings, such as Marmite, Savita or similar products to which no cooking salt is added. Instructions on the subject are given in this book. It is surprising how the sense of taste will then change and gain by the appreciation of natural flavors.

MEAT—OUR POINT OF VIEW

No meat is served in the Bircher-Benner Clinic since it is our opinion and experience that it does not assist the recovery of health. The resident patient will benefit by this experience for his whole life, for he will see how well nourished one can be, and how well people can feel without meat, and will realize that perfectly balanced menus are possible without it. Present-day cookery in Europe and the United States is still entirely centered around meat as the chief part of any meal; everything else appears to the trained chef or expert housewife as a supplement to a menu. A complete change of ideas is wanted here, for no type of food can lead to such harmful eating habits as meat. We have seen again and again that a diet containing a good deal of meat will tempt most people to eat more. As the intake of food nowadays is altogether far above the physiological requirements, it is often necessary to get a patient used to a reduced intake for the improvement of a condition. This can usually be achieved more successfully if meat is omitted.

Statistical investigation by the Swiss Commission on Food in War has demonstrated the general effect of meat in increasing the appetite and so the intake of food altogether. In contrast to this, many slimming diets do use relatively large quantities of meat with the object of diminishing the general desire for food. This has, however, been considered a fallacy and a return has been made to slimming diets which are based on a small intake of protein. Also in America it is believed that 'the prescription of "high protein diets" increases the tendency of eating too much instead of reducing this tendency as it was expected.' The low protein diets improved results considerably.

Our point of view has been strengthened by the newest modern development—the industrialization of meat, fish and egg production. This has resulted in a much more strained and diseased metabolism in the animals and an often prohibitively high load of toxins, antibiotics and pesticides. Furthermore, osteoporosis (weakening of bones and cartilages), a widespread and distressing disorder found in affluent populations, has been traced mainly to excess meat consumption (See A. Wachman and D. S. Bernstein, *Harvard Lancet* 7, 549 and 956, "Diet and Osteoporosis").

We have constantly seen a meatless and fishless diet to be more successful in bringing about that change which causes the palate to return to natural food instincts as it becomes accustomed to less strong seasoning. We lay great stress on this readjustment of the palate because it is an important aid to a lasting improvement. Some doctors and hospitals, in taking over our diet, have tried to 'improve on it' by adding meat. This, however, has always resulted in reducing rather than increasing the effects. In order to bring about such a major readjustment of the diet the whole menu must be built up differently. Meat should appear only as an accessory, or as an exception. From our point of view the healthy may occasionally add meat and fish to their normal diet if they wish. They will find suitable recipes elsewhere. None has been included here, but a variety of suggestions for planning meals without meat can be found in the chapter on menus.

DAIRY PRODUCTS

We consider milk an addition to the diet, not a main food. Its reputation as an 'ideal form of nourishment' is merited only within limits, provided healthy cows are fed on organi-

cally grown grass and it can be used unboiled and preferably
unpasteurized. In many countries it comes from animals kept
under unnatural conditions, wrongly fed and frequently diseased, and may only be drunk after boiling or pasteurizing.
Such milk lacks too many of those therapeutic qualities for it
to be included in any remedial diet. In normal diet it plays the
part of a valuable supplement, particularly as a means of supplying easily digested protein of excellent biological value
with a high calcium and Vitamin B_{12} content. It also facilitates
the preparation of other foods. The same applies to milk products. We prefer mild cottage cheese to the matured, salted
kinds; yogurt, sour milk and butter-milk to boiled cow's milk
(mainly on account of its fermenting properties and consequently favorable effect on the intestinal bacteria). The
preferably unsalted butter used should be fresh (see section
'Fats and Oils,' dealing with butter, vegetable fats and oils, p.
18).

SOIL FERTILIZATION

It cannot be a matter of indifference whether food has been
grown on healthy, humus-rich soil or in a field that has been
deprived of all its humus and trace elements, or has even been
treated with chemicals or liquid animal manure only. To ensure the growth of wholesome plant tissue and also for protec-
tion against disease, cultivated plants and vegetables require
a balanced, slow, steady feeding of nutritious substances
which humus-rich soil alone can guarantee.

It has been shown in many countries that enriching the soil
with good humus, combined with balancing the ecological factors in agriculture, restores the resistance of plants to plant
diseases, pests and fungi after three to four years. Heavy
chemical fertilizing (in widespread use today) has been
proved to deplete the soil of humus (a regulator), which in
turn causes prevalence of disease and pests. The increase of
plant diseases necessitates the increased use of poison sprays
with its implicit risk to human health. (See *Silent Spring* by
Rachel Carson.)

The difference between the two types of fertilization becomes apparent in the keeping qualities of the products, in
their flavor and their remedial qualities. Whenever possible,
therefore, we make use of vegetables fertilized with compost
for our patients' menus. In this respect the safest method of
all is to supply one's needs from one's own garden, from absolutely fresh and ripe fruit and vegetables. We are trying, in
particular, not to use green vegetables which have been treated

with chemicals, especially with nitrogen, and make every effort to replace them by those which have been compost grown.

How Much Food Do We Need?

A well-balanced diet with a large proportion of uncooked food seems to be more economically utilized by the system; by this greater economy in the working of the metabolism, the protein, fat and carbohydrate intake go further. This deliberate economy is one of our aims; it conserves strength and protects the organs from premature depreciation and enables us to remain youthful and supple, even in old age. Consequently most metabolic processes function very wastefully and the organism becomes prematurely aged and diseased.

'Too much food,' as Dr. Bircher-Benner taught us, 'improves neither health nor efficiency but, on the contrary, leads to premature old age and illness.' It can now be estimated to what extent average over-consumption of food has become a habit as a result of devitalized nutrition. Careful tests have shown that about half as much again is eaten than is either necessary or expedient in order to maintain health and efficiency. Furthermore, investigations carried out for twenty years at the McCay School of Cornell University showed that the prevention of senile disease, the prolongation of life, and the retention of youthful vigor in old age (if natural food is eaten) depend on avoiding such over-consumption.

The art of cooking, therefore, should not consist, as is customary today, of offering dishes containing too many concentrated foods that pass as rapidly as possible into the bloodstream. People should not be induced to eat and drink too much, but rather the reverse. All foods should and must be rich in natural fluids, in fibrous bulk, vitamins and mineral salts, but not particularly rich in calories. A pleasant sensation of satiety should follow as soon as the limit of capacity is reached.

We must also select foods with a protracted satiation curve —that is, foods which will keep us satisfied over a long period —to stifle any longing for snacks between meals. For instance, wholewheat dishes and uncooked fruit dishes have such a curve, whereas the usual Continental breakfast with coffee and white rolls has a short, rapidly falling one. The American breakfast, on the other hand, contains too many calories and over-concentrated foods (e.g. eggs) but nevertheless, owing to its quickly falling curve, requires a coffee break during the morning. Consideration has also been given to this point in the recipes and menus to be found later. Experience has repeatedly shown that the kind of meals we advocate lead to prompt and agreeable satisfaction of appetite without any feeling of heaviness. They also relieve the innate greed plaguing so many people and the longing for food between meals.

THE SENSE OF TASTE AWAKES

Nature has provided us with a wonderfully delicate and precise organ with which to select our food correctly—the palate. But today it is hardly given a chance. We devour what is put before us, at the same time thinking of many other things during a meal. And yet, as a fundamental biological function of primary importance, eating requires calm and serious concentration. The palate should be given the chance to test and appraise the taste of the food. If this happens regularly it will gradually be noticed that, apart from the overpowering, but fleeting, first sensation of taste, a second more intensive but also more subtle one—caused by fresh and unprocessed foods—will come to the fore. The basic nutritional instinct with which man was originally equipped in the same way as animals, but which has continually been submerged by stimulants, will then awake. It is a reliable guide to the return to wholesome food.

'INCOMPATIBLE' FOODS

Some nature-cure régimes disapprove of the use of certain groups of foods at one and the same meal, and consider them unwholesome. These teachings are to some extent controversial. However, it is often stipulated that fruit and cereals should not be eaten at the same meal.

Such opinions are most likely based on some observations which we ourselves have also made. We have tried to study this problem in detail but neither have we found sufficient facts which could be considered scientifically conclusive, nor have we found in our own clinical experience sufficient reasons for giving such general rules for the feeding of healthy people or invalids. Therefore, we do not feel justified in renouncing in principle all those natural, time-honored and valuable, tasty combinations of healthy foods, such as 'potatoes and cream cheese,' 'milk and cereals,' 'apples and bread,' which are all forbidden by these schools of thought. Such combinations are found particularly in the diets of the healthiest people in food geography or history.

The combination of cereals and fruit in particular is considered an especially happy one by us. The nutty spicy taste of whole wheat, oats and rye, combined with the aroma and juicy flavor of fruit, makes a particularly refreshing and stimulating mixture, while the vitamins of both supplement each other. The organic acids of uncooked fruit sometimes cause discomfort to sensitive digestions but the carbohydrates and 'swelling properties' of the grain help to make them more digestible.

The incompatibility of certain foods is, according to our opinion, something which has to be considered very carefully with each individual invalid by examining his reactions in each particular case. But it is really concerned with the invalid diet of the individual patient, not with the general teaching of dietetics.

'Rejuvenating,' 'Slimming' and 'Fattening' Foods

We know of no panacea, contributing more to the restoration and conservation of fresh and youthful vigor, than a correctly planned uncooked diet in conjunction with whole-grain and green-leaf food. We also know of no diet that conquers obesity better, more lastingly and with less danger than that advocated in this book, not even the high protein diets enriched by excessive quantities of meat and dry milk powder as promoted by some schools of thought. Abnormal emaciation can also be cured with raw foods. Their success in such cases is due to an adjustment of extremes of weight by restoring glandular functions to normal. Also dull, lifeless skin receives a better blood supply and becomes beautiful, fresh and clear.

Order and Number of Meals

The chapters on 'Menus' contain a large selection of menus for the midday meal in which cooked foods figure in addition to uncooked. In these menus the cooked foods assume their correct position, i.e., secondary in importance and in order. No meat dishes will be found, but none the less delicious menus. Well-balanced combinations of food make up a meal, achieving perfect satisfaction and a sense of well-being for those who eat it. Anyone acquainted with the cooking at the Bircher-Benner Clinic knows that the promises made are fulfilled. The main meal of the day is shifted to midday, breakfast and supper being light, frugal meals, in which raw, fresh foods predominate. Breakfast is of this type particularly, since such food is beneficial to the organism immediately after a night's rest. A heavy breakfast adversely affects the whole day.

The menu recommended here, although light, satisfies for some considerable time and provides enough energy until mid-day. The evening meal also avoids everything which might be too filling or heavy, in order to ensure early and deep sleep. Anyone accustomed to a different régime will soon discover how well this change of diet makes him feel.

This food plan prohibits the eating of between-meal snacks by the healthy adult. Frequent meals are in no sense conducive to health since they not only encourage immoderate eating but also disturb the metabolic rhythm. One main meal and two lighter, simpler ones are advisable: the type of food described in this book makes it easy to dispense with snacks. The history of nutrition shows that such intermediate meals were formerly unknown; they became popular only when whole-grain dishes with milk, such as porridge and frumentry, were replaced by tea and coffee, white bread and jam, and highly-processed cereals which immediately but only temporarily satisfy.

If we succeed in making the basic maxims described here a necessary part of our daily life, allow them indeed to become second nature to us, then it is of little importance if the last course of the main meal should consist of some sweet dish two to four times weekly, or if we now and then use white flour or make a few exceptions on some festive occasion. Not only do we survive such lapses better, but are usually eager to return to our new way of life, which makes us feel so much fitter and more active.

The recipes given have been tested with the most meticulous care. Really first-class dishes can be prepared if their directions are carefully followed. May this book promote the health and well-being of a great many people and, in particular, that of the younger generation.

PART I

THE BIRCHER-BENNER APPROACH TO
GENERAL NUTRITIONAL PROBLEMS

Dr. Bircher-Benner anticipated many of the later nutritional discoveries at the beginning of his clinical work on which his diet teaching and dietotherapy are based. He had already realized the relative values of uncooked fruit and vegetables before vitamins were discovered and the importance of minerals appreciated. The methods he suggested for preparation of fruit and vegetable dishes were later confirmed by growing knowledge of these nutrients. Even nowadays, microbiological findings, and even the new physics, help to explain the practical and clinical results of the Bircher-Benner diet for which no explanations have hitherto been available.

There is still, however, divergence of opinion between some of the generally accepted schools of thought and the Bircher Clinic regarding certain nutrients. Therefore, the underlying nutritional conceptions of this book—based on the experience of Dr. Bircher-Benner and the more recent work of his successors—are explained in the following paragraphs, for the benefit of those readers who are interested in studying the theoretical side before starting on the practical part—the recipes and menus.

1. PROTEIN REQUIREMENTS

The generally accepted opinion on nutrition favors a diet with a high protein intake and requires a considerable portion of this protein to be of animal origin (meat, fish, eggs, cheese, milk), which is generally considered to be of better quality than vegetable protein. This opinion is based on a great deal of scientific research which, however, was mainly carried out on animals which increase their weight much more quickly than human beings and, therefore, probably need protein of a different nature. For example, the white rats which are often used for these experiments increase their weight and bulk much more quickly than humans, and therefore require more protein for growing. Again, in these animal experiments the speed of growth was used as the sole criterion for the quality of the protein, while the effect of the protein on a fully grown animal was not taken into account. The growth of the animal can be speeded up by a special intake of protein, but eventually an unfavorable state of health results.

Some of the experts on protein research have recently reverted to the opinion, which the Bircher-Benner Clinic has always upheld, that an economical consumption of protein daily is preferable to a high one. C. M. McCay of Cornell has shown that a lifetime of first-rate health and efficiency can be achieved on an economical protein intake. Besides, once the period of growth of a human being is ended, a different quality of protein is required.

The great value which used to be attributed to animal protein is not entirely justified and protein derived from meat is by no means of the highest value. The daily protein consumption should be 50 grams rather than 100 grams and in a therapeutic diet—except for a few conditions—should be lower still for limited periods. It is, however, necessary to use supplementary protein combinations of the highest value, to which we will refer later on. The apparent therapeutic value of animal protein is in reality only due to a temporary stimulation, and the effect does not last. This is indeed a burden on the metabolism. If a specially high protein diet is indicated, it is successfully provided by milk protein in fermented form, such as yogurt or cream cheese added to the protein contained in green vegetables, whole cereals and nuts.

The Food and Nutrition Board of the International Research Council in Washington has reduced the quantity recommended for the country's consumption of protein to nearly half what is usual, and the International Congress of Gerontologists (March 1956) has also requested a similar reduction of the quantities suggested for protein and fat.

A gradual change of opinion—towards the Bircher-Benner point of view—has also taken place regarding the relative qualities of protein. It has been shown that the term 'biological value of protein,' which was established by Thomas in 1909 and has been used up to the present, did not take into account several factors and therefore further research became necessary. On the basis of the revised scale, the green-leaf and whole-cereal proteins were rated higher than hitherto in relation to the protein of meat, eggs and milk. It has also been established that the nature of individual types of protein is not of so decisive a value as hitherto believed. One kind of protein is very rarely taken alone, and, as soon as several proteins are combined, the one or two supplementing will either improve or reduce the total value. The new supplemented value could be either higher up or lower down the scale than the individual values of the component proteins.

For example, cocoa lowers the value of a protein combination considerably. In an animal experiment the addition of only 4 per cent of cocoa to a protein combination reduced the utilization of the protein to about 30 per cent. On the other hand, a combination of whole-grain and green-leaf protein is an extremely valuable one, which apparently can only be equalled by the combination of milk and potato protein. The relatively low protein content of both green leaves and potatoes is, therefore, of no consequence as a small quantity of each (1 : 9) is sufficient in order to increase the value of a large quantity of milk and whole-grain protein.

Research done at the Max Planck Institute for Nutritional Physiology since 1967 has led to definite evidence that protein combinations of purely vegetable protein or mixed vegetable and other protein have consistently higher value as protein than meat, milk and egg protein. Furthermore, vegetable protein has proved to be of much higher value in combination with a diet containing regular quantities of uncooked fruit and vegetables than in combination with the same quantity of cooked food. Protein requirements as low as 35 and even 25 grams per day (instead of 70 grams) have been proven capable of sustaining full vitality, stamina, health and growth (E. Kofranyi, *Ernährungs-Umschau*, 17, 402–404, Oct. 1970). And extremely low intake of protein, which in the long run would be inadequate by itself, is able to keep a person in good health for many months if taken in an unheated, uncooked and unprocessed state; while the same quantity if heated and cooked, and taken in combination with a mainly cooked diet, would soon cause symptoms of hunger edema.

The generally accepted ideas on protein ignore the fact that the speed of digestion plays an important part, particularly in the case of proteins. The power to absorb the components of proteins through the walls of the intestines, is bound to a given speed. In the case of a larger protein consumption a surplus floods the intestines and cannot be utilized as protein should be. Instead it is only used to produce thermo-energy (specific-dynamic effect). This causes the metabolism to be accelerated by stimulating the sympathetic nervous system in a similar way as does the caffein in tea or coffee. This, however, imposes a special strain on various organs; for instance, owing to the specific-dynamic effect the liver has a considerable amount of additional work to do. This effect must be understood as the result of an emergency reaction because the organism must at all costs get rid of the surplus protein. This constantly recurring emergency-reaction to such stimulation gives a false feeling of strength, which is sometimes increased in the case of meat with the aid of extractive substances and substances derived from roasting. It is, however, in fact, a constant stress, as explained by Selye. This research worker has shown in his well-known animal experiments that rats which were fed on low protein and low sodium diets (low in cooking salt) showed more resistance to other types of 'stress' than those rats which were fed on a diet rich in protein and salt. The considerably reduced need for oxygen and calories during the protracted period of peak efficiency necessary for climbers in high altitudes, is one of the interesting consequences of avoiding the acceleration of the metabolism caused by a surplus of protein.

A diet economical in protein therefore will help to avoid the diseases of old age, while one low in protein will, as a rule, help to regain and maintain health.

2. FATS AND OILS

The average consumption of fats nowadays is excessive and should be reduced in the interests of health. Preferably only fats and oils of high biological value should be used; most of the usual commercially produced fats are of low value biologically.

The biological value of fat and oil is based on several factors; most of these factors are contained:

(1) in the Essential Fatty Acids, the important E.F.A. factor, which are now considered to contain vital, highly active principles; combined with vitamins they can be found above all in the germ of all cereals, in nuts and, in very high concentration, in salad oils extracted from sunflower seeds and linseed by a cold process.

(2) in the content of fat-soluble Vitamins A, D and E. Their absorption however depends on E.F.A. A high content of Vitamins A and E can be found in summer butter, particularly when cattle have been grazing on mountains; or in vegetable oils of first (virgin) extraction only.

(3) in the digestibility of a fat. This depends on its being heated as little as possible during processing. Fresh butter, olive oil and those vegetable fats processed with low heat are therefore preferable from the digestive point of view.

3. ESSENTIAL FATTY ACIDS

E.F.A. FACTOR

During recent years this nutritional factor has come very much to the fore. Its importance was proved on the Continent when it was realized that a diet supplying an adequate fat intake, but fat without these active principles, eventually produced the same diseases as a fat-free diet.

Every fat or oil contains fatty acids. Among these are inactive or 'saturated' acids and active or 'unsaturated' ones. The active ones are of the greatest importance for health, while the inactive ones are a burden to the organism as they may have to be desaturated by it before they can be used. Those acids which are only slightly 'unsaturated' are still included in the inactive group, while those which are twice or three times more active or unsaturated (such as linolenic and linoleic acids) are considered essential to life. For some time the active acids were called 'Vitamin F' on the Continent, though this term is not technically quite correct. In the United States the technical term is E.F.A. (Essential Fatty Acids) and we shall use this abbreviation in the following paragraphs.

These E.F.A. are missing, either wholly or in part, from the fats of animals bred for fat, such as bacon, lard and suet, etc. Furthermore, those cooking fats which are hardened (hydrogenated) during processing, and those oils which are extracted by a heating process and then refined, are lacking in E.F.A., and it is these which are almost exclusively on sale nowadays. The E.F.A. can, however, be found in small quantities in butter, milk and olive oil and in larger quantities in nuts, soya beans and wheat germ. Breast milk contains considerably more E.F.A. than cow's milk. Of all vegetable oils mentioned in the previous section as the best sources of E.F.A., linseed and sunflower oil are known to be particularly rich in E.F.A., provided they are extracted without heating and the first extractions only (virgin oil) used.

The human organism needs E.F.A. in order to utilize to the full the fat-soluble Vitamins A, D and E, and particularly the precursor of A (carotene). Quite a number of vegetarians in the northern countries suffered from a slight Vitamin A and E.F.A. deficiency during rationing because they often had only skimmed milk, no nuts, no natural butter and no wholewheat bread with an adequate content of wheat germ. E.F.A. helps the body to increase the vitality of the individual cell, to get rid of superfluous fat deposits and to assist in overcoming some skin diseases (eczema, boils, psoriasis, milk scurf and others). It also plays a part in the treatment of two serious intestinal diseases (celiac disease and sprue).

Vitamin E and the E.F.A. have to be taken in a relative proportion as they supplement each other and an intake of one without the other might have unfavorable results. It is advisable, therefore, to take them if possible only in natural products such as whole grains, wheat germ and nuts, in each of which these two factors are contained in their relative proportions. A deficiency of E.F.A. can best be made up by the use of carefully processed sunflower oil in salad dressings on all salads and uncooked vegetables (or if available specially processed linseed oil), both very rich in E.F.A. They should not, however, be used in cooking as their highly active principles can lead to the production of harmful substances through excessive heating such as roasting and baking.

For all practical purposes the following directions should be observed. To take cereals in the form of whole grains, uncooked or cooked; to include nuts regularly in the daily diet; to make a special effort to obtain, and not to mind paying a higher price for, a good vegetable oil, e.g. sunflower oil of first extraction by a cold process. The total intake of fats and oils can be reduced when using oil of such first-class quality.

4. VITAMINS

The administration of synthetic vitamins and vitamin concentrates should, strictly speaking, be a matter for the physician only. It is often resorted to for the rapid adjustment of certain vitamin deficiencies or for bridging over impaired assimilation (caused by damage to the walls of the intestines or to the intestinal bacteria), until such time as normal vitamin absorption is restored. However, we always make it our special concern in the case of an invalid diet to provide the body with a complete and abundant selection of vitamins and trace elements, supplied in natural foods so that no lack of as yet unrecognized factors can affect the result. There are probably not yet recognized links between individual vitamins, and these are in turn linked with other nutrients and mineral substances. Jointly administered, their action is in many respects better and more powerful. One-sided effect is avoided, and the harmonious functioning of physical processes is best ensured. Vitamin pills, even combinations, risk disturbing the balance. Excess Vitamin C is harmless and may be useful (excess intake is rapidly excreted) but Essential Fatty Acids introduced heavily without adequate amounts of Vitamin E are harmful, just to give one example of a possible imbalance. As soon as the critical phases of an illness have been overcome, it is of the first importance to dispense with synthetic vitamins and concentrates, and to rely entirely on the natural abundance of vitamins in foods, above all in uncooked food. This principle has been considered in every possible way in the recipes contained in this book.

For this purpose it may be of value to know something about the natural content of certain vitamins to be found in individual foods.

VITAMIN A AND CAROTENE

Vegetable foods contain the precursor carotene (pro-vitamin A), animal foods chiefly the vitamin itself, though some of them, e.g. egg yolk, butter, also contain carotene with Vitamin A in varying proportions. Normally, carotene is converted by the body into Vitamin A completely and without difficulty, provided there is no marked deficiency of unsaturated fatty acids. There is no danger of such deficiency if the diet contains nuts, wholewheat bread and whole cereal foods (containing the germ), and natural oils and fats, such as cold-pressed oil and some nut-cream products. However, carotene utilization in the body may become altogether insufficient, and even an abundant intake of green vegetables and carrot juice may in no way keep pace with Vitamin A requirements, if cooking is done solely with margarine, butter (which may then contain practically no unsaturated fatty acids), animal fats and devitalized oils, particularly if no wheat germ is present in the bread, and no nuts are available. It has often been said that animal foods only can ensure an adequate supply of Vitamin A. This is not true. For instance, not the slightest signs of Vitamin A deficiency were found among the farming population of Java. On the contrary, although their diet consists of whole rice, some green vegetables and fruit, no butter or milk and practically no eggs or meat, an exceptionally good Vitamin A balance was found. The carotene content of green leaves, together with that of rice germ and the high percentage of unsaturated fatty acids contained in the latter, were adequate within the framework of a wholly natural diet.

It is important to have an adequate supply of Vitamin A chiefly to ensure the health of skin, eyes, hair, nails and all mucous membranes; for resistance to infection, the utilization of fat, and for the functioning of the thyroid and liver. The adrenal glands (those endocrine glands which have recently received so much attention since they supply natural cortisone, the hormone ACT which is effective against alcoholism, and probably other equally important hormones) require a particularly abundant supply of Vitamins A and C in order to remain healthy and to function properly. Considerable quantities of Vitamin A are also necessary to enable Vitamin C to be fully utilized, and are furthermore, advisable in many cases of eye weakness and disorders, of inadequate functioning of the thyroid gland and emaciation.

It should be realized that staple foods of animal origin (except liver) are in general not very rich in Vitamin A. Only egg yolk and butter, and to a lesser degree milk and bacon, contain a moderate amount of the vitamin, and this only during the warm seasons of the year. Compare the fact that carrots stored during the winter actually increase their carotene content, whereas animal foods are comparatively poor suppliers of it during the winter. An abundant supply is best assured by the consumption of carrots and green leaves. A few figures will make this clear. Carrots, for instance, contain 6–12 mg. of carotene per 100 gm., spinach 4·38 mg. of Vitamin A, spinach beet 3·07 mg., corn salad (lamb's lettuce) 2·76 mg., curly kale 2·16 mg. Egg yoke contains 2·8–5·5 mg., while white of egg contains 0·0 and butter 0·74 mg. of carotene and 0·6–2·7 mg. of Vitamin A according to the season. Among fruits, ripe apricots contain 2 mg. of carotene, blueberries and cherries 1 mg., and rose hips 5 mg.

Once the vitamin content and the quantity necessary daily for human health are known, it is no difficult matter to compile a menu containing an adequate, even a plentiful daily supply, sufficient to satisfy the most exacting demands:

7 oz. carrots	18 mg. vitamin A.	
7 oz. spinach	11 mg.	"
7 oz. tomatoes	4 mg.	"
2½ cups milk	5 mg.	"
1½ tablespoons butter	¼ mg.	"

In sumer nearly 3 lb. of butter and in winter nearly 6½ lb. would have to be consumed to obtain corresponding amounts of this vitamin!

VITAMIN C

For some time the standard of daily requirement of Vitamin C was considered to be 50 mg. This is no longer correct today. Far less is necessary in order to prevent scurvy. In the mesotrophic state a human being can live almost entirely without Vitamin C and, although he shows no signs of avitaminosis, he will develop diseases of old age and degenerative phenomena.

50 mg. daily is not, however, sufficient in order to maintain perfect health. According to leading research workers, an average intake of 100 mg. per day is necessary, that is, a constant saturation with Vitamin C, particularly if the body is to retain its youthfulness in old age.

In order to achieve this, it is essential to give sufficient attention to the Vitamin C supply which, despite our vitamin-conscious age, is not present in adequate quantities in present-day nutrition. A test made on Swiss soldiers in 1941 (at a time when the diet was still rich in vegetables) proved that only 11 per cent of the men showed a normal C-saturation.

With the exception of liver, animal foodstuffs are, in general, practically or totally deficient in Vitamin C, as are the cereal foods, bread, pastries, biscuits, indeed all farinaceous foods, and even whole-grain foods. On the other hand, 70–75 mg. Vitamin C are found in 100 gm. of germinated cereal grains. This suggests valuable possibilities if fresh vegetable foods should be unobtainable. It is well known that green vegetables, rose hips and fresh fruit of the sea-buckthorn (*Hippophae rhamnoides*) also contain a large quantity of the vitamin.

More than the entire daily requirement is found, for example, in:

peppers	100–200 mg. per 100 gm. or 3½ oz.
sprouts	121 mg.
curly kale	101 mg.
black currants	100–160 mg.
rose hip pulp	400–1500 mg.

The following are also especially rich in Vitamin C:

cauliflower	91 mg.
broccoli and red cabbage	65–81 mg.
Savoy	54–77 mg.
spinach	61–72 mg.
French spinach	68 mg.
spinach beet	64 mg.
cornsalad (lambs' lettuce)	58 mg.
white cabbage	43–52 mg.
kohlrabi	52 mg.
long radishes	50 mg.
fresh walnuts	45 mg.

but not the pale hearts of lettuce.

The following fruits are specially rich in Vitamin C:

strawberries	69–89 mg.
oranges	43–80 mg.
lemons	40–70 mg.
grapefruit	50–56 mg.

Comparatively good sources of Vitamin C are:

Hamburg parsley root	39 mg.
New Zealand spinach	39 mg.
turnips	29 mg.
purslane salad	28 mg.
onions	17–25 mg.
leeks	23 mg.
green beans	18–23 mg.
outdoor cucumbers	17 mg.
endive salad	17 mg.
dandelion salad	17 mg.

One-fourth lb. of fresh tomatoes contains 22 mg., which seems a small amount until one realizes that ¾ lb. are quickly eaten. The rather moderate C-content of new potatoes also gains in importance in view of the fact that potatoes are cheap and that large quantities can be eaten. As potatoes are stored the Vitamin C content steadily drops, and by the end of the season may be less than 5 mg. per 100 gm.

These amounts of Vitamin C can be destroyed in a number of ways, so that only a small part of the intake may prove really effective. The content in leaf vegetables, such as spinach, drops to one-fifth after several days' storage in a warm place, which refrigeration, of course, could prevent. In potatoes it drops to half after 2 months' storage in a cellar; to one-third after 4–6 months. In most cases 25 per cent of the C-content is destroyed in the first minutes of cooking. A large part is dissolved in the cooking water. Many metals, for instance copper saucepans, destroy the vitamin to a great extent. Vitamin C in the intestines may be destroyed by unbalanced intestinal flora before it can be absorbed into the bloodstream.

Fruit and vegetables are best eaten raw and gathered from one's own garden shortly before they are required. Once they are in contact with the digestive juices they are protected from further loss. It should also be borne in mind that cutting up foods in the kitchen and exposing their tissues to air hastens the destruction of Vitamin C and, therefore, in order to avoid this loss, care should be taken to follow closely the directions given in this book.

Constant saturation of the system with Vitamin C has many favorable effects on health. There is a saving of glycogen in the liver and this organ is better protected. Also recovery after bodily fatigue is more rapid. The protein contained in the various foods is better utilized since activation of the protein-splitting enzymes is induced by this vitamin. The toxic action of poisonous substances is reduced, tendency to bleeding decreased and resistance to infection increased. A number of organs require a particularly good supply of Vitamin C in order to function efficiently: the eyes, all endocrine glands, especially the pituitary gland and the adrenal glands, the brain, the heart, the lungs and the insulin-producing pancreas. Vitamin C has also an anti-allergic action.

In case of necessity saturation can also be achieved by Vitamin C tablets. However, fresh uncooked foods, which also supply all the other vital substances, are a necessary foundation for most of the combined and cumulative effects which are the result of the joint action of some of these substances. Without raw food this action would not be achieved. If, as so frequently occurs, the intestinal flora have become unbalanced (para-coli), all the vitamin tablets in the world will be of no avail. On the other hand, if the Vitamin C is supplied in the form of fresh fruit and raw vegetables, these foods, in general, are able to regenerate rapidly the intestinal flora by the help of the enzymes of the living plant cells. It is only with the aid of Vitamin P (the bioflavinoids), which can be found combined with Vitamin C only in natural foods, that Vitamin C is able to develop its most effective action on cellular tissue.

VITAMINS OF THE B GROUP

There is increasing recognition that it is essential to ensure a supply of the entire B complex (which has not as yet been fully investigated) in the form of natural foods, rather than to attempt to take any single element of the B complex alone. This should not be a difficult matter if the directions given in this book are carefully followed. To this group belong those factors which are not essential to life but are essential to health, and which Dr. W. Kollath of Rostock University (at present at Freiburg) has grouped together under the name auxons. If this group is missing the result will be 'mesotrophy' (semi-nourishment), another term coined by Kollath; he considers this to be an aplastic-consumptive deficiency disease, in fact a lowered state of health. This condition was discovered by him and corroborated in the course of animal experiments by nutritionists in Stockholm and Munich. It allows a normal span of life but at a lower physiological level. This meso-trophic state causes numerous degenerative alterations, such as dental and osseous decay, and a pathogenic condition of the intestinal flora, which subsequently causes the other vita-mins and minerals (apart from B, calcium phosphate, traces of zinc and the animal protein factor) to lose their efficiency to a large extent. This loss can only be prevented, and to a certain extent compensated, by that group of lesser-known and less-essential vitamins, the auxons (pantothenic acid, para-aminobenzoic acid, folic acid, inositol, choline, biotin and Vitamins K and T). If this auxon group is abundantly supplied, the human body is able to thrive and to attain the highest degree of health without animal protein (a fact which may be of vital importance in cases of allergy). An ample supply of auxons is best ensured by a diet containing sufficient quantities of raw green vegetables, whole-grain products and nuts, such as are suggested in this book. Buttermilk and the germ of cereals increase the auxon supply still further. It is of interest to note that folic acid, a vitamin of the auxon group, which is so important for the formation of blood, is contained most abundantly in New Zealand spinach.

Vitamin B_{12} is supplied by milk. It is an excellent source but is not indispensable if well-balanced intestinal flora are work-ing normally. Should this not be so, normal functioning can be quickly restored by following a diet on the lines of this book, alternating with periods on an entirely raw diet under medical supervision. After prolonged doses of sulfonamides and antibiotics, however, the administration of colivaccines may often be necessary (in about 30 per cent of all cases) to restore the intestinal flora to normal. It is probably wiser not to take Vitamin B_{12} concentrates for any length of time, and in-stead to meet Vitamin B_{12} requirements from milk, raw vege-tables and whole grains, helped of course by a healthy func-tioning of the digestion.

Foods rich in Vitamin B_1

Vegetables	curly kale, savoy, Brussels sprouts, lettuce, cress, beans, soya beans, peas, carrots, red peppers.
Fruit	apples, apricots, plums, bananas, raspber-ries, grapefruit.
Nuts	peanuts, hazelnuts (filberts), almonds, wal-nuts.
Cereals	wheat, rye, oats, rice, sweet corn, baker's yeast.
Animal food	egg yolk.

Foods rich in Vitamin B₂

Vegetables	curly kale, savoy, kale, lettuce, endive, cress, spinach, nettle leaves, beans, peas, cauliflower.
Fruit	apricots, peaches, plums, pears.
Nuts	peanuts, almonds, walnuts.
Cereals	wheat, rye, oats, barley, rice.
Animal foods	milk, eggs (especially egg yolk).

Foods rich in anti-pellagra factor

Vegetables	spinach, endive, nettle leaves, peas, soya beans, carrots, cauliflower, Brussels sprouts, tomatoes.
Fruit	dried apricots, dates, peaches, plums, apples, bananas.
Nuts	peanuts, almonds.
Cereals	wheat, rye, barley, oats, rice, sweet corn.

Foods rich in pantothenic acid

Vegetables	beans, peas, carrots, cauliflower, curly kale, soya beans, nettle leaves.
Nuts	peanuts, walnuts.
Cereals	wheat, rye, barley, oats, rice, sweet corn.
Animal food	whole egg.

Foods rich in Vitamin B₆

Vegetables	dried beans and peas, potatoes, curly kale, lettuce, corn salad, soya beans, tomatoes.
Fruit	bananas.
Nuts	peanuts.
Cereals	wheat, rye, barley, oats, rice, sweet corn.
Animal food	egg yolk.

Foods rich in folic acid

Vegetables	beans, spinach and all green vegetables (see above).
Nuts	peanuts.
Cereals	wheat, sweet corn.

Foods rich in biotin

Vegetables	dried beans and peas, cauliflower, spinach.
Fruit	peaches, bananas, raspberries.
Nuts	peanuts.
Animal food	whole egg.

VITAMIN D

Foods rich in Vitamin D

A wide variety of plants, especially cereal germ and green leaves, also yeast, supply the pro-vitamin D or precursor, which changes into the actual Vitamin D in the body when the skin is exposed to sunlight.

Milk, butter, eggs contain the complete Vitamin D.

VITAMIN E

A plentiful supply of this vitamin is necessary to ensure healthy development of the reproductive functions, to protect mother and child during pregnancy and to utilize fully the intake of carotene and E.F.A. (highly unsaturated fatty acids, see p. 19). Vitamin E is most abundant in green leaves and is to be found in:

cabbage	6 mg. per 100 gm. (or ¼ lb.)
lettuce	6 mg.
cereal germ:	
wheat germ	30 mg.
sweet corn germ	16 mg.
wheat grains	2·3–5·4 mg.
sweet corn grains	1·3–3·6 mg.

Normal daily requirements are estimated at 2 mg. and during pregnancy at 5 mg.

Foods rich in Vitamin E

	wheat germ oil, peanut oil, soya oil, if fresh and left unprocessed.
Vegetables	curly kale, savoy, cress, lettuce, nettle leaves, peas.
Cereals	in all cereal grains, especially in the germ.

VITAMIN K

The vitamin essential for coagulating the blood.

Foods rich in Vitamin K

Vegetables	curly kale, green cabbage, spinach and nettle leaves.

5. MINERAL SUBSTANCES

The mineral substances in food have many varied and im-

portant tasks to fulfil in the body. They have, quite unjusti-
fiably, been considered to be of less importance since the
development of the disproportionate vitamin publicity. However, the experience gained in wartime has proved that much
greater attention must be given to them.

Mineral substances are essential for building the body,
especially the bones and teeth. Another—no less important—
function is the regulation of the acid-alkali balance in the
blood and tissues, of the osmotic pressure and swelling po-
tentiality of the protein molecule. A third task is the activation
of the processes of fermentation connected with enzymes. The
following elements are at present considered to be of vital
importance:

Hydrogen, oxygen, carbon, nitrogen, *phosphorus, calcium,*
sulphur, chlorine, *iodine, sodium, potassium, magnesium,
iron, copper, zinc, manganese, cobalt,* vanadium and *fluorine.*
Those in italics are the mineral salts of particular importance
to the dietician. They are abundant in vegetables and fruit.
Potassium, calcium, sodium and iron, in addition to phosphorus, are plentiful in vegetables, especially in leafy ones. Long
before the 'vitamin era' vegetables and fruit were considered
valuable from a therapeutic point of view on account of this
mineral content and together with the vitamin reserves they
supply essential nourishment.

Professor H. C. Sherman, member of the National Research
Council (the authoritative body on questions of diet in the
U.S.A.) wrote on the subject, 'We also have the clinical proof
that people who live more on fruit, vegetables and milk, suffer
less from senility and degenerative diseases in old age.'

It is not a simple matter to give specific figures for the
mineral content of vegetables, for they vary considerably according to habitat, quality and method of fertilization of the
soil, climate, hours of sunshine, rainfall, etc. Fertile lowlands
with a copious rainfall usually yield ample harvests but vegetables deficient in minerals, whereas dry soils well provided
with minerals often yield poor harvests but products rich
in mineral substances. The stage of growth at which the vegetables are gathered is also an important factor—many of
them are more valuable when still in the young, tender and
juicy stage, others when fully ripe; the mineral content is
also subject to fluctuation in the course of a single day, therefore harvesting should, preferably, be carried out in the early
morning. The figures showing the mineral content (given below) must, therefore, be regarded only as an approximate
average, capable of considerable variation.

Cooking may cause substantial loss of minerals. It is essential therefore to make use of the cooking water whenever possible since more than half of the minerals will be transferred to the water in the process of scalding and boiling. Vegetables which are steamed or stewed in fat (sautéed) suffer the smallest loss.

The quantity of mineral substances eventually reaching the alimentary tract to be absorbed by the body depends on their relationship to each other which also governs their full utilization. It is not enough to know how many mineral substances have been taken, but whether their absorption is being secured. This requires thorough mastication, healthy intestinal conditions and altogether a moderate diet (not over-plentiful). This particularly concerns the calcium-phosphorus group.

CALCIUM-PHOSPHORUS

The element calcium follows in importance immediately after the four main elements which build up the body: carbon, oxygen, hydrogen and nitrogen. It takes first place among the alkaline-forming minerals. Calcium not only plays an important part in building the bony structure of the body but also as a neutralizing agent for harmful acids. It appears, moreover, to fulfil a vital task as a constituent of the cell nucleus. It is particularly important to have an abundant supply of calcium with food during the period of growth in order to build up the bones. It has also been found that a good reserve of calcium while young keeps the adult youthful for a longer period. Even in the adult, however, the bony tissue is not something constructed once and for all, but is continually being re-formed and renewed. The calcium requirement of the adult is estimated by Lehnartz at 1–2 gm., by others at about 0·8 gm. daily. It is not possible to give definite figures for the total requirement, since it depends largely on the composition of the diet as a whole, and especially on the proportion of calcium in relation to the phosphorus consumed at the same time. The less the diet is overloaded with a surplus of acid-forming foods (meat, cheese, eggs, dishes made with white flour, refined sugar and fats), the less the need for calcium to neutralize this surplus. The more the diet follows the lines indicated in this book the more easily can the normal requirement of calcium be met. Thus the danger of calcium deficiency decreases, and with it the chances increase for the maintenance of good, strong bones and sound teeth. It has been shown in long-term experiments that a daily average of about ¼ gm. of calcium is sufficient to maintain a favorable calcium balance if the diet consists mainly of vegetables. Children, pregnant women and nursing mothers, however, need a considerably larger supply of calcium with their food.

As mentioned above, it is important that calcium and phosphorus be supplied in a favorable proportion in the food. This proportion may vary considerably without any disturbing influence on growth or calcification of the bones, but the maximum mineral content and the greatest powers of resistance and efficiency of the bones are only attained if the proportion of calcium to phosphorus is about 1 : 1·7. This is the approximate proportion found in nuts and berries. The proportion is comparatively unfavorable in all cereal products since it veers too far towards phosphoric acid:

wholewheat bread	1 : 4
oat flakes	1 : 4·6
macaroni	1 : 7
yellow peas	1 : 7
white rolls	1 : 8

very unfavorable in meat:

beef	1 : 27

and less in fish. As a compensation for cereal products, therefore, many foods with a more satisfactory proportion of calcium to phosphorus must be consumed, as for instance:

oranges	1 : 0·5
lemons	1 : 0·7
lettuce	1 : 0·6
radishes	1 : 0·7
cow's milk	1 : 1·0
cheese	1 : 1·4
dried figs	1 : 1·17
cauliflower	1 : 1·0
celeriac	1 : 1·0
carrots	1 : 1·1 etc.

Vegetables, herbs, fruit and milk are also in this respect the ideal supplement to bread.

The citric acid to be found in orange juice enables the body to utilize a greater quantity of calcium than the calcium content of the orange juice itself. It is assumed that the citric acid in the juice transforms the calcium of other food in the intestines into readily soluble citrates, thus creating more favorable conditions for absorption. The action of Vitamin D seems to improve the absorption of those calcium salts which are difficult to assimilate, so that the body can make better use of them.

On the other hand, there are substances contained in foods which supply calcium compounds (so-called 'calcium robbers') which are not otherwise readily available, such as oxalic acid and phytin. The latter is present in the outer layers of the cereal grain, but this is no reason to eschew whole-grain bread, because if the dough is correctly prepared phytin is largely destroyed and can have no effect whatever. Even if the dough is incorrectly prepared, the phytin is nearly all destroyed in the intestines by coli-bacteria. Furthermore, if a diet is based on the directions given in this book, the calcium requirement is reduced to such an extent, as already explained, that even a certain amount of phytin action cannot affect the adequate supply, as comparatively large quantities of calcium are contained in the vegetables, green leaves, milk and milk products, suggested in our diet.

Foods very rich in calcium
Gruyère (Swiss) cheese, soft cheese and sesame seeds } 1½–½ gm. in ¼ lb. of substance

Foods rich in calcium
almonds, black radishes, kohlrabi leaves, dried figs and cucumbers } ½–⅕ gm. in ¼ lb.

Foods comparatively rich in calcium
peanuts, walnuts, egg yolk, ripe beans, lemons, milk, tangerines, leeks, curly kale, lettuce, cauliflower, endive, celery } ⅕–1/10 gm. in ¼ lb.

Phosphorus and calcium are the most important fundamental substances for the formation of bones and teeth, comprising a total of 80 per cent of the bony structure. Adults require at least 0·9 gm. of phosphorus daily, children and young people 1·3 gm., pregnant women and nursing mothers 1·5 gm. The correct proportion of phosphorus to calcium is here of decisive importance.

Foods rich in phosphorus (in which the proportion to calcium is favorable)
Gruyère (Swiss) cheese and other hard cheese } 2·3 gm. per cent. P_2O_3

peanuts, almonds, walnuts, hazelnuts (filberts), ripe beans, ripe peas, lentils	1·1–0·5 gm. per cent.
hen's eggs (without shell), currants, globe artichokes, curly kale, Brussels sprouts, kohlrabi, white cabbage, salsify, raisins, dried figs, milk	0·5–0·2 gm. per cent.
grapes, celery leaves, cauliflower, potatoes, horseradish, celeriac, lettuce, dates, bananas, oranges	0·2–0·1 gm. per cent.

MAGNESIUM

Magnesium also plays a decisive part in the formation of bones and teeth, though in a far smaller quantity. Seventy per cent of the magnesium present in the body is stored in the bones. The daily requirement amounts to 0·3 gm; the rate of absorption by the intestines is similar to that of calcium. It is generally assumed that the daily food supplies enough magnesium. However, more recent research shows that a comparatively generous supply of magnesium may have a significant influence on health. Important foods containing magnesium are:

almonds, peanuts, hazelnuts (filberts), ripe beans, black radishes, millet, oats, sweet corn, rye, wheat, barley, cucumbers, rose hips	0·2–0·1 gm. per cent magnesium
walnuts, onions, tomatoes, dates, figs, raisins, Gruyère (Swiss) cheese	0·1–0·05 gm. per cent magnesium

IRON

Iron belongs to the most important bio-elements, being a necessary constituent of hemoglobin, muscle protein (myoglobin), various enzymes, the blood plasma and the body cells. The adult body requires 12 mg. of iron daily (children 12–15 mg., pregnant women and nursing mothers 15 mg.), though the daily quantity most favorable to health would appear to be considerably larger. The research carried out at the Peckham Health Centre in England has shown that an incipient form of anemia is common today, especially among women, and is frequently connected with the well-known 'housewife's fatigue'.

It was found possible to cure this condition with a plentiful supply of iron.

A particularly large amount of iron is required in early childhood, by girls during puberty, by pregnant women, and by all those who have lost blood or suffer from feverish illnesses.

Many cases of iron deficiency, especially in girls of 13–18, at which age anemia easily develops as a result of rapid growth and menstruation, can be cured by a correct choice of foods. Owing to present-day eating habits, nearly every young girl has a tendency to anemia due to iron deficiency. This may have a lasting effect on their later life, which can be avoided if the diet is planned as suggested.

It can never do any harm to take plenty of iron with food, as all surplus above actual requirement is eliminated.

The best sources of supply of nutritional iron are fruit, vegetables and cereals in their whole-grain form, though not, however, if the bran is removed. Apples, pears, bananas, red currants, cherries, grapes, apricots, plums and damsons are recommended for supplying hemoglobin in the youthful organism. It is, however, not only their iron content, but also the presence of other substances that promote the absorption of iron in the organism. The saponin in spinach, for instance, has such an effect. Milk is poor in iron but after drinking milk the utilization of iron from other food is greatly improved.

Foods rich in iron

celeriac	500 mg. per cent.
cream cheese	66 mg. per cent.
tangerines	57 mg. per cent.
spinach (if fresh and organically-grown) honey, turnips, whole rice, peanuts, hazelnuts, black radishes, dried green rye (for soups), leeks, lettuce, oat flakes, Jerusalem artichokes, kohlrabi, lentils, horseradish, endives, salsify, rye	50–20 mg. per cent.

SODIUM, POTASSIUM AND THE WATER METABOLISM OF THE BODY

Sodium and potassium, the chief representatives of a specific group of minerals, are so distributed in the body that potassium compounds (potassium phosphate and potassium bicarbonate) predominate in the cells and blood corpuscles, and sodium compounds (common salt and sodium bicarbonate) in the blood fluid and tissue fluids outside the cells. The more each group predominates in its own sphere the greater the tension between them, the more powerful the functioning of the vital processes in the organism, the better the general health. On the other hand, the more their contrasting characteristics are intermingled and equalized, the feebler will be the functioning of the vital processes, the slower the cell respiration and the lower the body's powers of resistance and regeneration. As already stated elsewhere, only fresh raw plant nutrition is capable of permanently strengthening this tension between the sodium and potassium groups.

About 70 per cent of the human body consists of water: 5 per cent of which is in the blood fluid, 50 per cent in the cellular fluid and 15 per cent in the fluid between the cells and blood vessels. This extra-cellular fluid, which surrounds all the tissues, is of particular importance, as it is the internal environment in which all the tissues live, in the same way as the organism as a whole lives in the external environment. It is, in fact, the *Lebensraum*, the native soil that ensures the nourishment of the cells, absorbs and eliminates all their metabolic products, keeps the temperature of the cells stable and generally acts as a safety valve. It is due to the stability of this wonderful regulation, this *milieu intérieur* (Claude Bernard), that the human system is able to exist in comparative independence of external influences. It intercepts and softens, as it were, the impact of the outer world.

As long as good general health is maintained, the composition and quantity of the body fluids remain largely stable. However if, for instance, large quantities of salt are used in the preparation and consumption of food for any length of time, disturbances may result from the retention of surplus salt in the fluids of the body. At the same time, water would also be retained in order to maintain the correct solution of salt in the body fluid. There is a close connection between mineral and water metabolism. If water is lost by the body for any reason, for instance as a result of perspiration or diarrhea, there is a corresponding elimination of common salt (possibly also of potassium). If, conversely, the salt consumption is intentionally decreased by a salt-free raw diet, a corresponding elimination of water can be observed.

In practical life it can be of great value to be able to eliminate water retained in the body, by decreasing the salt intake contained in food. This is best achieved by the consumption of foods as low as possible in sodium and as rich as possible in potassium. A salt-free, uncooked plant diet is by far the best for this purpose. The effect of such a diet can be increased by specially selecting foods for their sodium and potassium content, because even fruit and vegetables show considerable variations. In milk, for example, the sodium-potassium proportion is 1 : 4; in potatoes 1 : 40; in rice 1 : 100, and in bananas as much as 1 : 400. However, in spite of its potassium surplus, milk produces no elimination of water unless the milk's salt has been specially removed. Some foods containing sodium and potassium in a proportion of over 1 : 20, are listed below in order of their eliminative effect.

In 100 gm. (or ¼ lb.) of fresh substance	mg. potassium	mg. sodium	K : Na
bananas	400	1	400 : 1
cherries	280	1	280 : 1
tangerines	460	2	230 : 1
wheat (whole grain)	430	2	215 : 1
pears	180	1	180 : 1
oats	340	2	170 : 1
lemons	460	3	153 : 1
curly kale	560	4	140 : 1
black currants	260	2	130 : 1
oranges	250	2	125 : 1
red currants	110	1	110 : 1
rice	100	1	100 : 1
Brussels sprouts	380	4	93 : 1
sorrel	360	4	90 : 1
kohlrabi	260	5	52 : 1
ripe peas	820	17	48 : 1
filberts	620	13	48 : 1
parsnips	390	9	43 : 1
potatoes	460	1–30	40 : 1
almonds	840	23	37 : 1
broccoli	400	24	25 : 1
plums	220	10	22 : 1
green beans	220	10	22 : 1
dried figs	970	46	21 : 1

If the above list is carefully studied it will be seen how easily a full diet can be combined with a high potassium and low sodium content. Suggestions for diet days with a surplus of alkali-forming foods for the purpose of removing the surplus water retained in the tissues, which is often one of the factors responsible for obesity, will be found in another chapter, on p. 312.

Neither orange nor lemon juice is acid-forming as many

people think, but alkali-forming, that is, it has a surplus of alkalis. Organic acids, such as citric acid contained in lemons, are burned in the system and the remaining mineral substances have a powerful alkali-forming action.

6. TRACE ELEMENTS

Apart from the above-mentioned mineral substances, which are needed by the body in fairly large quantities, there are some of which only very small traces are present in the body. These are called trace elements and include iodine, copper, cobalt, manganese, vanadium, zinc and fluorine. What part each of these trace elements plays in the human organism is a question only partly solved, and much research still remains to be done. Trace elements are found in drinking water, as well as in food.

IODINE

This element is stored by the thyroid, which requires it to produce the thyroid hormone. If there is a deficiency of iodine in the diet, the iodine content of the thyroid, normally 40 mg. per cent, drops. A content of only 10 mg. per cent causes the thyroid to degenerate noticeably and goiter results. The iodine requirements of the adult are presumed to be 0·15 mg. daily, though this amount may prove quite insufficient during puberty, pregnancy, breast-feeding and infectious diseases.

In Switzerland goiter was widespread in the 1920's. As a result of the introduction of iodized cooking salt, it has become rare in its visible form, but in its milder, barely visible forms, as a hypo-function of the thyroid, it has not yet entirely disappeared. It is still especially noticeable in those regions where few vegetables are eaten and the cooking water thrown away. This sub-normal functioning of the thyroid is not a matter of indifference to the mental and physical efficiency of the human race. Among other things, eggs, whole-grain rye and wheat and lettuce are rich in iodine.

Even more important than the iodine content is the amount of Vitamin A (or carotene) supplied to the body. The better the supply of Vitamin A, the less iodine is needed by the thyroid. Even a salt-free diet, provided it is rich in carotene, can sufficiently replenish the iodine stored in the thyroid.

COPPER

Copper serves to help build up hemoglobin and some enzymes. Daily requirements amount to about 2 mg. In some circumstances, the supply contained in food may drop to 1 mg.

Important foods containing copper

egg yolk	22 mg. per cent.
rye (whole-grain)	4–30 mg. per cent.

Comparatively rich in copper . . . .

filberts	
almonds	
walnuts	1·2–1·0 mg. per cent.
red currants	
peas	
lentils	
dried figs	0·7–0·4 mg. per cent.
dates	
bananas	
blackberries	
apricots	
raisins	
plums	
cherries	
potatoes	0·2–0·1 mg. per cent.
cauliflower	
kohlrabi	
radishes	
asparagus	
spinach	

COBALT

The discovery of the cobalt-bearing Vitamin B_{12} has shown the vital importance of this trace element. Tomatoes are very rich in cobalt.

MANGANESE

This vital element, essential for the production of various enzymes in the system (daily requirements 2–3 mg.) is also found most abundantly in plant food, above all in:

nuts	
oats	
rye	
wheat	5–2 mg. per cent.
sweet corn	
beans	

Cloves are rich in manganese as is shown by the dark blue color of their ashes.

ZINC

Daily requirements 5–20 mg. Zinc is also a component of many enzymes, so that disturbances in growth and metabolism result if it is absent. However, since requirements are easily met, deficiency signs are comparatively rare.

Generally speaking, vegetables are very rich in mineral substances as compared to animal foodstuffs, or even fruit. Their content of alkaline-forming mineral components greatly outweigh the acid-forming ones. Their potassium content is particularly high. For this reason they were suspected for some time of encouraging the growth of cancer, since tumors contain much potassium. In reality, the organisms's resistance to cancer is strengthened by as great a surplus as possible of the potassium supply over that of sodium—in other words, by nutrition rich in vegetables and fruit, especially in their uncooked state. This preponderance of the potassium group entails slower growth of the more valuable cells, whereas a greater tendency towards the sodium group produces more rapid growth of primitive cells.

A rich and well-balanced supply of minerals and particularly of trace elements, is best assured by a fruit, vegetable, wholegrain and milk diet, provided it comes from soil which is either fertile and well-cultivated or enriched with properly prepared organic compost.

The minerals in foods have a considerable influence on the utilization of other nutrients, therefore a harmonious mixture of all of them produces the best results.

PART II

THE PRACTICAL PART:
RECIPES AND MENUS

EDITOR'S NOTES ON VARIOUS INGREDIENTS

Fats and Oils

Vegetable cooking fat, made from clarified butter and vegetable fat, is used in many recipes. It is usually mixed with nut
butters. To prepare: melt ⅓ butter over low heat, stir when it
begins to rise until it becomes clear and the sediment sinks.
Remove from heat. While still hot add ⅓ vegetarian cooking
fat (see below) and ⅓ vegetable oil. Stir until liquefied then
pour into earthenware jar. Cover with greaseproof paper when
cool.

Vegetarian cooking fat is a mixture of ground nuts and palm
kernel oils, purified, deodorized and non-hydrogenated.

Various non-hydrogenated margarines are now available for
those concerned about the effect of fatty acids on chronic
heart conditions, coronary thrombosis and disturbances of
the metabolism.

Plain Flour

When flour is mentioned in these recipes, it always refers to
wholewheat flour.

Salt

The use of salt often leads to exaggerated usage. The less
salt used, the better, and in certain conditions a salt-reduced
or salt-free diet is recommended. Herbs are a good substitute.
If salt is used, add it during cooking, since a little salt goes a
longer way than when it is added afterwards.

Sea salt, which contains minerals in their natural balance,
is preferable to the highly refined and processed table salts.

Uncooked dishes, particularly raw salads, should not be
salted. The flavor of lemon and herbs in the dressing will provide the necessary seasoning. When dishes are cooked, how-

ever, a little salt may be added, as minerals are lost in the cooking. To avoid salting more than necessary it is best to taste any mixture at the latest stage before cooking—or even after cooking, in some cases—and adjust the seasoning.

Sugar

For the same reasons brown sugar is preferred to white sugar for most recipes. Brown sugar refers to raw brown unrefined sugar, available at most health food stores.

Cream Cheese

When cream cheese is specified in ingredients, the recipe given on page 63 should be used. If substituting the store-bought variety, ask for creamed cottage cheese.

Flavorings

No artificial flavorings or substitutes are used at the Bircher-Benner Clinic or recommended for use in this book. The flavor of sweet or a few bitter almonds is infinitely better than the flavor of almond extract, and vanilla beans are so much better in flavor than vanilla extract. Beans are easy to handle and can be used several times, if cooked in milk, taken out and dried again. Or small parts of a pod can be cut off and the black beans scraped into the food to be flavored. Beans can also be kept in clean, dry screw-top jars with sugar. If kept in a dry place and shaken occasionally, the sugar will have absorbed the flavor and some of it can be used for flavoring. More sugar can be added to the jar as the flavor will intensify in time.

Agar-Agar

Agar-Agar is a natural pulverized jellying agent derived from seaweed, and is a complete substitute for gelatine. It is odorless, flavorless and makes a clear jelly. Fruit or vegetable juices can be jellied without heating them to more than blood heat, thus retaining most of the value of the juices.

Sauté

Before beginning to use the recipes for cooked food it would be advisable to study some of the methods and cookery terms which are used in this book. There is, for instance, the term 'sauté', frequently mentioned because it is the best description of the first stage of 'stewing vegetables in their own juice'. This method is used with most of the cooked vegetables because it retains more flavor in vegetable cookery and makes it more attractive.

Sauté is a French cooking term, now frequently adopted in American cookbooks, depicting stewing in butter, oil or fat. It is shallow frying in a heavy iron (glazed with enamel), shallow-sided, lidded saucepan or heavy frying pan. The foods are put into the pre-heated fat (not too hot) and tossed until their own juices 'sweat out'; then the lid can be added and 'stewing in their own juice' begins. The steam of the fat and juice helps to make the food tender in a short time. A heavy pan, which must be frequently stirred or shaken, is necessary to prevent sticking and burning, and a well-fitting lid when the 'stewing' begins.

1. RECIPES

BIRCHER MUESLI:

RAW FRUIT PORRIDGE

Originally this dish was simply called 'fruit diet dish'. At Bircher-Benner's it was known everywhere as 'the dish'—no need to say which! It appeared on the table so frequently, and so much as a matter of course, that it had become, as it were, the epitome of nutrition, somewhat similar to the 'daily bread' of former times.

What Dr. Bircher-Benner did was to reintroduce an old custom of his native country with this Bircher Muesli. At one time it had been usual in the fruit-growing parts of Switzerland to eat a kind of fruit porridge for lighter meals, especially the evening meal. It consisted of fruit, various cereals and milk. The old English frumenty (wheat) and Scottish porridge (oats) are based on the same tradition. Fruit according to season—apples, pears, berries, or dried fruit—with wheat, oats or barley and milk, usually unboiled and fresh from the cow, made one of the oldest and most natural of dietetic combinations with nuts to crown a pefect whole. In those days people had strong teeth and the cereals were often eaten in whole grain. Real Muesli was also known in Switzerland, berries being mixed with oatmeal and milk.

When Dr. Bircher-Benner started practicing, this old tradition was almost forgotten. Fruit, especially fresh fruit, had fallen into disrepute in Switzerland. A mere luxury, and a dangerous one at that, fruit was eaten only as dessert or a sweet and even then preferably stewed and sweetened. Most of it, indeed, was converted into alcoholic-cider, fruit-wine, or spirits. People with delicate digestions avoided fresh fruit like poison though, in fact, they were the people who needed it most of all. This prevailing attitude forced Dr. Bircher-Benner to find some way of making the consumption of fresh fruit once again a popular daily habit, not only among those still in possession of strong teeth but also among the many whose powers of mastication were weakened.

Bircher Muesli was his solution. It met with such approval that Dr. Bircher-Benner's patients began serving it at home; friends and acquaintances asked them for the recipe and it became widely popular long before its preparation was first described in a booklet.* Many restaurants started serving Muesli. In Lausanne and Geneva guests often ask for *un birche* when they have no idea where the dish originated. It may happen that quite unexpectedly a Muesli is offered in a shepherd's hut in the High Alps or on a tropical plantation. Henry Ford was said to have become a devotee of Muesli, while a professor in Milan offered it to his guests under the name *Dolce Sorpresa* (Sweet Surprise). In England it is called often simply 'Swiss Breakfast'. In fact, it has once again become something approaching a Swiss national dish.

Present-day Muesli is more subtle and appetizing than the old peasant food. Its composition conforms to our knowledge of modern nutritional science; it is surprisingly refreshing, tasty and complete in itself, all nutrients being present in correct proportions.

As a rule, Bircher Muesli is eaten at the beginning of breakfast and the evening meal, in accordance with the basic Bircher-Benner principle that the keenest edge shall be taken off the appetite with fresh, raw food, before anything else is eaten.

It is by no means difficult to make a good Bircher Muesli. Many people, guided by preconceived ideas that Muesli is a cereal dish, think that the cereal part is the most 'nourishing' part and should therefore predominate.

Muesli will turn out successfully, and be of the greatest value, if the following three points are borne in mind:

Firstly, it must not be forgotten that Muesli is primarily a fruit dish. Porridge or any similar cereal dish is good, too, but a mixture of porridge and mashed apple is not very pleasant. In Muesli, fruit is the principal food, every other ingredient being merely an addition. Therefore, no more oatflakes or cereal grains should be used than are given in the recipe, i.e., one tablespoonful per person. The taste of the fruit must not be swamped by the taste of the cereal. The dish should be light and fruity—a real fruit dish. The spoon should not be able to stand upright in it!

* *Fruit Dishes and Raw Vegetables*, published by the Wendepunkt Press in 1924 (English translation, The C. W. Daniel Company Ltd., 1926, revised translation 1946).

Secondly, whenever practicable the Bircher Muesli must be freshly made, the fruit in it as fresh from the garden or store-room as possible. It is not a dish that can be made in advance and then kept until it becomes grey-brown and musty. It is essential that Muesli should always be prepared immediately before a meal and that no more be made of it than will be finished up at that meal. The basic mixture can be prepared beforehand in a bowl but the apples must be grated into it at the very last moment, preferably just when everyone is sitting down to table. When grating the apples, strong pressure should be used to prevent the apples from becoming too mushy. Each apple should be mixed quickly and well into the basic mixture to avoid discoloration. If a mechanical mixer is used, roughly chopped apples or other fruit can be placed in the container together with the other basic ingredients, but the mixer should not be started until everyone is ready, and even then for a few seconds only, so that the Muesli does not become too mushy. On the whole, up till now no really satisfactory way of producing Muesli mechanically has been found.

Muesli does not take long to prepare and even a busy housewife can usually find the time to make it, particularly if it becomes a daily routine. There is, however, a tendency to upset the proportion of ingredients and Muesli can lose its value by becoming a cereal dish instead of a fruit dish! This applies especially when making Muesli from some of the valuable ready-made Muesli packs which are now available at health stores and some supermarkets all over the country. Only fresh fruit and milk or yogurt need be added. A deep-frozen variety, if carefully prepared, can be of good quality.

Thirdly, it should be noted that Muesli belongs to the beginning of a meal and not to the end. It can, of course, be served as a dessert, garnished with whipped cream and canned cherries, but such is not its aim. The fresh raw substances it contains can be better utilized when the stomach is still empty. Eaten at the end of a substantial meal its therapeutic powers may have too dynamic or even opposite effects from those to be expected.

The fruit used should be varied according to the season, and nowadays there is usually an abundant variety of fruit throughout the year from which to choose. Most kinds of fruit may be used, save for the very watery. Especially recommended are apricots, peaches, strawberries, blueberries, blackberries, currants, especially black currants, raspberries, plums and loganberries. If apples are used, a suitable variety must be chosen, white-fleshed, juicy and rather sour.

The cereal need not always consist of rolled oats or oatmeal or oatflakes. The more variety the better. Soaked, fresh whole-wheat grains, soya flakes, millet flakes, mixed flakes, wheat germ, germinated wheat, etc., may be used.

The milk part of the ingredients may also be varied: top of the milk, cream, yogurt, nut cream or almond purée (see p. 60) replacing the condensed milk. Sweetened condensed milk has the advantage of blending well with the slightly sour fruit and the lemon juice. It can be condensed at a sufficiently low temperature, owing to the preserving qualities of its sugar content, for its biological value to be preserved. Moreover, the milk used is undoubtedly of first-class quality. One advantage of unsweetened condensed or evaporated milk is its lack of sugar, but this is offset by the fact that it is too liquid and does not bind the other ingredients together so well as the sweetened variety. However, it may be used if a sugar-free diet is required (for example, in diabetes and certain gastro-intestinal disturbances) unless yogurt—becoming more and more popular—is preferred for this purpose. Cream (if permitted), sweetened with a little honey, can also be used. Another excellent combination is two parts of yogurt and one part of cream or top of the milk.

The nuts should always be sprinkled on top and not mixed in with the Muesli. They improve the taste and the nutritional value, but may be omitted, especially if the cereal ingredient consists of fresh wholewheat grains or cereal germ.

MUESLI

All the Year Round

The original recipe for Muesli, worked out by Dr. Bircher-Benner, should be considered a prescription rather than a recipe. If closely followed it will not only provide the best balance of essential nutrients, but experience has also shown that people will not become tired of it, if regularly taken once or twice per day—something which may easily happen if richer and more elaborate versions are offered.

Any apple which is juicy, tart and white-fleshed is recommended. A combination of eating and cooking apples often yields the best results. For example, any of the following, alone or in combination: Cortland, McIntosh, Rhode Island Greening, Northern Spy, Winesap, Jonathan, Gravenstein.

Later on in the season, when home-grown apples tend to become dry and tasteless, their flavor can be improved by the addition, just before serving, of some freshly-grated orange or lemon peel, orange juice or rose hip purée.

BASIC RECIPE

Note.—Before any of the following Muesli recipes can be prepared, the rolled oats or oatmeal must be soaked beforehand for 12 hours. It is not necessary to soak the quick-cooking varieties if they have to be used. They are, however, not so valuable since heating processes have been used in their manufacture. The less heat a cereal has undergone, the greater will be its value.

For 'D' see note on page v.

I D. APPLE MUESLI   I D.

Ingredients:

Per person:

1 tablesp. rolled oats (or 1 tablesp. medium oatmeal) soaked for 12 hrs. in 3 tablesp. water	1 tablesp. sweetened condensed milk
1 tablesp. lemon juice	1 large apple (or 2–3 small ones)
	1 tablesp. grated filberts or almonds

Method:

1. Mix lemon juice and condensed milk to a smooth cream.
2. Add to oats, stirring thoroughly.
3. Wash apples, wipe with cloth and remove tops, cores and any blemishes.
4. Using a two-way or Bircher grater,* grate apple into mixture, stirring frequently to prevent discoloring.
5. Sprinkle nuts over the finished dish and serve immediately.

Note: 1–2 tablesp. water or orange juice can be added if required, depending on the variety of apple used and the length of time they have been in storage.

Instead of 1 tablesp. rolled oats, the following can be used: 1 teasp. rolled oats, previously soaked, and 1 teasp. cereal grains. These should be soaked in water 12 hr., then rinsed through a sieve and in cold water, and used either whole, coarsely ground, crushed or prepared in electric blender. Alternatively cereal flakes such as wheat, rice, barley, rye, millet, buckwheat or soya or dried wheat flakes (possibly mixed with yeast flakes for Vitamin B) may be used. Most of these are obtainable at health food stores or leading grocers.

* Available at health food stores.

2 D. APPLE MUESLI WITH ALMOND PUREÉ   2. D.

(Muesli without animal protein: for Vegans and in cases of allergy.)

Ingredients:

Per person:

1 tablesp. rolled oats (or 1 tablesp. medium oatmeal) soaked for 12 hrs. in 3 tablesp. water

1 tablesp. Almond Purée diluted in 3 tablesp. water

1 tablesp. lemon juice

1 tablesp. honey or brown sugar

1 large apple (or 2–3 small ones)

1 tablesp. grated filberts or almonds

Method:

1. Put the Almond Purée into a china bowl and add the water drop by drop.

2. Stir constantly until the mixture becomes whitish and emulsified, then add to the oats.

3. Add the lemon juice and honey or brown sugar and stir thoroughly.

4. Prepare and add the apple as in Basic Recipe No. 1 D.

5. Sprinkle nuts over the finished dish and serve immediately.

3 D. APPLE MUESLI WITH YOGURT   3 D.

(For slimming diets and for those who cannot tolerate milk. Tarter in flavor, stimulates digestion.)

Ingredients:

Per person:

1 tablesp. rolled oats (or 1 tablesp. medium oatmeal) soaked for 12 hrs. in 3 tablesp. water

4 tablesp. yogurt

1 teasp. lemon juice

1 tablesp. honey or 1½ tablesp. brown sugar

1 large apple (or 2–3 small ones)

1 tablesp. grated filberts or almonds

Method:

1. Mix the yogurt to a smooth consistency with lemon juice.

2. Add to the oats, stirring well, and mix in the honey or sugar.

3. Prepare and add the apple as in Basic Recipe No. 1.

4. Sprinkle nuts over the finished dish and serve immediately.

4 D. APPLE MUESLI WITH CREAM   4 D.

(Specially enriched dish for those wanting to put on weight.)

(For diabetics on a low fat diet unsweetened condensed or evaporated milk or yogurt should be used, or an excellent unsweetened but not tart Muesli can be made by using 2 tablesp. yogurt plus 1 tablesp. top of the milk or cream, omitting lemon juice and honey; substitute orange juice when permitted.)

Ingredients:

Per person:

1 heaped teasp. rolled oats (or 1 teasp. medium oatmeal) soaked for 12 hrs. in 1–2 tablesp. water

4–6 tablesp. cream
1 teasp. lemon juice
1 tablesp. honey
1 large apple (or 2–3 small ones)
1 tablesp. grated filberts or almonds

Method:

1. Add cream, lemon juice and honey to the oats and mix thoroughly.

2. Prepare and add apple as in Basic Recipe No. 1 D.

3. Sprinkle nuts over the finished dish and serve immediately.

5 D. MUESLI MADE FROM SOFT OR STONE FRUIT   5 D.

(Especially rich in Vitamin C.)

Ingredients:

As for Basic Recipe No. 1 D, substituting for the apple:

¾ cup strawberries, *or* raspberries, loganberries, red and black currants, blackberries, blueberries

or ½ lb. (or about ¾ cup crushed fruit) cherries, peaches, apricots, plums or greengages

Method:

For Soft Fruit

1. Select, wash and hull soft fruit.

2. Crush with fork or wooden spoon.

Continue as Basic Recipe, Method 1, 2 and 5.

For Stone Fruit

1. Select, wash and stone.

2. Chop up or reduce to pulp in electric blender.

Continue as Basic Recipe No. 1 D, Method 1, 2 and 5.

6 D. MUESLI MADE FROM FRUIT MIXTURES   6 D.

Any of the following mixtures can be used:

strawberries and raspberries

strawberries, raspberries and red currants

strawberries and apples

black currants and apples

blackberries and apples

apples with finely chopped orange or tangerine

apples and bananas

plums, peaches or apricots, etc.

Note: Apricots and plums should be avoided by anyone suffering from gastric and intestinal complaints.

Method:

For preparation of Basic Mixture, see Recipe No. 1 D, Method 1, 2 and 5.

7 D. MUESLI MADE FROM DRIED FRUIT   7 D.

If no fresh fruit is available Muesli can be prepared from dried fruit, i.e. apple rings, prunes, dried pears or apricots (*not* dried figs, dates or raisins).

Ingredients:

Per person:

As for Basic Recipe No. 1 D, omitting apple.

½ cup dried fruit, washed and soaked for 12 hrs.

Method:

1. Put the soaked fruit through a clean, well-galvanized or enameled mincer or Moulin-Légumes, or an electric blender.

2. Add this purée to the Basic Mixture—see Recipe No. 1 D.

Note: Care must be taken that the dried fruit is of good quality, without preservative or bleaching agents, otherwise troublesome gastric and intestinal disturbances may result.

RAW VEGETABLE SALADS AND DRESSINGS

The following four principles must be observed in the preparation of raw vegetables:

1. *Freshness*

The ideal vegetables are sun-ripened, organically grown, compost-fertilized, from one's own garden.

Raw vegetables should, if possible, be prepared just before they are intended to be eaten, so that no wilting and loss of juice takes place. After they have been chopped, grated or shredded they should not be exposed to the air for too long but should be mixed immediately with the dressing to prevent oxidizing.

2. *Quality*

Leaf and root vegetables should be young, tender and of good color. They should, whenever possible, have been grown on soil fertilized with compost and be free of plant diseases.* This is specially important in the case of invalid diet.

3. *Thorough Cleaning*

The instructions given below on the cleaning of vegetables must be followed exactly, to get rid of any worms and to avoid infection with colibacilli.

Compost-grown vegetables, and those grown without chemical or animal manure, do not contain any worm eggs.

4. *Well-balanced mixtures*

Whenever possible, every raw vegetable dish should combine roots-fruit-leaves. Invalid diet, in particular, should always include green leaves. The dressing used for the same raw vegetable salad should also be varied as much as possible.

Bright and harmonious colors make the salad dishes more attractive and increase the pleasure of eating.

Herbs, radishes and young carrots, etc., are effective as decorations when, for special occasions, a more festive air is wanted. Not more than three raw vegetables, however, should be served for any single daily salad, more attention being paid to variety during the course of the day. Too much variety can have a bad effect on the digestion.

CLEANING OF LEAFY VEGETABLES

Cabbage and cos lettuce, endive, kale, white cabbage, red cabbage, etc., separate the leaves' remove brown and imperfect parts and leave to soak for 1 hr. in slightly salted water (1 handful to about 6 qt. water). Rinse several times, if possible washing each leaf separately under the tap. Drain well in wire basket or clean cloth.

Special care must be taken with the preparation and washing of corn salad or lamb's lettuce, spinach, dandelion, lettuce, cress, sprouts and similar small leafy salads. Remove any little roots and tough parts and rinse thoroughly.

Halve chicory, remove outer leaves and wash well.

CLEANING OF ROOT VEGETABLES

Carrots, beetroots, turnips, radishes, kohlrabi, celeriac and salsify. Scrub roots with a brush under running water. Peel

* See p. 10.

and put immediately into cold water to which salt and lemon juice have been added (half a lemon or squeezed out peel to about 6 qt. water), so that vegetables do not lose their fresh color.

CLEANING OF VEGETABLE FRUITS

Tomatoes, cucumbers, zucchini, green and red peppers. Wash and, if necessary, peel and cut up into small pieces.

Peel cucumbers starting from the center, working towards the ends. Cut off bitter ends. Tender cucumbers need not be peeled.

Use only very young, tender zucchini for salad; do not peel. Green peppers are less sharp than the red variety. Cut peppers in half and remove the seeds, score thick parts and soak in water if too sharp.

With cauliflower cut into florets, remove imperfect parts, scrape stalk lightly and put into salt water. Scrape celery and cut away tough parts. Halve leeks, remove bad parts and rinse thoroughly. Halve fennel and wash.

SPECIAL METHODS OF CLEANING

If there is any doubt as to the growing and hygienic handling of any fruit or vegetables, or their freedom from bacteria, the following methods of cleaning must be observed:

1. In order to destroy any worm eggs and insects, put vegetables into a diluted salt solution (1 handful cooking salt to about 6 qt. water). The salt solution dissolves the protein layer by which the worm eggs are attached and subsequent rinsing of the vegetables removes them.

2. Bacteria, colibacilli and fungi, which are not harmful to healthy people, particularly in northern countries, can be removed with citric acid or vinegar. The vegetables, particularly leafy ones, should be left in a solution of 2 oz. citric acid to about 2 pt. water for 15 min. Rinse well afterwards under running water. If the citric acid solution is strained and set aside it can be used three or four times.

3. Put root vegetables and vegetable fruits in a colander or sieve and dip into boiling water for ten seconds. The outer layer is thus freed of any bacteria while the vegetables remain raw inside.

4. Vegetable and fruit juices can be practically freed of bacteria if lemon juice is added (one-fifth of the total quantity of juice).

5. To prevent any danger of amoebic infection in the tropics, dip the prepared vegetables into a chloride of lime solution

(5 gm. = ⅙ oz. to 2 pt. water), then wash well in boiled water, to remove all traces of it.

Various Methods of Cutting Up the Vegetables

Cabbage lettuce, cos lettuce, lamb's lettuce, dandelion, cress, watercress	Leave whole or halve largest leaves.
French endive, chicory	Cut into ¼-in. strips.
Spinach, leeks, peppers, celery, fennel	Shred.
Kale, white and red cabbage, Brussels sprouts	Shred finely.
Carrots, beetroots, turnips, celeriac	Grate with two-way grater or preferably Mouli-grater.
White radishes, salsify, kohlrabi	
Cucumbers, squash, radishes, cauliflower	Slice very finely or grate with Mouli-grater.

SALAD DRESSINGS

8 D. FRENCH DRESSING   **8 D.**

Ingredients for mayonnaise:
Per person:
1 tablesp. oil   some grated onion or garlic
1 teasp. lemon juice   1 teasp. fresh or ¼ teasp. dried green herbs*

Method:
Mix all ingredients together thoroughly, stirring vigorously to break up the oil.

9 MAYONNAISE DRESSING   **9**

Ingredients: for mayonnaise
1 egg yolk   lemon juice according to
1 cup oil   taste

Method:
1. Whisk yolk.
2. Add oil drop by drop, whisking continuously (the oil should not be too cold or too warm).
3. Add lemon juice when mixture becomes too thick.

Note: Above quantity is sufficient for 6–8 portions, or even more if more oil is added. It will keep for days in a cool place.

* About the use of herbs, fresh or dried, see 'Culinary Herbs,' p. 211.

Dressing:
Per person:
1 tablesp. mayonnaise   some onion (and garlic if
1 teasp. lemon juice   liked)
                          1 teasp. fresh or ¼ teasp.
                          dried green herbs

Method:
Mix all ingredients thoroughly together.

10 D. MAYONNAISE DRESSING WITH SOYA FLOUR   10 D.

(For Vegan diet and when animal protein should be avoided soya flour replaces egg.)

Ingredients for mayonnaise:
3 level tablesp. soya flour   1 cup oil
9 tablesp. water   4½ tablesp. lemon juice

Method:
1. Mix the soya flour and water to a smooth paste.
2. Add oil and lemon juice alternately, very slowly, then whisk well.

Dressing:
Per person:
Same mixture as for mayonnaise dressing. Make as above.

11 CREAM DRESSING   11

Ingredients:
Per person:
3 tablesp. cream   some onion (and garlic if
1 teasp. cream cheese   liked)
1 teasp. lemon juice   1 teasp. fresh or ¼ teasp.
                            dried green herbs

Method:
Whisk all ingredients thoroughly together.

12 D. YOGURT DRESSING   12 D.

(For a low fat diet.)

Ingredients:
Per person:
3–4 tablesp. yogurt   1 teasp. fresh or ¼ teasp.
few drops lemon juice   dried green herbs
some onion (and garlic if
liked)

Method:
Whisk all ingredients thoroughly together.

13 D. ALMOND PURÉE   13 D.

(*For Vegan diet and when animal protein should be avoided.*)
Ingredients:

Per person: some onion (and garlic if
1 tablesp. Almond Purée   liked)
4½ tablesp. water   1 teasp. fresh or ¼ teasp.
1 teasp. lemon juice   dried green herbs (if
                                 liked)

Method:
   1. Add drops of water to Almond Purée until it becomes
whitish and of a creamy consistency.
   2. Add remaining water and mix all ingredients together
slowly and thoroughly.

SUGGESTED RECIPES FOR DRESSING SALADS
AND RAW VEGETABLES*

Raw Vegetables	Preparation	Dressing	Flavoring	
Cabbage lettuce	Use whole leaves	French dressing	Chives, onion	14
Lettuce (thinnings)	Use whole leaves	French dressing	Chives, onion	15
French endive	Cut in ½-in. strips	French dressing or mayonnaise	Chives, onion, parsley†	16
Cos lettuce	Use leaves whole or shredded	French dressing or mayonnaise	Sweet basil, marjoram‡	17
Lamb's lettuce	Use whole leaves	French dressing or mayonnaise	Onion	18
Cresses	Use whole leaves	French dressing or mayonnaise	Onion	19
Spinach	Shred	French dressing or mayonnaise	Peppermint	20
Cabbage: white cabbage, savoy, sprouts, sauerkraut	Shred finely	French dressing or mayonnaise	Lovage, savory, thyme, caraway seeds	21
Tomatoes	Slice or dice	French dressing or mayonnaise	Basil, thyme, dill	22
Cucumbers	Slice finely	French dressing or mayonnaise	Dill	23

* For cleaning and cutting of vegetables, see Raw Vegetables, pp.
49–50.
† A moderate quantity of chives, parsley and onion may be added to
every dish of raw vegetables.
‡ For use of herbs, see 'Culinary Herbs,' p. 211.

Raw Vegetables	Preparation	Dressing	Flavoring	
Fennel	Slice finely or chop	French dressing or mayonnaise	Onion, chives	24
Peppers	Shred finely	French dressing or mayonnaise	Chives	25
Large black or white radishes	Slice or grate	French or cream dressing	Chives	26
Small red radishes	Grate or slice finely	French or cream dressing	Chives	27
Celery	Shred finely	French or cream dressing	Onion, chives	28
Squash or zucchini	Slice finely or grate roughly	French dressing or mayonnaise	Dill, basil	29
Carrots or other roots	Grate finely	French or cream dressing	Marjoram, lovage	30
Celeriac	Grate finely	Cream or French dressing	Basil, thyme	31
Beetroots uncooked	Grate finely or roughly	Cream dressing or mayonnaise	Lovage, thyme, caraway seeds	32
Cauliflower	Separate florets, grate stalks	Cream dressing or mayonnaise	Basil, marjoram, walnuts	
Chicory	Cut in ½-in. strips, shred	Cream or French dressing	Tarragon, marjoram	33
Jerusalem artichokes	Grate	Cream dressing	Thyme, lemon balm	34
Kohlrabi	Grate or chop finely	Cream or French dressing	Thyme, lovage	35
Red cabbage	Shred or grate finely	Cream or French dressing	Some grated apple, caraway seeds, lovage	36
				37

38   MIXED RAW VEGETABLES   38

Chicory with diced tomato—oil dressing or mayonnaise.
Peppers and fennel—oil dressing.
Fennel, chicory and diced tomato—mayonnaise.
Fennel, carrots or other roots—cream dressing.
Tomatoes and peppers—oil dressing or mayonnaise.

39   STUFFED RAW TOMATOES   39

Stuffed with:
     Cucumber—oil dressing or mayonnaise.
     Celery or celeriac—cream dressing.
     Cauliflower—cream dressing.
     White cabbage—mayonnaise.

40 D.   GERMINATED CEREAL GRAINS   40 D.

(Containing high content of Vitamin E and the B group and providing an all-round strengthening effect.)

Wheat, rye, oats, barley (whole grains).

1st day: Evening. Wash grains in sieve under running water and put in a bowl. Cover with water. Keep at room temperature near stove or radiator.

2nd day: Morning. Rinse and spread out to dry on a flat plate. Keep at room temperature near stove or radiator.

3rd day: Morning. Rinse and spread out to dry on a plate. Evening. Place in a bowl and cover with water. Keep at room temperature near stove or radiator.

The grains should by now have developed ½–¾ in. long sprouts.

Specially advised for Children:

Coarsely ground cereal grains, soaked and mixed with bananas, honey and water.

SAUERKRAUT

Sauerkraut is cabbage pickled in salt and spices; it is a very valuable raw vegetable, particularly in winter, as it is rich in Vitamin C. It is easier to digest when raw than when cooked. If sauerkraut is cooked occasionally, its flavor and digestibility can be improved by adding finely cut fresh sauerkraut.

A recipe is given below for making sauerkraut at home. Firm cabbages, preferably compost grown,* are used. This is a good way of using up any surplus in the garden. When made at home the sauerkraut will contain less salt than the commercially pickled, and sea-salt only can be used.

41 HOME-MADE SAUERKRAUT   41

Ingredients:

4 lb. cabbage (when prepared)

1 oz. coarse sea-salt

1 handful caraway and juniper berries *or* mixed sauerkraut herbs and spices containing caraway seeds and juniper berries

dill

mustard seeds

sticks of horse-radish (if available)

* See p. 10.

Method:

1. Remove outer leaves and stalks.
2. Shred cabbage, preferably using a wooden shredder with two blades, or an electric shredder.
3. Using a large earthenware jar (preferably with straight sides), put layers of cabbage alternately with layers of salt, caraway, juniper, etc.
4. Press down each layer with fists or a wooden masher until liquid rises and covers the cabbage.
5. Repeat this until the container is full.
6. Cover with a clean cloth, then a wooden lid or a plate.
7. Put a heavy clean stone on top to press the lid firmly down.
8. Leave for 4 weeks; occasionally ladling out the rising liquid and washing the rim of the jar and the lid.

Note: After four weeks the sauerkraut is ready for use and can be eaten raw or cooked. At intervals of one week the cloth, lid and stone must be washed. If the top layer of sauerkraut becomes soft and discolored, it must be removed.

As long as these instructions are carried out with care, the sauerkraut can be kept until the warmer weather, usually about the beginning of April or longer according to season.

41 D. SAUERKRAUT SALAD   41 D.

Ingredients:

sauerkraut

caraway seeds ⎫ when using
juniper berries ⎬ canned
        ⎭ sauerkraut

1 chopped onion

1 shredded apple
juice of 1 lemon
2 tablesp. oil

Method:

1. Loosen sauerkraut (particularly if using canned).
2. Cut up and mix with all the ingredients except the lemon and oil.
3. Add the lemon and oil and mix thoroughly.
4. Serve with corn salad or watercress, and with any variety of uncooked root salad.

FRESHLY EXPRESSED FRUIT AND VEGETABLE JUICES AND CEREAL CREAMS

Juices are uncooked food rich in vitamins and minerals in a form which is liquidized by some mechanical means; they are meant either to be an addition to or special enrichment of the diet; they are of considerable value in cases where roughage (cellulose) must be avoided, or in the case of gastro-intestinal conditions.

It should, however, be realized that the whole fruit and vegetable are, without exception, of greater value, and in the long run cannot be replaced by juices. As soon as permissible, a return should therefore be made to whole fruit and raw vegetables.

Many types of juice extractors are obtainable for squeezing out the fruit and vegetable juices. These include the small hand-model, the juice-extracting attachment of an electric food-mixer, or electric blender. If the hand type is used, the fruit or vegetables must first be cut up. Before squeezing, apples, pears, and all root vegetables should be finely grated; leaf vegetables and herbs should be finely chopped.

42 D.   FRUIT JUICES   42 D.

Serve immediately after extracting. Delay of any kind causes loss in value.

(a) UNMIXED FRUIT JUICES (without any addition):
Oranges, tangerines, grapefruit, apples, pears, grapes, strawberries, raspberries, red currants, loganberries, blueberries, peaches, apricots, plums.

(b) MIXED FRUIT JUICES:
Oranges, tangerines, grapefruit,
or
Soft fruit juice with apple juice.
Soft fruit juice with peach, apricot or plum juice.
Bananas, mashed and whisked, with orange, soft fruit, peach or apricot juice.
Additional ingredients as required or prescribed:
Lemon juice, brown sugar, honey, cream, yogurt, Almond Purée, linseed, cream of rice,* or barley* (for gastro-intestinal conditions).

43 D.   VEGETABLE JUICES   43 D.

Served fresh, they have a high vitamin and mineral content. Each juice has its own special value (see chapter on mineral substances and vitamins).

(a) UNMIXED VEGETABLE JUICES:
Tomatoes, carrots and other roots, beetroot, white radishes, cabbage, celeriac, potatoes, all leaf, root and tuberous vegetables.

* Available at health food stores.

(*b*) MIXED VEGETABLE JUICES:

In our experience, the best mixtures are:

Carrots, tomatoes, spinach (in equal proportions).

Tomatoes and carrots.

Tomatoes and spinach.

Other mixtures (and vegetable cocktails) can be combined according to individual taste.

For a change, add to the mixture before extracting, some sorrel, tender nettles, chives, parsley, tender young celery or celeriac leaves or root. Other leaf vegetables which may be added include: white or green cabbage, lettuce, endive, lamb's lettuce, dandelion. In spring, special additions of dandelion, sorrel and nettle juice are suggested and other herbs may be added, all of which may be fresh or dried green and added before extraction. In latter case allow them to permeate the juice before extracting.

Additional supplementary ingredients:

Per glass (about 6–8 oz.):

1 tablesp. cream, some lemon juice, perhaps a little fruit pulp or juice; or cream of linseed, rice or barley. (See below.)

(*c*) POTATO JUICE:

Use well-cleaned, if necessary peeled, potatoes. Use no unripe, greenish or sprouting ones.

Prepare like carrot juice. Does not taste very pleasant, but may be suggested by a doctor.

44 D.   CEREAL CREAM AS SUPPLEMENT   44 D.
TO JUICES

One-third of cereal cream can be added to raw juices. It neutralizes tart fruit flavors and is advisable for babies and in gastro-intestinal conditions.

(*a*) CREAM OF RICE OR BARLEY*

Ingredients:

1 heaping teasp. rice or rice flakes or barley flakes or meal	1 cup water

Method:

1. Mix cereal with the cold water.
2. Bring to the boil.
3. Cook for 5 minutes, stirring constantly.
4. Allow to cool.

* Available at health food stores. Barley and oat flakes are mostly organically grown.

(*b*) CREAM OF LINSEED

Ingredients:

 1 tablesp. linseed   1 cup water

Method:

 1. Wash linseed in a sieve under running water.

 2. Boil in the water for 10 minutes.

 3. Strain and allow to cool.

The daily quantity of cereal cream for babies or gastro-intestinal patients can be prepared at one time, then put into a thermos flask and added to each freshly prepared raw juice as required.

VARIETIES OF MILK (including Soya) AND SOYA BEANS

NON-DAIRY AND DAIRY PRODUCTS
PLANTMILK

Milk made from nuts, and vegetable milk.

MILK MADE FROM NUTS

45 D. NUT OR ALMOND MILK   45 D.

 (*A vegetable protein-fat-food; mucilaginous; soothing.*)

Ingredients:

1 tablesp. Almond Purée	¾ cup water *or* ¾ cup water and ¼ cup fruit juice which will produce slight thickening
1 teasp. honey	

Method:

 1. Mix Almond Purée and honey together with whisk.

 2. Add water drop by drop continually whisking or stirring well.

ALMOND MILK FROM FRESH ALMONDS

   (*Particularly easy to digest.*)

Ingredients:

1½ tablesp. peeled almonds (do not use bitter almonds	1 teasp. honey ¾ cup water

Method:

 1. Mix in electric blender or mixer.

 2. Strain if necessary.

46 D. PINE KERNEL MILK 46 D.

(*Extremely rich in easily-digestible fat and vegetable protein.*)

Ingredients:

1½ tablesp. washed pine ¾ cup water
kernels
1 teasp. honey

Method:
Prepare like Almond Milk.

47 D. SOYA MILK 47 D.

1. Wash and dry soya beans.
2. Crush in nut mill or Mouli-grater or electric blender.

Ingredients:

1 cup soya beans (soaked water to mix
for 2 hrs. in) 1 tablesp. sugar
7½ cups water pinch of salt

Method:
3. Soak soya beans for 2 hr.
4. Boil for 20 min. in soaking water, stirring constantly.
5. Rub through a sieve or Moulin-Legumes.
6. Add water until of same consistency as cow's milk.
7. Add sugar and salt; and allow to cool.

Editor's Notes: There is available in America a 'ready for use' Plantmilk in powder form made from specially processed Soya. It can be made into a smooth milk or cream by the addition of water and it can be used for babies as well as for adults. The name of this milk is 'Soyamel,' and full instructions for its uses are given on each can.*

SOYA BEANS

The soya bean has become increasingly popular in recent years in United States and European cookery, after having been widely grown in China for centuries. Owing to its pleasant taste and health value it may be considered a welcome and enriching addition to our kitchen.

It belongs, however, to the most highly concentrated of natural foodstuffs, being richer in fat and protein than nuts and meat; so that over-nourishment can result from using too much of it. In spite of its higher concentration, this danger is, nevertheless, not so great as in the case of meat. The stimulat-

* Available at health food stores.

ing substances of meat induce a desire for more meat, whereas the appetite is soon appeased with soya dishes. Furthermore, soya protein is a plant protein of extremely high biological value and is particularly rich in lecithin and the important unsaturated fatty acids (E.F.A.). The same applies to soya oil. The high vitamin content—especially of the B group and Vitamin E—of the soya bean is remarkable. Even more remarkable is its richness in mineral salts, particularly calcium and iron. It also contains a surplus of alkalis.

Nevertheless, concentrated soya dishes should only be served as an exception. Soya flour should be used more as an addition and enrichment, specially for binding. For this purpose soya flour can replace eggs completely, for example in pancakes and cakes.

The low starch content of the soya bean makes it very valuable in a diabetic diet.

If possible, fully ripe soya beans of the light yellow kind, or whole soya flour, should be chosen.

For preparation of soya milk, see above recipe, No. 47 D. Other soya recipes are Nos. 67 D, 264 D, 267 D, and 417 D.

DAIRY MILK PRODUCTS

48 D. YOGURT   48 D.

(*Yogurt is the purest, most efficacious and easily digestible way of supplying dairy milk protein. It stimulates the digestion.*)

Ready-prepared yogurt can be used if a good quality can be obtained from a dairy or a health food store.

There is some kitchen equipment available which makes it possible to produce yogurt at home. The makers' directions must be closely followed.

Ingredients:
5 cups (2½ pt.) milk   ½ cup yogurt

Method:
1. Bring milk to the boil. Cool to 100° F.
2. Whisk yogurt together with milk.
3. Pour into a glass receptacle.
4. Cover with muslin and a lid.
5. Place in padded hay box.
6. Cover with blanket or cushion.
7. Leave in warm place for 24 hr.
8. Store in refrigerator until required.

48 SOUR MILK, CURD, SOUR CREAM AND CREAM CHEESE 48

Ingredients:

5 cups or 2½ pt. *unpasteurized* T.T .(tuberculin-tested) or *pasteurized* milk (Should give about ¼ lb. curd.)

Method:

1. Pour milk into basin (preferably shallow to give a wide surface) and cover lightly.

2. Stand in warm, but not sunny, place in the kitchen, near the stove.

3. Allow to get sour and firm (consistency of junket); according to temperature this will take 2–3 days.

4. This can now be eaten and used as sour milk with brown sugar and wholewheat crumbs on the top, or whisked and used like yogurt, or made into cream cheese as follows:

5. Skim off the cream and put aside in a small cup or basin for cooking.

6. Place the skimmed milk in a warmer place (on top of warm but *not hot* stove) and allow the liquid whey to get separated.

7. When the whey has satisfactorily separated from the milk, and not before, pass the whole contents of the basin through a muslin bag and allow to drip. Do not remove the curd from bag before all the liquid has been drained.

Note: The sour cream should not be removed from the milk before it has become absolutely firm, as milk which has not finished the souring process, as well as milk which has been left standing for too long, is less digestible, while sour milk products prepared at the right moment are excellent aids to digestion.

As quick souring should always be aimed at, the process can be hastened, particularly in cool weather, by adding to the basin of fresh milk a spoonful of sour milk of the previous souring and beating it well together. This should be done as soon as possible after the milk has been poured out, as it is important that the milk should not be disturbed once souring has begun. If it is necessary to move the basin, this should be done as gently as possible. If no sour milk is available, a little sour cream curd or yogurt will also help towards the quick increase of souring agents. In winter one of these additions is essential to get the souring process started at all.

CREAM CHEESE

After the sour cream has been removed from the sour milk and the solid contents made into curd by draining off the whey, the solid substance of curd (which should not contain any whey if properly done) can be used immediately for cream cheese or can be kept for a few more days and used for various recipes. Cream cheese to be used as a spread or in combination with salad or potato dishes is made in the following way:

Pass curds through a sieve and add gradually *fresh* cream or top of fresh milk, stirring well all the time until a thick creamy consistency is achieved. Add a little salt and chopped chives, spring onions, onion green or nasturtium (freshly chopped or dried green). It can also be flavored with caraway seeds if liked. As a sweet the thick mixture can be flavored with sugar and ground cinnamon or fruit juice or purée and served in individual dishes. If the *sour* cream is put back into the curd after sieving, a much tarter flavor is obtained, which usually is not so popular with children. To introduce cream cheese for the first time it is wiser to mix it with fresh cream.

49 MANY-FLAVORED CREAM CHEESE DISH 49

Ingredients:

4–5 oz. curd	Some vegetable stock *or*
¾ cup milk	½ teasp. Marmite
Potatoes steamed in their jackets	½ teasp. tomato purée
	½ teasp. caraway
1 pinch salt	2 teasp. mixed copped herbs
1 tablesp. chopped chives	such as basil, thyme, parsley and garlic (if liked)

Method:

1. Whisk curd with milk or top of the milk until creamy.
2. When smooth divide into five different portions.
3. Mix well chopped chives into portion 1.
4. Dissolve Marmite with a little warm water or use vegetable stock, and whisk well into portion 2.
5. Whisk Tomato Purée into portion 3.
6. Mix caraway well with portion 4.
7. Add mixed herbs (whether finely chopped fresh or dried green) and mix well into portion 5.
8. Arrange five portions, each different in color, attractively on a flat dish.
9. Serve with potatoes in their jackets.

Note: All these cream cheese mixtures can be served by slitting open large cooked potatoes in their jackets and piping the cream cheese along the slit.

See Recipe No. 193 D.

SOUPS

The use of vegetable stock is suggested for the soup and vegetable recipes. However, since it is not usually possible to prepare such a stock every day, vegetable and yeast extracts such as Marmite can be used instead. For saltless or salt-reduced diets saltless Marmite is available. These yeast extracts, available at health food stores, are rich in Vitamin B, e.g. glutathione and lecithin.

Cream improves and refines every soup and vegetable dish although milk can be used instead.

50 D. VEGETABLE STOCK 50 D.

Vegetables according to season, for instance celery, carrots and other roots, some cabbage or kohlrabi, leeks, tomatoes, celeriac and onions. The tougher but still sound parts may also be used, as well as potato peel.

Ingredients:

1 tablesp. vegetable cooking fat (p. 40) or sunflower oil
1 onion
2 carrots or other roots
1 cup shredded or diced celery or celeriac
cabbage
spinach beet leaves
4 or 5 qt. cold water
lovage, basil or other fresh or dried herbs
½ bay leaf
salt (only for a normal diet)

Method:
1. Melt fat.
2. Halve onion, with skin, and brown cut surface in fat.
3. Cut vegetables in small pieces.
4. Add to the onion and stew gently for at least ¼ hour, covered with a lid.
5. Add cold water, simmer for 2 hr.
6. Season according to taste.

51 D. CLEAR VEGETABLE BROTH 51 D.

Ingredients:

2½ qt. vegetable stock
Marmite or other yeast extract to taste
1 level tablesp. butter
chives or parsley
salt

Method:
Pour hot vegetable stock over all other ingredients.

ADDITIONS TO SOUPS

52 BUTTER DUMPLINGS 52

Ingredients:

3 tablesp. butter	salt
¾ cup flour	chopped fresh or dried green
milk	herbs as desired
1 beaten egg	stock

Method:

1. Melt butter and fry flour in it.
2. Add milk, beat till mixture leaves sides of the pan.
3. Mix beaten egg, herbs and salt with hot paste.
4. Scoop out small dumplings with teasp. Add to boiling stock and simmer for 5 min.

53 FLOUR DUMPLINGS 53

Ingredients:

¾ cup milk or water	¾ cup flour
1 level tablesp. vegetable	1 beaten egg
fat	salt

Method:

1. Bring milk or water and cooking fat to the boil.
2. Sieve flour and salt and add all at once to the boiling milk.
3. Beat the egg into the hot paste.
4. Put into pastry tube and force balls the size of a filbert onto a cookie sheet.
5. Bake in slow oven (300°) until pale fawn or simmer in boiling stock 5 min.

54 CHEESE DUMPLINGS 54

The same as No. 53 but with the addition of 2 tablesp. grated cheese.

55 PANCAKE STRIPS 55

Ingredients:

4½ tablesp. flour	¾ cup milk/water
½ of an egg	salt
	1 tablesp. vegetable fat

Method:

1. Make thin pancake mixture.
2. Fry 3–4 pancakes, cut into thin strips.

56 RIBELI 56

Ingredients:

7½ tablesp. flour   salt
1 egg

Method:

1. Make firm paste with flour, egg and salt, allow to dry out.
2. Grate on flat grater into boiling stock.
3. Bring again to the boil.

57 DICED EGG CUSTARD 57

Ingredients:

1 large or 2 small eggs   salt
½ teasp. cornstarch   ¾ cup warm milk
                           nutmeg

Method:

1. Beat up egg, cornstarch, salt and a grating of nutmeg.
2. Add to warmed milk, beat.
3. Put into buttered baking dish or cups, cover and steam gently in hot water till firm.
4. When cool, turn out and chop up into small cubes.

58 FARINA DUMPLINGS 58

Ingredients:

2 tablesp. butter   salt
¾ cup fine farina   nutmeg
1 egg

Method:

1. Cream butter.
2. Mix farina, egg, seasoning and nutmeg thoroughly with the butter and leave to stand for ½ hr.
3. Scoop out small dumplings with teasp., add to boiling stock and simmer for 15–20 min.

59 GOLDEN CUBES 59

Ingredients:

2 slices wholewheat bread   5–6 tablesp. milk
1 beaten egg   1½ tablesp. vegetable fat

Method:
1. Cut bread into equal squares.
2. Mix egg and milk, pour over bread and allow to soak up.
3. Melt fat.
4. Fry cubes until golden yellow.

60 D. TAPIOCA SOUP WITH VEGETABLES 60 D.

Ingredients:

1½ oz. tapioca
5 pt. vegetable stock
1 tablesp. vegetable fat
1 small carrot, diced
1 piece celery or celeriac, diced

½ leek, shredded
salt
Marmite or other yeast extract
parsley, chives or mixed herbs (soup mixture)

Method:
1. Boil vegetable stock, slightly salted.
2. Stir tapioca into it.
3. Melt fat in another pan.
4. Sauté vegetables in it.
5. Add to vegetable stock and cook for ½ hr.
6. Add Marmite and herbs to finished soup.

The vegetables may also be finely shredded as for Julienne soup.

61 D. CLEAR RICE SOUP 61 D.

Ingredients:

1 heaping tablesp. vegetable fat
½ onion, chopped
1 small carrot
piece of celery or celeriac, finely cut

½ finely cut leek
4½ tablesp. rice
5 pt. vegetable stock
chives

Method:
1. Melt fat.
2. Fry onion in it.
3. Sauté all vegetables together.
4. Add rice and stock and cook for 15–20 min.
5. Add chives to the finished soup.

62 D. THICK RICE SOUP 62 D.

Ingredients:

1 heaping tablesp. vegetable fat
1 piece celery or celeriac, finely cut
1 small carrot, finely cut
½ leek
4 tablesp. rice

3 tablesp. flour
5 pt. vegetable stock
salt
3 tablesp. cream
chives

Method:
1. Melt fat.
2. Sauté vegetables in it.
3. Add rice and sauté together.
4. Sprinkle flour over all.
5. Add stock and seasoning and cook for 30 min.
6. Add cream and chives to finished soup.

63 D. ITALIAN RICE SOUP 63 D.

(*For light diets:* without cheese.)

Ingredients:

2 tablesp. vegetable fat
1 cup finely diced vegetables (carrots, onions, celery)
1 lb. finely shredded spinach

almost 1 cup rice
5 pt. water
salt
1 level teasp. butter.
2–3 tablesp. cheese (if permitted)

Method:
1. Melt fat.
2. Sauté diced vegetables in it until slightly browned.
3. Add spinach and stew till juice has condensed.
4. Add rice, water and salt and cook for 20 min.
5. Place butter in tureen or soup bowls and pour soup in.
6. Sprinkle cheese over.

64 D. CREAMED RICE SOUP 64 D.

Ingredients:

5 pt. vegetable stock
approx. ¾ cup rice flour
1 tablesp. flour
cold water

½ cup milk
salt
1½ tablesp. butter
4½ tablesp. cream
chives to taste

Method:
1. Bring stock to the boil.
2. Blend rice and flour to a smooth cream with some cold water.
3. Add to the boiling stock and season.
4. Add milk and cook for ½ hr., stirring frequently.
5. Put butter, cream and chives into tureen or soup bowls and pour soup over.

65 D. CREAM SOUP, 1   65 D.

Ingredients:

1 heaping tablesp. vegetable fat	salt
	3 tablesp. cream
⅓ cup wholewheat flour	chives to taste
5 pt. vegetable stock	

Method:
1. Melt fat.
2. Sauté flour in it lightly.
3. Add stock and salt and cook for ½ hr., stirring frequently.
4. Put cream and chives into tureen or soup bowls and pour soup over.

66 D. CREAM SOUP, 2   66 D.

Ingredients:

⅓ cup flour	4½ tablesp. cream
1¼ pt. milk	1 teasp. butter (if liked), *or*
3¾ pt. vegetable stock	1 egg yolk
salt	

Method:
1. Blend flour with some of the cold milk.
2. Bring vegetable stock to the boil.
3. Add blended flour and rest of milk to the boiling stock.
4. Season and cook for ¼ hr., stirring frequently.
5. Put cream, butter or egg into tureen, add boiling soup and whisk.

66*a* D. HERB SOUP   66*a* D.

Prepare cream soup as in Recipe Nos. 65 or 66 above, add fresh chopped or dried green herbs such as lovage, basil, tarragon, according to taste.

67 D. SOYA SOUP 67 D.

Ingredients:

1 heaping tablesp. vege-
table fat
½ onion
¼ cup flour
1½ tablesp. soya flour

3¾ pt. vegetable stock
1 tomato, peeled and diced
salt
cream (if allowed)

Method:

1. Melt fat and sauté onion.
2. Sauté flour and soya flour in it.
3. Add tomato, stock and salt.
4. Cook fo ¼ hr., stirring frequently.
5. Add cream if used.

68 D. CREAM OF ROLLED OAT SOUP 68 D.

Ingredients:

1 heaping tablesp. vege-
table fat
1½ tablesp. flour
⅓ cup rolled oats
5 pt. vegetable stock

1 piece celery or celeriac
salt
4½ tablesp. cream
chives if liked

Method:

1. Melt fat, and brown flour and oats lightly in it.
2. Add vegetable stock, celery and salt and cook for 1 hr.
3. Pour through strainer.
4. Put cream in tureen or soup bowls and pour soup on to it. Add chives if used.

69 D. OATMEAL SOUP 69 D.

(*For light diet:* without croûtons.)

Ingredients:

1 heaping tablesp. vege-
table fat
9 tablesp. fine oatmeal
3¾ pt. vegetable stock
1 piece of celery or ce-
leriac

salt
3 tablesp. cream
chives if liked

Method:

Prepare as for Recipe No. 68. Serve with croûtons of fried bread.

70 D. OATMEAL GRUEL (Cream of Oats)   70 D.

(*For special diets.*)

Ingredients:

7 tablesp. (approx.) rolled oats	salt
5 pt. cold water	butter or cream (if allowed)

Method:

1. Cook rolled oats in the water with salt for 30–40 min.
2. Sieve and add butter or cream if allowed.

71 D. OAT GROATS SOUP   71 D.

Ingredients:

1 heaping tablesp. vegetable fat	piece celery or one-quarter celeriac
½ onion, chopped	salt
9 tablesp. groats	Marmite or other yeast extract
8¾ cups water	3 tablesp. cream (if liked)
1¼ cups milk	

Method:

1. Melt fat and sauté onions in it until golden.
2. Add groats and sauté until golden brown.
3. Add water, milk, celery and salt and cook for 1 hr.
4. Put yeast extract and cream in tureen or soup bowls and pour soup over them.

72 D. BARLEY SOUP   72 D.

Ingredients:

1 heaping tablesp. vegetable fat	8¾ cups water
½ chopped onion	1¼ cups milk
1 cup finely shredded leeks, carrots, celery or celeriac	salt
	3 tablesp. cream
	nutmeg
½ cup (approx.) barley	chives

Method:

1. Melt fat and sauté onion in it.
2. Add leeks, carrots, celery and sauté together.
3. Add barley, water and milk and salt.
4. Cook for 1½ hr., stirring from time to time.
5. Add cream, nutmeg and chives and serve.

73 D. BARLEY MEAL SOUP   73 D.

Ingredients and method as for Recipe No. 69, substituting barley meal for oatmeal.

74 D. FARINA SOUP   74 D.

Ingredients:

6 tablesp. farina	1 egg
5 pt. stock	nutmeg
salt	chives
3 tablesp. cream	

Method:

1. Stir farina into boiling stock and add salt.
2. Cook for ½ hr., stirring frequently.
3. Put cream and egg into tureen and pour the boiling soup on to them.
4. Whisk well adding nutmeg and chives.

75. VAUDOIS FARINA SOUP   75

Ingredients:

1 heaping tablesp. vegetable fat	5 pt. vegetable stock
4½ tablesp. farina	1½ tablesp. cream
1½ tablesp. wholewheat flour	1 teasp. butter
1 plateful cabbage, finely shredded	1 tablesp. chopped parsley

Method:

1. Melt fat.
2. Sauté the farina and wholewheat flour in it.
3. Add cabbage and sauté until cabbage loses its crispness.
4. Pour in the stock and cook altogether for ½ hr.
5. Put cream and butter into tureen, pour soup over and add the chopped parsley.

76 BREAD SOUP   76

Ingredients:

3 tablesp. vegetable fat	5 pt. vegetable stock
1 chopped onion	salt
3 slices wholewheat bread cut in cubes)	caraway seeds (if liked)
2 tablesp. wholewheat flour	1 oz. cream
	some chopped celery leaves

Method:
1. Melt fat and sauté onion in it.
2. Add bread and wholewheat flour and sauté altogether.
3. Add stock, salt and caraway seeds and cook for ½ hr.
4. Sieve if necessary.
5. Put cream into tureen or soup bowls and pour soup over it.
6. Add chopped celery leaves.

77 CHEESE SOUP 77

Ingredients:

1 heaping tablesp. vegetable fat	4½ tablesp. cheese (half of it Parmesan)
9 tablesp. flour	3–4 tablesp. cream
8¾ cups vegetable stock	some Marmite or other yeast extract
1¼ cups milk	
salt	1 teasp. butter

Method:
1. Melt fat and sauté flour in it.
2. Add stock, milk and salt and cook for 20 min.
3. Mix cheese, cream, Marmite and butter in tureen.
4. Pour soup over them and whisk altogether till smooth.

78 BROWNED WHOLEWHEAT SOUP 78

Ingredients:

6 tablesp. wholewheat flour	salt
6 tablesp. flour	1 tablesp. butter
5 pt. cold water	3 tablesp. cream (optional)
1 onion, whole	3 tablesp. grated Parmesan cheese
1 teasp. caraway seeds (if liked)	

Method:
1. Roast flour until chestnut brown, then cool.
2. Add the cold water gradually to the flour until smooth.
3. Add onion, caraway seeds and salt and cook for ½ hr. Remove onion.
4. Put butter, cream and cheese into the tureen and pour soup over it.

79 TOMATO SOUP, 1

Ingredients:

1 heaping tablesp. vege-
table fat
½ onion
1 small carrot
1 piece celery or celeriac
½ leek
1 clove of garlic
some rosemary

4 tomatoes
6 tablesp. flour
8¾ cups vegetable stock
some tomato pureé if necessary
1 teasp. butter
3 tablesp. cream
chives

Note: Cook 1 tablesp. rice or tapioca with soup if desired,
or add fried bread cubes before serving or serve separately.

Method:

1. Melt fat.
2. Cut up all vegetables (except tomatoes) into small
pieces and sauté well in the fat.
3. Add tomatoes.
4. Sprinkle flour over the mixture and sauté all together.
5. Add the stock and cook for ½ hr. Sieve.
6. Put the butter and cream into a tureen, pour the soup
over and garnish with chives, or add these before serving.

80 D. TOMATO SOUP, 2 80 D.

Ingredients:

2 lb. ripe summer toma-
toes
salt
1 teasp. sugar

1 teasp. lemon juice *or* 3–4
tablesp. cream
herbs according to taste
(fresh or dried)

Method:

1. Dice tomatoes, add salt and sugar, and bring to the boil.
2. Sieve.
3. Add lemon juice or cream and serve soup hot or cold
garnished with herbs.

81 D. CARROT SOUP 81 D.

Ingredients:

1 heaping tablesp. vege-
table fat
½ onion, chopped
4 large carrots, chopped
7½ tablesp. flour
8¾ cups vegetable stock

1¼ cups milk
salt
1 teasp. caraway seeds (if
liked)
celery leaves or lovage
3 tablesp. cream

Method:
1. Melt fat and sauté onion and carrots in it.
2. Sprinkle flour over the mixture and sauté lightly.
3. Add stock, milk, salt and herbs and cook for ½ hr. Sieve.
4. Put cream into tureen or soup bowls and pour soup over it.

82 D. SPINACH OR SPINACH BEET SOUP   82 D.

Ingredients:

1 heaping tablesp. vegetable fat	1¼ cups milk
	salt
½ onion, chopped	1 plate finely chopped spinach
1 clove of garlic, chopped	
7½ tablesp. flour	some peppermint leaves
1 plateful chopped spinach	3 tablesp. cream (optional)
	nutmeg
8¾ cups vegetable stock	

Method:
1. Melt fat and sauté onion, garlic and flour in it.
2. Add spinach and sauté all together.
3. Add stock, milk and salt and cook for 20 min.
4. Mix raw finely chopped spinach with peppermint leaves.
5. Add to the finished soup and do not allow to boil again.
6. Put cream and nutmeg into tureen or soup bowls and pour soup over it.

83 D. CELERIAC SOUP   83 D.

Ingredients:

1 heaping tablesp. vegetable fat	5 pt. vegetable stock
	salt
½ onion, chopped	¼ bay leaf
1 stick celery or medium celeriac, finely chopped	lovage
	3 tablesp. cream
6 tablesp. flour	nutmeg

Method:
1. Melt fat.
2. Sauté onion.
3. Add celery and sauté.
4. Sprinkle flour over the mixture and sauté all together.
5. Add stock, salt and herbs and cook for ¾ hr.
6. Sieve.
7. Put cream and grated nutmeg into tureen or soup bowls and pour soup over it.

84 CAULIFLOWER SOUP 84

Ingredients:

1 small cauliflower
1 heaping tablesp. vege-
table fat
4½ tablesp. flour
5 pt. vegetable stock
salt

¼ bay leaf
basil (very little)
some Marmite or other yeast
extract
3 tablesp. cream

Method:

1. Cook cauliflower florets carefully, separately.
2. Cut uncooked stalks into small pieces.
3. Melt fat and sauté flour in it.
4. Add small pieces of stalk and sauté together.
5. Add stock, salt, bay leaf and basil and cook for ¾ hr.
6. Sieve.
7. Put cooked florets, cream and yeast extract into soup shortly before serving. Do not allow to boil again.

85 D. CHERVIL SOUP 85 D.

Ingredients:

1 heaping tablesp. vege-
table fat
½ onion, chopped
3 medium-sized potatoes,
diced

3 tablesp. flour
5 pt. vegetable stock
salt
2 tablesp. chopped chervil
3 tablesp. cream

Method:

1. Melt fat and sauté onion in it.
2. Add diced potatoes and sauté.
3. Sprinkle flour over the mixture and sauté all together for a few minutes.
4. Add stock and salt and cook for ½ hr.
5. Sieve.
6. Put chervil and cream into tureen or soup bowls and pour soup over them.

For another version: Sauté onions and chervil in melted fat and then proceed from Method No. 3. (Leave out potatoes and do not sieve.)

86 D. SPRING SOUP 86 D.

Ingredients:

1 heaping tablesp. vegetable fat
6 tablesp. flour
8¾ cups water or vegetable stock
salt
½ onion

a few small celery leaves
1 young carrot
some small spinach leaves
lovage, sorrel, nettle or dandelion leaves
1¼ cups milk
3 tablesp. cream

Method:

1. Melt fat and sauté flour lightly in it.
2. Add stock and salt and cook for ½ hr.
3. Chop onion, herbs and vegetables finely, add to the soup and simmer for a few minutes.
4. Add milk.
5. Put cream into tureen or soup bowls and add soup.

87 CREAM OF LEEK SOUP 87

Ingredients:

1 heaping tablesp. vegetable fat
1 large leek, cut up coarsely
9 tablesp. flour

5 pt. vegetable stock
salt
3 tablesp. cream
1 egg yolk, if desired

Method:

1. Melt fat and sauté leek in it till tender.
2. Sprinkle flour over it.
3. Add stock and salt and cook ½–¾ hr.
4. Sieve.
5. Put cream and yolk of egg (if used) into tureen and pour soup over them.

88 ONION SOUP 88

Ingredients:

1 heaping tablesp. vegetable fat
2 large onions, cut in strips
7½ tablesp. flour
5 pt. water

salt
Marmite, or other yeast extract
3 tablesp. cream
nutmeg
basil

Method:
1. Melt fat and sauté onion in it till tender.
2. Sprinkle flour over it.
3. Add stock and salt and cook ½–¾ hr.
4. Sieve.
5. Put cream and yolk of egg (if used) into tureen and pour soup over them.

89 D. POTATO SOUP   89 D.

Ingredients:

1 heaping tablesp. vegetable fat	3 tablesp. flour
1 leek	5 pt. water
1 piece celery or celeriac	1½ tablesp. cream
½ carrot	marjoram
4 medium-sized potatoes, cut up	chives

Method:
1. Melt fat, cut vegetables into pieces and sauté well.
2. Sprinkle flour over the mixture and sauté.
3. Add water and cook for ½ hr.
4. Sieve.
5. Put cream and herbs into tureen or soup bowls and pour soup over.

90 POTATO AND LEEK SOUP   90

Ingredients:

1 heaping tablesp. vegetable fat	salt
1 leek, shredded finely	Marmite, Vecon, or other yeast extract
3 tablesp. flour	basil, marjoram, etc.
5 pt. vegetable stock	3 tablesp. cream
3 medium-sized potatoes, cut up in small pieces	

Method:
As for Recipe No. 87; cook until tender, do not put through a sieve.

91 BROWN POTATO SOUP   91

Ingredients:

4½ tablesp. flour	salt
5 pt. water	marjoram
3 medium-sized potatoes, sliced	caraway seeds (if liked)
	3 tablesp. grated cheese

Method:
1. Roast flour to a chestnut brown.
2. Add a little cold water and mix well.
3. Add gradually to remaining water.
4. Add potatoes, salt, herbs, and cream if desired, and cook until soft.
5. Put cheese into tureen or soup bowls and pour soup over it.

---

92 CABBAGE AND POTATO SOUP   92

Ingredients:

1 heaping tablesp. vegetable fat	4 potatoes, sliced
½ onion, chopped	5 pt. water
1 plateful cabbage, finely shredded	salt
	dill or caraway seeds
3 tablesp. flour	1 oz. cream

Method:
1. Melt fat and sauté onion.
2. Add cabbage and sauté gently until soft.
3. Sprinkle flour over the mixture and sauté together for a short time.
4. Add potatoes, water and salt and cook for ½ hr.
5. Add dill and caraway to season.
6. Put cream into tureen or soup bowls and pour soup over it.

---

93 BEAN SOUP   93

Ingredients:

Prepared cream soup as in Recipes No. 65 D *or* 66 D.

1 heaping tablesp. vegetable fat	summer savory
1 clove of garlic	¼ cup water
½ lb. beans, shredded diagonally	salt

Method:
1. Melt fat.
2. Sauté chopped garlic in it.
3. Add shredded beans and summer savory and sauté.
4. Add water and salt and cook until soft.
5. Add to cream soup.

94 PEA SOUP   94

Ingredients:

½ lb. dried yellow peas
2½ pt. water
1–2 potatoes
2½ pt. vegetable stock
salt
1 heaping tablesp. vege-
table fat
½ onion, chopped

½ leek
1 small carrot
1 piece celery or celeriac
1½ tablesp. flour
3 tablesp. cream
chives, parsley or other herbs
2 tablesp. fried bread cubes

Method:

1. Soak peas in the water for 12 hr.
2. Cook peas and potatoes in soaking water for 1–1½ hr. (or in pressure coker) until tender.
3. Sieve and add stock.
4. Melt fat and sauté the onion and then the finely shredded vegetables in it.
5. Sprinkle flour over the mixture and sauté.
6. Stir in sieved soup, gradually, add salt to taste.
7. Cook gently for 20 min.
8. Put cream and herbs into tureen or soup bowls and pour soup over it.
9. Serve with fried bread cubes.

95 D. MINESTRA   95 D.

(*For special diets:* without cheese.)

Ingredients:

1 heaping tablesp. vege-
table fat
½ onion, chopped
½ lb. celery or celeriac
1 leek
some celery leaves
1 plateful spinach beet
leaves

5 pt. water
salt
lovage or thyme
1 clove garlic
¼–½ cup noodles or rice
1 teasp. butter

Method:

1. Melt fat and sauté onion in it.
2. Shred vegetables and leaves finely and sauté gently together.
3. Add water, seasoning and herbs and cook for ½ hr.
4. Add garlic and noodles and cook for another 15–20 min.
5. Add butter to improve flavor.

Ingredients:

1 heaping tablesp. vegetable fat
1 tablesp. chopped onion
½ leek, shredded
½ celery stalk, shredded, *or* ¼ celeriac, diced
1 small carrot, diced
2–3 cabbage leaves, shredded
1–2 diced potatoes
some spinach or spinach beet leaves

1 handful cooked beans
2 ripe tomatoes *or* 1 teasp. tomato purée, diluted
5 pt. water
lovage, thyme, or other herbs
salt
1 cup noodles or rice
1 tablesp. butter
3 tablesp. grated Parmesan cheese

Method:

1. Melt fat and sauté onions in it.
2. Add all vegetables and sauté together.
3. Add tomatoes or purée and sauté again.
4. Add water, herbs and salt and simmer for 1 hr.
5. Add noodles or rice and cook with the mixture for the last 15 min.
6. Put butter and grated cheese into tureen and pour soup over.

Vegetables can be varied according to season and personal taste. Diced squash, zucchini, pumpkin, tips of wild asparagus, green beans, etc.

VEGETABLES

The same basic rules for preserving the nutritive value and for careful preparation which are suggested for raw vegetables (see p. 49), apply also to cooked vegetables: cleanliness, freshness and care in preparation.

Nearly all vegetables can be cooked in their own steam and juice, or with a very little vegetable stock (see Sauté, p. 41). If vegetables have to be cooked for a short time in salted water, the water can be used for sauces or soups; only water in which asparagus has been cooked should not be used as it is not wholesome. When, or where, fresh vegetables are difficult to obtain, deep frozen ones may be used instead.

Times of cooking, measures and weights cannot always be given exactly as they vary according to the freshness and size of the vegetables, and the appetites of those eating them. Some ingredients may be added or omitted according to taste.

IT IS EXTREMELY IMPORTANT TO USE ONLY VERY LITTLE

COOKING SALT WITH ALL DISHES. SALT CAN BE REPLACED BY
THE ADDITION OF SUBTLY BLENDED CULINARY HERBS.

Steaming and Stewing Vegetables in their own Juice

Steaming is easiest with the aid of a special double-sided
pan, in which food is slowly cooked in steam until tender. The
vegetables retain their aroma and nutritive value because
overheating is not possible and valuable substances do not
dissolve into water. A tiered steaming pan is a great help to
the busy housewife, since foods can be cooked in it without
supervision.

For stewing in its own juice, a special glazed stewing pan
with a heavy bottom and a well-fitting lid is required. A little
oil or vegetable fat must first be heated in the pan and the
food tossed or sautéd in it, then covered with a well-fitting lid
until its own juice 'sweats out' (see p. 41). The vegetables
can then be stewed in it until tender. Vegetables without much
juice of their own are first sautéd lightly until they produce
their own juice, then a little boiling water or vegetable broth
should be added. They can be cooked for five minutes over
strong heat, then the heat should be reduced and the vegetables simmered gently for 20–40 minutes until tender, always
covered by a well-fitting lid.

Flavor and aroma are much better preserved by this method
of preparation and the dishes are, consequently, more appetizing and more valuable.

97 D. SPINACH, WHOLE LEAVES, I   97 D.

Ingredients:

3 tablesp. vegetable fat	nutmeg
1 small onion, chopped	Marmite or other yeast ex-
1 garlic clove, chopped	tract
2 lb. young spinach	1 tablesp. butter ⎫
salt	1 tablesp. grated ⎬ optional
	cheese ⎭

Method:

1. Melt fat and sauté onion and garlic in it until golden.
2. Pick over spinach, remove thick stalks, wash and drain.
3. Add to the onion and cook gently over low heat in a
covered pan, with a little salt.
4. Add nutmeg and Marmite to taste.
5. Add 1 tablesp. hot butter and 1 tablesp. grated cheese if
liked and not on Light Diet.

Note: Overgrown winter spinach should be blanched for a
short time in salt water or it will taste bitter.

98 D. SPINACH, WHOLE LEAVES, 2   98 D.

(*Especially good for salt-free diet.*)

Ingredients:

2 lb. spinach	2 tablesp. currants
1 heaping tablesp. vegetable fat	some water if necessary salt
½ onion, chopped	
2 tablesp. pine kernels	

Method:

1. Place washed spinach in a saucepan, cover and cook over very low heat.
2. Melt fat and sauté the onion gently in it until golden yellow.
3. Add spinach and cook for a short time.
4. Add the pine kernels, currants, and water if necessary.
5. Cook gently all together.

99 D. SPINACH PURÉE, 1   99 D.

Ingredients:

2 lb. spinach	1 cup milk or vegetable stock
1 heaping tablesp. vegetable fat	salt, nutmeg
1 small onion, chopped	3 cups raw spinach
1 garlic clove	peppermint leaves
1 heaping tablesp. flour	3 tablesp. cream (if liked)

Method:

1. Pick over spinach and remove any thick stalks.
2. Place it in a saucepan, cover, steam over low heat until the water collects.
3. Drain and keep water for later use.
4. Mince or chop spinach finely.
5. Melt fat, sauté onion and garlic in it.
6. Add flour, and sauté.
7. Add milk or stock, smooth and cook for 15 min.
8. Add spinach and seasoning.
9. Chop raw spinach and peppermint leaves or put through the blender.
10. Add this to the cooked spinach just before serving; do not allow to boil again.
11. Add cream to enrich the dish.

100 D. SPINACH PURÉE, 2   **100 D.**

Ingredients:

2 lb. spinach
½ tablesp. vegetable fat
½ onion, chopped
3 tablesp. cream

1½ teasp. fresh butter
nutmeg
3 cups raw spinach
peppermint leaves

Method:

1. Pick over the spinach and remove any thick stalks.
2. Place spinach in a saucepan, cover and steam over low heat until water collects.
3. Drain.
4. Mince or chop spinach finely.
5. Melt fat and sauté onion in it.
6. Add spinach and heat up all together.
7. Add cream, butter and seasoning.
8. Chop the raw spinach and peppermint leaves very finely or put through a blender.
9. Add to the cooked spinach just before serving.

101 D. LETTUCE   **101 D.**

Ingredients:

5 medium-sized cos lettuce
7½ pt. salted water
3 tablesp. vegetable fat

1 onion, chopped
1¼ cups vegetable stock
4½–6 tablesp. cream

Method:

1. Halve and wash the lettuce.
2. Cook gently in salted water.
3. When partly cooked but still firm put into a colander to drain.
4. Place in a baking dish.
5. Melt fat, sauté onion in it until golden and pour over lettuce.
6. Add stock and bake in medium oven (350°) 30–40 minutes.
7. Pour cream over just before serving.

102 D. ENDIVES   **102 D.**

Take 5–6 endives and prepare as in Recipe No. 101 D.

103 D. CHICORY   103 D.

Ingredients:
  1¾ to 2 lb. prepared   salt
    chicory   some drops of lemon juice,
  1 heaping tablesp. vege-   if desired
    table fat   some hot butter
  ¼ cup milk or cream
  ½ cup vegetable stock

Method:
  1. Make crosswise incision in chicory stalks.
  2. Heat cooking fat in a heavy saucepan and put in chicory
in layers.
  3. Add milk and stock, cover and cook for ½ hr.; salt if
necessary.
  4. Add lemon and hot butter just before serving.

104 CHICORY POLONAISE   104

Ingredients:
  1¾ to 2 lb. chicory
  1 egg, hard-boiled   1 teasp. fresh butter

Method:
  1. Prepare chicory as in Recipe No. 103 D.
  2. Chop egg finely and sprinkle over finished chicory.
  3. Melt butter and pour over just before serving.

105 D. STALKS OF SPINACH BEET, I   105 D.

(*For Light Diet:* Use 4½ tablesp. cream instead of Béchamel
                    Sauce.)

Ingredients:
  1¾ lb. stalks   some drops lemon juice
  1 heaping tablesp. vege-   salt
    table fat   Béchamel Sauce (Rec. No.
  1 cup vegetable stock   299)

Method:
  1. Cut stalks into 2-in. long pieces.
  2. Sauté in the fat.
  3. Add stock, lemon juice and salt and cook over low heat
until tender (½–¾ hr.).
  4. Add Béchamel Sauce, enriched with egg yolk, and mix
well together.

Ingredients:

2 lb. stalks
3 tablesp. vegetable fat
salt

some drops of lemon juice *or*
6 tablesp. milk
1½ cups vegetable stock

Method:

1. Cut stalks into 4-in. long pieces.
2. Sauté in the fat.
3. Add lemon juice or milk to preserve the color.
4. Add stock, taste and salt, cover with a lid and cook gently until tender—about ½–¾ hr.
5. Arrange on a flat dish like asparagus.
6. Serve with Sauce Remoulade, Recipe No. 320.

The stalks can also be sprinkled with grated cheese and hot butter poured over if desired.

107 D. CELERY   107 D.

(*For Light Diet:* Without cheese, use 4½ tablesp. cream instead, if permitted.)

Ingredients:

1 large bunch of celery
 (about 10 stalks)
some drops of lemon juice
 or 6 tablesp. milk
3 tablesp. vegetable fat

2 cups vegetable stock
salt
grated cheese } optional
hot butter }

Method:

1. Cut celery into about 3-in. long pieces and add lemon juice or milk.
2. Melt fat and sauté celery in it, then cover with lid.
3. Add stock, taste and salt, and cook until tender (½–1 hr.).

Sprinkle with grated cheese and pour hot butter over the finished dish before serving, if desired, but it then no longer remains a D dish.

108 D. SWEET OR FLORENCE FENNEL, 1   108 D.

Ingredients:

4 large or 6 small fennel
 (swollen stem bases)
1 heaping tablesp. vege-
 table fat
½ onion, chopped

½ cup milk
1 cup vegetable stock
salt
3 tablesp. cream

Method:
1. Cut away any tough parts of fennel, halve and wash.
2. Melt fat and sauté onions in it until golden.
3. Add fennel and sauté all together.
4. Add milk and stock, taste and salt, cover and cook until tender (¾ hr.).
5. Add cream just before serving.

109 SWEET OR FLORENCE FENNEL, 2   109

Ingredients:

4 large or 6 small fennel (swollen stem bases)	½ cup milk
	1 tablesp. flour
1 heaping tablesp. vege-	½ cup cream
table fat	3 tablesp. grated cheese
½ cup vegetable stock	

Method:
1. Melt fat, sauté fennel in it.
2. Add stock and milk and cook gently until tender.
3. Mix flour and cream and add to the cooked fennel.
4. Bring to the boil.
5. Sprinkle the grated cheese over the finished fennel before serving.

110 D. CELERY STALKS   110 D.

(*For Light Diet:* Without cheese, if desired use 3 tablesp. cream instead.)

Ingredients:

1 medium-sized celery stalk	salt
	2–3 tablesp. cheese (if per-
5 pt. water	mitted)
1 cup milk	2–3 tablesp. butter

Method:
1. Prepare celery stalk and cut into finger-length pieces.
2. Bring the water and milk and salt to the boil and cook celery in the liquid until soft (about 1 hr.).
3. Drain and arrange on a serving dish.
4. Sprinkle with cheese, if used, and pour hot butter over the finished dish.

III D. CARROTS III D.

Ingredients:

1½ tablesp. vegetable fat
1 small onion, chopped
1¾ lb. carrots (about 14 carrots)

1–1½ cups vegetable stock
rosemary

Method:

1. Melt fat and sauté onion in it.
2. Slice carrots and add to the onions.
3. Pour stock on to the vegetables, add rosemary.
4. Cover and cook for ¾ hr.

112 CREAMED CARROTS, 1 112

Ingredients:

½ tablesp. vegetable fat
1¼ lb. carrots (about 10 carrots)
1 tablesp. vegetable fat
1 tablesp. flour
1½ cups milk

1½ cups water or vegetable stock
salt
marjoram, chives or parsley

Method:

1. Melt ½ tablesp. vegetable fat.
2. Slice carrots finely and sauté in the fat until they are nearly cooked.
3. Melt 1 tablesp. vegetable fat, stir flour into it.
4. Gradually add milk and water, or vegetable stock, to make a thin sauce.
5. Add carrots, salt and herbs to season.
6. Cook gently all together until carrots are cooked.

113 CREAMED CARROTS, 2 113

Ingredients:

1¼ cups vegetable stock
1¼ lb. carrots (about 10 carrots)
salt
1 heaping tablesp. vegetable fat
1 tablesp. butter

4½ tablesp. flour
2 cups milk or vegetable stock
salt
1 small bay leaf
2–3 tablesp. cream, if liked

Method:

1. Shred or slice carrots and cook until soft in the vegetable stock, add salt.

2. Make a Béchamel sauce with the ingredients given (Recipe No. 299), season with salt and bay leaf.

3. Pour sauce over the cooked carrots, add cream if desired, and serve.

114 D. PEAS AND CARROTS   114 D.

(For Light Diet: Use only sweet, young peas.)

Ingredients for Peas:	*Ingredients for Carrots:*
½ tablesp. vegetable fat	½ tablesp. vegetable fat
¼ onion, chopped	¼ onion, chopped
1½ cups shelled peas	6 carrots, sliced, or
½–1 cup vegetable stock	shredded
salt	½–1 cup vegetable stock
pinch of sugar	salt

Method:
1. Melt fat for the peas, sauté onion in it.
2. Add peas, stock and seasoning, and simmer until cooked.
3. Melt fat for the carrots, sauté onion in it.
4. Add carrots, stock and seasoning and simmer until cooked.
5. Mix peas and carrots in one saucepan or arrange alternately on a serving dish.

115 D. PEAS   115 D.

(For Light Diet: Use only sweet, young peas.)

Ingredients:

2 tablesp. vegetable fat	salt
½ onion, chopped	pinch of sugar
6 cups shelled peas	1 tablesp. butter
1–1½ cups vegetable stock	

Method:
1. Melt fat and sauté onion in it.
2. Add peas, stock and seasoning, simmer until cooked.
3. Serve with hot butter poured over the finished dish.

116 D. PEAS, FRENCH STYLE   116 D.

Ingredients:

2 tablesp. vegetable fat	3 cups shelled peas
½ onion, chopped	1 cup vegetable stock
1 head of lettuce,	salt
shredded	

Method:
1. Melt fat and sauté onion in it.
2. Add other ingredients and simmer gently until the peas are cooked.

117 PEAS WITH PEARL ONIONS 117

Ingredients:

2 tablesp. vegetable fat	salt
¼ lb. pearl onions	pinch of sugar
4½ cups shelled peas	chopped basil

Method:
1. Melt fat and sauté onion in it.
2. Add peas, salt and sugar; cover and simmer until cooked.
3. Sprinkle chopped basil over the finished dish before serving.

118 SUGARPEAS (EDIBLE-PODDED PEAS) 118

Ingredients:

2 tablesp. vegetable fat	pinch of sugar
1 onion, chopped	1–1½ cups vegetable stock
3½ cups sugarpeas	parsley or lovage
salt	

Method:
1. Melt fat and sauté onion in it.
2. Add sugarpeas, salt and sugar and sauté all together.
3. Add vegetable stock and herbs, cover and simmer ½–1 hr. (if preferred the herbs can be sprinkled over the finished dish).

119 GREEN BEANS 119

Ingredients:

2 tablesp. vegetable fat	salt
1 onion, chopped	1½ cups vegetable stock
1 clove garlic	summer savory
2 lb. beans	parsley

Method:
1. Melt fat and sauté onion and garlic in it.
2. Add beans and sauté together.
3. Add stock and herbs, taste and salt, cover and cook gently for 1 hr.
In place of vegetable stock 4 diced tomatoes can be used, adding a little stock if too dry.

120 DRIED GREEN BEANS   120

Ingredients:
As Recipe No. 119, without fresh beans
¼ lb. dried beans

Method:
1. Soak beans overnight.
2. Drain well, but retain soaking water.
3. Prepare as in Recipe No. 119, using the water in which
the beans were soaked instead of stock. Cooking time may be
longer.

121 CELERIAC   121

Ingredients:
1 heaping tablesp. vege-   1½ cups vegetable stock
  table fat   salt
1 small onion, chopped   4½ tablesp. cream
1½ lb. sliced celeriac
1 teasp. lemon juice *or*
  4½ tablesp. milk

Method:
1. Melt fat and sauté onion in it.
2. Cut celeriac into thin small slices.
3. Sauté with the onions.
4. Add lemon juice or milk and stock and cook until tender
(½–¾ hr.). Add salt to taste.
5. Add cream before serving to improve flavor.

122 CELERIAC WITH BÉCHAMEL SAUCE   122

Ingredients:
1¼ lb. celeriac
other ingredients as in Recipe No. 121

Method:
1. Prepare as in Recipe No. 121.
2. When finished mix with Béchamel Sauce, Recipe No. 299,
and serve.

123 CELERIAC SLICES WITH SAUCE HOLLANDAISE   123

Ingredients:
1½ lb. celeriac   2½ pt. water
½ cup milk   salt

Method:

1. Peel and cut celeriac into quarters.
2. Add to the milk and water and cook until tender.
3. Cut into ½-in. slices and arrange these in rows on a hot dish with slices overlapping.
4. Pour Sauce Hollandaise, Recipe Nos. 314 or 315, over vegetables shortly before serving.

124 D. SCORZONERA OR SALSIFY (OYSTER PLANT)   124 D.

(*For Light Diet:* Mix with a little fresh butter or cream, and fresh or dried herbs if desired.)

Ingredients:

1½ lb. scorzonera or salsify (peeled and prepared)
1 heaping tablesp. vegetable fat
½ cup milk
1 cup vegetable stock
salt

Method:

1. Cut salsify into 3-in. long pieces.
2. Melt fat and sauté salsify in it.
3. Add milk, stock and salt, cover and simmer for 1 hr.
May be served with Béchamel Sauce, Recipe No. 299.

125 SCORZONERA OR SALSIFY POLONAISE   125

Ingredients:

1½ lb. salsify
1 egg, hard boiled
1 teasp. butter
chives, parsley or other herbs

Method:

1. Prepare salsify as in Recipe No. 124.
2. Chop egg finely and sprinkle over the salsify.
3. Melt butter and spread with herbs over finished dish.

126 D. BEETROOTS   126 D.

(*For Light Diet:* Make without flour.)

Ingredients:

1½ lb. beetroot
salted water
1 heaping tablesp. vegetable fat
½ onion, chopped
½ cup vegetable stock
pinch of sugar
1 tablesp. lemon juice
¼ bay leaf
1 tablesp. caraway seeds
salt, if necessary
1 tablesp. flour
cold water
3 tablesp. cream

Method:

1. Wash carefully, cut off root-tips and leaves about ¾ in. above roots—without damaging the skin.

2. Cook in salted water until tender (2–3 hr.) (25 min. in a pressure cooker).

3. Pour cold water over beetroots.

4. Peel and cut into fine slices.

5. Melt fat and sauté onion in it.

6. Add beetroot and all other ingredients except the flour and cream, mix well.

7. Simmer for ¼ hr.

8. Blend flour with a little cold water and add to the mixture to bind (if desired).

9. Pour in cream just before serving.

127 BEETROOTS, STUFFED   127

Prepare in the same way as kohlrabi, Recipe No. 163.
Cooking time for beetroots, however, is about 2 hr.
Serve with Herb Sauce, Recipe No. 301.

128 D. JERUSALEM ARTICHOKES   128 D.

(*For Light Diet:* Without sauce.)

Ingredients:

1¾ lb. Jerusalem arti-chokes	1 small onion
1 heaping tablesp. vege-table fat	3 tablesp. cream
	sweet basil

Method:

1. Cook like potatoes in their skins. Recipe No. 191.

2. Peel and slice.

3. Melt fat and sauté onion in it, add Jerusalem artichokes and sauté together.

4. Add cream to enrich and basil to season.

These can also be served with Béchamel Sauce, Recipe No. 299, and grated cheese.

129 D. TOMATOES AS A VEGETABLE   129 D.

Ingredients:

2 tablesp. vegetable fat	1 clove garlic
1 small onion, chopped	salt
1¾ lb. peeled tomatoes (6 or 7)	herbs

Method:
1. Melt fat and sauté onion in it.
2. Cut up tomatoes and add to onion.
3. Cook gently to reduce a little.
4. Add garlic and salt and cook until tender.
5. Sprinkle liberally with chopped parsley or other herbs before serving.

Note: If tomatoes will not peel easily, pour boiling water over them and leave for 2–3 min.

130 D. TOMATOES, BAKED   130 D.

Ingredients:

1¼ lb. tomatoes (approx. 5)   1½ tablesp. butter
salt

Method:
1. Halve tomatoes and put in a baking dish.
2. Sprinkle with salt.
3. Put a dab of butter on each tomato and bake for about 15 min. in a moderate oven.

If desired a few more tomatoes may be chopped finely (or put through a blender), mixed with cream, brought to the boil, and poured over the baked tomatoes. Or pour scrambled eggs whisked with cream over them.

131 TOMATOES WITH CHEESE SLICES   131

Ingredients:

3 or 4 tomatoes   1 cheese slice for each to-
                                     mato

Method:
1. Prepare tomatoes as in Recipe No. 130 D.
2. Place a slice of cheese on each tomato.
3. Bake in a moderate oven until the cheese melts.

132 TOMATOES, STUFFED, I   132

Ingredients:

1¼ lb. tomatoes   Bread stuffing (Recipe No. 179)
salt   *or*
                                   Rice Stuffing (Recipe No. 178)
                                   butter

Method:
1. Halve, or cut off the top of tomatoes, and remove pulp.
2. Put in a baking dish and sprinkle with salt.
3. Fill each tomato with stuffing, and put a dab of butter on each one.
4. Bake in a moderate oven (350°) for about 10 min.

133 D. TOMATOES, STUFFED, 2   133 D.

(*For Light Diet:* Without Cheese.)

Ingredients:

8 small or 4 large tomatoes	1 chopped clove garlic
1 oz. rice	1½ tablesp. butter *or* olive oil
chopped basil	grated cheese, if liked

Method:
1. Cut tops off tomatoes and remove inside pulp.
2. Mix rice with chopped or strained pulp, herbs and salt.
3. Fill tomatoes with mixture and put a dab of butter or a drop of oil on each.
4. Cover with the cut-off tops and sprinkle with cheese if used.
5. Bake in a hot oven (400°) for about 30 min.

134 TOMATOES   134

Ingredients:

8 smallish tomatoes	vegetable stock
3–4 hard-boiled eggs	gherkins
salt	cress
mayonnaise Recipe No. 9	radishes

Method:
1. Slice tomatoes and eggs, place alternately on a dish so that they just overlap.
2. Sprinkle with salt.
3. Dilute mayonnaise with vegetable stock and pour over the tomatoes.
4. Garnish with gherkins, cress and radishes if liked.

135 D. TOMATOES A LA PROVENCE   135 D.

Ingredients:

1¼ lb. tomatoes	6 tablesp. cream *or*
salt	1 large onion, chopped
3 tablesp. breadcrumbs	3 tablesp. parsley
3 tablesp. grated cheese	

Method:

1. Cut tomatoes in half and put in a baking dish.
2. Sprinkle salt over them.
3. Mix breadcrumbs, cheese and cream and put a spoonful on each tomato, *or* sprinkle onion and parsley over them.
4. Bake in a moderate oven.

136 D. ZUCCHINI OR SQUASH, I   136 D

(*For Light Diet:* Without sauce or cheese.)

Ingredients:

1¾ lb. zucchini	rosemary, dill, parsley
4½ tablesp. oil	vegetable stock, if necessary
salt	Tomato Sauce, or grated cheese

Method:

1. Select small zucchini, wash and cut off both ends.
2. Halve and put on a flat baking sheet.
3. Pour oil over and sprinkle with herbs.
4. Bake in a moderate oven or over gentle heat on top of the stove.
5. Add a little vegetable stock if too dry.
6. Serve with Tomato Sauce, Recipe No. 303, or sprinkle with grated cheese if liked.

137 ZUCCHINI OR SQUASH, 2   137

Ingredients:

3 tablesp. vegetable fat	salt
1 onion, chopped	rosemary, dill, parsley
1¾ lb. squash	vegetable stock if necessary

Method:

1. Melt fat, sauté onion in it.
2. Dice squash (removing pith and seeds of large squash) and add, with salt, to onion.
3. Cook all together very slowly, adding vegetable stock if mixture becomes too dry.
4. Season with chopped herbs just before serving.

If desired, ½ lb. of peeled diced tomatoes can be added and cooked with the squash.

138 ZUCCHINI OR SQUASH, STUFFED 138

Ingredients:

4–6 squash	3 tablesp. grated cheese
salt	vegetable stock
Bread Stuffing, Recipe No. 179	Tomato Sauce, Recipe No. 303, if liked

Method:

1. Halve squash and put in a baking dish.
2. Sprinkle with salt, cover with Bread Stuffing and top with grated cheese.
3. Pour in vegetable stock to a depth of ½–1 in., and bake in hot oven (400°) for ½ hr.

Serve with Tomato Sauce if desired. Larger squash can have their centers removed and the hollow filled with the mixture. When baking, turn squash several times.

139 ZUCCHINI OR SQUASH, FRIED 139

Ingredients:

1 lb. squash	salt
	flour

Method:

1. Cut squash into finger-length strips or ½-in. slices.
2. Spread out on a dish and sprinkle with salt.
3. Leave for a few min. to draw.
4. Dip into flour and fry immediately in deep fat.

140 SQUASH, FRENCH FRIED 140

These can be made exactly like French fried potatoes. Slice into hot fat and remove as soon as they have browned.

141 D. PEPPERS, GREEN OR YELLOW 141 D.

(Pepper dishes should be considered an additional rather than a main dish.)

Ingredients:

1½ lb. peppers	1 small onion, chopped
4½ tablesp. oil	salt

Method:

1. Remove pith and seeds carefully.
2. Slice peppers and put into a saucepan with the oil, onion and salt.
3. Cover and cook gently for ½ hr.

Ingredients:

4 large or 8 small peppers	vegetable stock
salt	1½ tablesp. grated cheese
Tomato Rice ingredients	1½ tablesp. butter
(½ of Recipe No. 227)	

Method:

1. Cut tops off small, or halve large peppers, remove pith and seeds.
2. Put the peppers in a greased baking dish.
3. Sprinkle salt over them.
4. Prepare Tomato Rice (see Recipe No. 227).
5. Stuff peppers with it.
6. Pour in stock to a depth of ½ in., sprinkle cheese over and dot with butter.
7. Bake in hot oven (400°) for ½ hr.

Note: Fully-grown peppers should be blanched in boiling salt water or soaked in cold water for 1 hr. before using.

143 PEPPERS STUFFED WITH SPAGHETTI OR NOODLES 143

Ingredients:

4 large or 8 small peppers	1 small onion, chopped
5–6 oz. spaghetti or noodles	¾ lb. tomatoes (about 3)
3½ pt. salt water	1½ tablesp. grated cheese
3 tablesp. oil	oil

Method:

1. Prepare peppers as in previous recipe.
2. Cook spaghetti for 15 min. in the salt water, cut into short lengths.
3. Heat oil and sauté onion in it.
4. Skin tomatoes, cut into dice, sauté with the onion.
5. Mix with spaghetti and cheese.
6. Fill the peppers and replace tops.
7. Put a little oil in a baking dish, place peppers in it, drop a little oil on each.
8. Bake in the oven or cook in a covered saucepan for ¾ hr., turning peppers several times.
9. Remove lids of peppers and serve.

144 D. PEPERONATA 144 D.

Ingredients:

½ lb. peppers	1 clove garlic
½ lb. squash	6 tablesp. oil
½ lb. eggplant	salt
½ lb. tomatoes	2–4 potatoes
1 large onion	

Method:

1. Halve peppers, remove pith and seeds and dice.
2. Prepare and dice squash and eggplant.
3. Skin tomatoes and cut into large cubes.
4. Chop onion and garlic and sauté in the oil.
5. Add other diced vegetables and sauté together.
6. Add salt.
7. Cut potatoes into ½-in. cubes, add to the other vegetables.
8. Cook very slowly for ½ hr. in a covered saucepan.

145 D. EGGPLANT 145 D.

Ingredients:

1 lb. (approx.) eggplant	salt
2 tablesp. vegetable fat	vegetable stock if necessary
1 small onion, chopped	

Method:

1. The eggplant should be washed and cut into cubes and can be peeled if liked.
2. Melt fat and sauté onion in it.
3. Add eggplant, cut into cubes, and cook until soft, only adding stock if necessary.

Garnish with baked tomatoes, Recipe No. 130 D., or with tomatoes as a vegetable, Recipe No. 129 D.

146 EGGPLANT AU GRATIN 146

Ingredients:

¾ lb. eggplant	3 tablesp. grated cheese
oil	breadcrumbs
2 tomatoes	1½ tablesp. butter
salt	

Method:

1. Wash eggplant and cut into slices.
2. Cook in oil until tender.

3. Put in a baking dish.

4. Slice tomatoes and put on top of the eggplant.

5. Sprinkle with cheese and breadcrumbs and dot with butter.

6. Bake for ½ hr. in a moderate oven (350°).

147 STUFFED EGGPLANT 147

Ingredients:

4–6 medium-sized egg-plant	Bread Stuffing, Recipe No. 179
	or
4½ tablesp. oil	Rice Stuffing, Recipe No. 178
vegetable stock	cheese, if desired

Method:

1. Peel and halve eggplant, scoop out a slight hollow in each.

2. Put in a baking dish with the cut side uppermost.

3. Brush each with oil. Pour in vegetable stock until half way up the eggplant.

4. Cover with a lid and cook in a moderate oven until semi-soft.

5. Stuff each eggplant, replace lid and finish cooking.

If liked sprinkle with grated cheese and finish cooking without the lid.

148 D. GLOBE ARTICHOKES, I 148 D.

(*For Light Diet:* Serve with Vinaigrette Sauce, Recipe No. 322 D.)

Ingredients:

4–6 artichokes	salt
5 pt. water	1 teasp. lemon juice

Method:

1. Prepare artichokes by cutting off stalks and removing hard lower leaves. Cut off tips of other leaves.

2. Halve, cut out flowers, wash well.

3. Rub cut surfaces with lemon juice.

4. Bring water to the boil, add artichokes and salt, and cook until tender (¾ hr. approx.).

5. Drain, arrange on a hot dish and cover with a napkin.

6. Serve with Hollandaise Sauce, Recipe No. 314, Remoulade Sauce, Recipe No. 320, or Vinaigrette Sauce, Recipe No. 322 D.

149 GLOBE ARTICHOKES, 2

Ingredients:

8–10 artichokes	1 lemon
salt	3–4 tablesp. oil
	4–8 oz. water

Method:

1. Remove hard parts of artichokes, wash and slice the remainder.

2. Rub with lemon and sprinkle with salt.

3. Heat oil, add artichokes, and cook gently in a covered pan until tender, adding water if necessary.

150 D. ROMAN ARTICHOKES

Ingredients:

8 small or 4 large arti- chokes	chopped peppermint leaves clove of garlic
lemon	oil
salt	water

Method:

1. Pull off all outer leaves of the artichokes until only the tender part remains.

2. Cut off the tips of the remaining leaves.

3. Peel stalk down to the pith and leave about 2 in. of it.

4. Rub with lemon, open out the leaves a little.

5. Sprinkle with salt, and put peppermint and garlic in the center.

6. Pour oil into a saucepan until the bottom is just covered.

7. Put in the artichokes, cover and cook in their own steam, turning them occasionally.

8. Then add water to half height of artichokes and steam until the water has evaporated.

9. Continue steaming in the oil only, for a short time.

151 D. ASPARAGUS

(*For Light Diet:* With Vinaigrette Sauce, Recipe No. 322 D.)

Ingredients:

2 lb. asparagus	*or* Hollandaise Sauce, Rec.
salt	No. 314
grated cheese	*or* Mousseline Sauce, Rec.
hot butter	No. 316
	or Mayonnaise, Recipe, No.
	317, *or* Vinaigrette, Rec-
	ipe No. 322 D

Method:

1. Wash the asparagus carefully without breaking.
2. Boil until tender for 20–30 min. with salt.
3. Take out with a skimming ladle and arrange on a hot dish, cover with a napkin.
4. Serve grated cheese and melted butter or the chosen sauce.

152 CORN ON THE COB   152

Ingredients:

6–8 ears of corn   salt
2½ pt. water   butter

Method:

1. Choose only ears where the corn is young and milky in color.
2. Remove leaves and silk.
3. Boil until tender (10–30 min. according to age).
4. Arrange on a hot dish covered with a napkin, serve with hot butter.

153 CAULIFLOWER   153

Ingredients:

1 medium-sized cauli-
   flower
2½ pt. water
salt
Béchamel Sauce, if desired

Ingredients for Cauliflower Polonaise

1 tablesp. fine bread-
   crumbs
1 hard-boiled egg
parsley
1½ tablesp. grated cheese
3 tablesp. melted butter

Method:

1. Cut off the cauliflower leaves and remove stalk close to the flower.
2. Cut into largish florets, peel stalk and keep tender leaves.
3. Put into cold salt water for 1 hr. Rinse well.
4. Cook until tender (20–30 min.); take out and drain well.
5. Arrange on a hot deep dish.
6. Serve with Béchamel Sauce, Recipe No. 299, poured over or as Cauliflower Polonaise made as follows:
7. Sprinkle fine breadcrumbs over the cauliflower, add finely chopped hard-boiled eggs, parsley and cheese.

8. Pour 3 tablesp. hot melted butter over.

Note: Cauliflower is the most easily digested of the cabbages and may therefore be eaten by those suffering from gastric disorders. For them it is advisable to prepare without a sauce, but add 1 tablesp. melted butter and a few breadcrumbs if desired.

154 BROCCOLI   154

Prepare in the same way as Cauliflower, Recipe No. 153.

155 BRUSSELS SPROUTS   155

Ingredients:

1 heaping tablesp. vegetable fat	butter, *or*
1½ lb. Brussels sprouts	Béchamel Sauce, Recipe No. 299
1 cup vegetable stock	

Method:
1. Melt fat and sauté sprouts in it.
2. Add stock and cook until tender (about ½ hr.).
3. Before serving pour a little melted butter over them or Béchamel Sauce if liked.

Note: Large or tough sprouts should be blanched before they are cooked.

156 CABBAGE   156

Ingredients:

3 tablesp. vegetable fat	basil or lovage
1 onion, chopped	Marmite or other yeast extract
2 lb. young cabbage	nutmeg
1 cup vegetable stock	caraway seeds
salt	

Method:
1. Melt fat and sauté onion in it.
2. Cut the cabbage into ½-in. wide strips and sauté with the onion.
3. Add stock gradually and simmer until tender.
4. Add salt, herbs and spices to taste.

Note: Blanch tough or old cabbage before cooking.

157 CABBAGE, CHOPPED 157

Ingredients:

1½ lb. cabbage
2½ pt. salt water
1 heaping tablesp. vege-
    table fat
½ onion, chopped
3 tablesp. flour

2 cups vegetable stock *or*
    ½ milk and ½ stock
3 tablesp. cream
Marmite or other yeast ex-
    tract
nutmeg

Method:

1. Cut cabbage into four.
2. Cook in the salt water until tender.
3. Drain well and chop finely.
4. Melt fat and sauté onion in it.
5. Sprinkle flour over onion and sauté.
6. Add stock and simmer for ¼ hr.
7. Add cabbage and bring to the boil again.
8. Add cream, Marmite and nutmeg.

158 CURLY KALE 158

Prepare and cook as in Recipe No. 157.

159 STUFFED CABBAGE LEAVES 159

Ingredients:

¼ cabbage
boiling salt water
Bread Stuffing, Rec. No.
    179 *or* Rice Stuffing,
    Rec. No. 178

1 heaping tablesp. vegetable
    fat
1 onion, chopped
vegetable stock
nutmeg
3–4 tablesp. cream

Method:

1. Blanch cabbage in the boiling water. Drain well.
2. Strip cabbage leaves from the stalk, allowing 2–3 leaves
for each stuffed leaf.
3. Put 2–3 tablesp. stuffing on each leaf, roll up lengthwise.
4. Put side by side in a flat casserole.
5. Melt fat, sauté onion in it.
6. Spread over cabbage rolls.
7. Pour in vegetable stock to just cover cabbage rolls.
8. Season with nutmeg and bake for ¾–1 hr. in a moderate
oven.
9. Pour cream over just before serving.

160 SOUR WHITE CABBAGE   160

Ingredients:

2 tablesp. vegetable fat	1 cup vegetable stock
1 onion, chopped	½ cup apple juice
1½ lb. white cabbage	salt
1½ tablesp. lemon juice	caraway seeds
1½ tablesp. flour	

Method:

1. Melt fat and sauté onion in it.
2. Shred cabbage and add to the onion.
3. Add lemon juice and sauté all together.
4. Sprinkle in the flour.
5. Add stock and apple juice and stir until smooth.
6. Add salt and caraway to taste, cover and cook gently for 1 hr.

161 COOKED SAUERKRAUT   161

Ingredients:

3 tablesp. vegetable fat	2½ cups vegetable stock
½ onion, chopped	1 raw potato, *or*
1 lb. sauerkraut	1 tablesp. flour

Method:

1. Melt fat and sauté onion in it.
2. Add sauerkraut, loosen with a fork and sauté for a short time.
3. Add stock, cover and simmer gently for ½–1 hr.
4. Grate potato into the sauerkraut, or stir in flour 10 min. before serving.

Note: How to make Sauerkraut at home and Sauerkraut Salad, see Recipe No. 41.

162 RED CABBAGE   162

Ingredients:

2 tablesp. vegetable fat	1 cup vegetable stock
1 onion, chopped	½ cup grape juice *or*
1½ lb. red cabbage	apple juice
1½ tablesp. lemon juice	salt
1 apple	2 apples
1½ tablesp. flour, if required	1 teasp. butter

Method:
1. Melt fat and sauté onion in it.
2. Add finely shredded red cabbage and sauté all together.
3. Add lemon juice and one apple cut into thin slices.
4. Stir in flour if the mixture appears too liquid.
5. Add stock and juice gradually and stir until smooth. Salt moderately. Cover pan and simmer until tender (1–1½ hr.).
6. Peel two apples, remove cores and cut into thick segments; brush with butter.
7. Place on a baking sheet in the oven.
8. Decorate red cabbage with the apples and dot with butter before serving.

163 KOHLRABI   163

Ingredients:

6 kohlrabi	salt
1 heaping tablesp. vegetable fat	kohlrabi leaves
1 onion, chopped	3 tablesp. cream
1–1½ cups vegetable stock	

Method:
1. Cut kohlrabi into quarters then slice finely.
2. Melt fat and sauté the vegetables in it.
3. Add stock, cover and cook gently for ½–1 hr.
4. Add salt to taste.
5. Chop some tender kohlrabi leaves or parsley and add with the cream just before serving.

164 KOHLRABI WITH HERBS   164

Ingredients:

The same as in Recipe No. 163	parsley, mint, onion green, tarragon, chervil, or mixture of green dried herbs
Béchamel Sauce, Recipe No. 299	

Method:
1. Cook the kohlrabi as in Recipe No. 163.
2. Add a large quantity of tender kohlrabi leaves, chopped. and a variety of herbs to taste.
3. Mix with Béchamel Sauce, Recipe No. 299.

165 KOHLRABI, STUFFED 165

Ingredients:

8 small kohlrabi	Bread Stuffing Rec. No. 179
3¾ pt. vegetable stock *or*	1½ tablesp. butter
salt water	1½ tablesp. cream

Method:

1. Peel kohlrabi and make a small hollow in each.
2. Parboil for ½ hr. then put in a baking dish.
3. Pour in vegetable stock to a depth of about 1 in.
4. Fill kohlrabi, put a dab of butter and cream on each.
5. Cook in a moderate oven for about ½ hr.

If desired, serve with Tomato Sauce, Recipe No. 303, or Herb Sauce, Recipe No. 301.

166 LEEKS 166

Ingredients:

1 heaping tablesp. vege-	salt
table fat	6 tablesp. cream
1¾ lb. prepared leeks	grated cheese
½ cup vegetable stock	

Method:

1. Melt fat, cut leeks into 4 in. pieces and add to the fat in layers.
2. Pour vegetable stock over and simmer until tender. Salt.
3. Add cheese and cream just before serving.

If preferred, cut leeks in half then into 1-in. pieces. Cook as above. Mix with Béchamel Sauce, Recipe No. 299, instead of cheese and cream.

167 ONIONS 167

Ingredients:

1 tablesp. vegetable fat	pinch of sugar
1¼ lb. onions	½–1 cup vegetable stock
salt	peas *or* Béchamel Sauce

Method:

1. Melt fat and sauté onions slowly in it; add salt and sugar.
2. Add stock and cook slowly for ¾ hr.
3. Garnish with peas or serve with Béchamel Sauce, Recipe No. 299.

168 CHESTNUTS AS A VEGETABLE 168

Ingredients:

2 lb. chestnuts	2½ cups vegetable stock
3 tablesp. vegetable fat	salt
3 tablesp. sugar	1½ tablesp. butter

Method:

1. Cut two slits, with a sharp knife, in the form of a diagonal cross on the flat side of the chestnut shells.
2. Place on a baking sheet in a hot oven until they split open; peel.
3. Melt fat, add sugar and brown it.
4. Add vegetable stock, chestnuts and salt.
5. Cook for ½ hr. until liquid has evaporated.
6. Add butter to the chestnuts before serving.

If preferred omit the sugar and sauté the chestnuts with chopped onion. Add vegetable stock and cook. Serve garnished with strips of fried onion.

169 PURÉE OF DRIED PEAS 169

Ingredients:

¾ lb. dried peas, yellow or green (soaked overnight)	salt
	2 tomatoes
	½ onion, chopped
2 small potatoes	1 teasp. butter
½ cup milk	1 slice of bread cut in cubes
½ cup cream	1½ tablesp. butter
vegetable stock if required	

Method:

1. Cook peas and potatoes in the water used for soaking, until quite tender, drain well and put through a sieve.
2. Add milk and cream to make a thick purée; add stock if required; salt.
3. Keep warm over boiling water.
4. Sauté tomatoes and onion in butter and use to garnish.
5. Fry bread cubes in remaining butter and serve with finished dish.

170 LENTILS   170

Ingredients:

¾ lb. lentils (soaked overnight)

2½ pt. vegetable stock

salt

1 onion with 3–4 cloves pressed into it

1 heaping tablesp. vegetable fat

1 onion, chopped

1 tablesp. flour

1½ tablesp. lemon juice *or* 3 tablesp. cream

Method:

1. Drain soaked lentils well.
2. Add vegetable stock, salt and onion with cloves, to the lentils.
3. Cook until tender.
4. Melt fat and sauté onion in it.
5. Sprinkle flour over lentils and add sautéed onion.
6. Add lemon juice or cream.

Note: Green lentils are preferable and this recipe is based on them.

171 WHITE (HARICOT) BEANS WITH TOMATOES   171

Ingredients:

¾ lb. beans (soaked overnight)

2½ cups vegetable stock

salt

1 heaping tablesp. vegetable fat

1 onion, chopped

½ lb. tomatoes

1 clove garlic

Method:

1. Drain soaked beans well.
2. Add stock and salt, and cook until tender.
3. Melt fat and sauté onion in it.
4. Skin and dice tomatoes, chop garlic, and add to the onions.
5. Add this to the bean mixture and cook all together for a few min.

If the finished dish appears too moist mix a tablesp. of cornstarch with a little cold water, add to the beans and cook until the mixture thickens.

Ingredients:

1 heaping tablesp. vegetable fat
1 onion, chopped
3 large stalks celeriac or celery
4 carrots
½ cup vegetable stock *or* milk and water

¼–½ lb. cauliflower
1–1½ cups peas or beans
¼–½ cup extra vegetable stock
¼–½ lb. spinach
1 teasp. butter
1 small onion, chopped

Method:

1. Melt fat and sauté onion in it.

2. Dice celeriac or celery and carrots and sauté with the onion.

3. Add ½ cup vegetable stock and cook gently until tender.

4. Cook cauliflower in a little stock, or milk and water, until tender.

5. Cook peas and beans in the vegetable stock over low heat, until tender.

6. Shred spinach and chop onion, cook together without adding any liquid.

7. Either mix all the cooked vegetables together or arrange in layers on a dish.

8. Melt butter and pour over.

Note: Any other vegetable may be used as desired.

Ingredients:

1½ lb. of any of the following vegetables can be used for Vegetables au Gratin:

spinach beet stalks	salsify
celery	Chinese artichokes
leeks	Jerusalem artichokes
cauliflower	celeriac
fennel	

Ingredients for Béchamel Sauce:

1 heaping tablesp. vegetable fat
3 tablesp. flour
2 cups vegetable stock *or* vegetable water

½ cup milk
salt
grated cheese
butter

Method:

1. Prepare vegetables and cook in their own juice according to the Recipes given for these vegetables.

2. Prepare Béchamel Sauce, Recipe No. 299.

3. Grease a baking dish and arrange chosen vegetable in it.

4. Add cheese to the sauce and pour over vegetable.

5. Put dabs of butter on top.

6. Bake in a moderate oven (350°) for ½ hr.

174 VEGETABLE FRITTERS 174

Prepare batter as in Recipe No. 328. Dip suitable sized pieces of any of the following vegetables into it and deep fry in hot vegetable fat, or oil, until golden brown.

Fritters of cooked vegetables:

Ingredients:	*Method:*
(a) cauliflower milk and water salt	Divide flowers into medium-sized florets. Cook in milk and water until tender, drain well.
(b) salsify	Cook until tender. Recipe No. 124.
(c) eggplant salt water	Bring to the boil in the salt water and drain immediately.
(d) carrots	Cook until tender: Recipe No. 111.
(e) celeriac	Cook until tender. Recipe No. 121, or cook in milk and water until tender.

Fritters of raw vegetables:

Ingredients:	*Method:*
(a) baby squash	Cut into slices.
(b) sage leaves	
(c) elderflowers	

(d) The vegetable fritters may be served with Rémoulade Sauce, Recipe No. 320, or with Tomato Sauce, Recipe No. 304, the elderflower fritters with sugar.

175 D. VEGETABLES SERVED IN SHELLS   175 D.

(*For Light Diet:* Without dumplings, Béchamel Sauce
and cheese.)

Ingredients:
Suitable combination of vegetables such as:
  cauliflower, Brussels sprouts and beans *or*
   carrots, celeriac and salsify *or*
    peas, asparagus and tomatoes *or*
   leeks, tomatoes and cauliflower, etc.
 Butter Dumplings, Recipe No. 52
 Béchamel Sauce, Recipe No. 299
 grated cheese

Ingredients for Butter
 Dumplings:
1½ tablesp. butter
6 tablesp. flour
¾ cup milk
1 egg
salt
chopped chives or parsley
 if liked
nutmeg

Ingredients for Béchamel
 Sauce:
½ tablesp. vegetable fat
2 tablesp. flour
¼ cup milk
½ cup vegetable stock
salt
grated cheese

Method:
 1. Prepare vegetables according to the various Recipes
given for these vegetables.
 2. Mix the chosen vegetables and put into greased shells.
 3. Prepare dumplings as in Recipe No. 52.
 4. Prepare Béchamel Sauce as in Recipe No. 299.
 5. Place small dumplings on the vegetables.
 6. Pour Béchamel Sauce over.
 7. Sprinkle with grated cheese.
 8. Bake in a hot oven for 10–15 min.

176 VEGETABLE PIE   176

Ingredients:
1 heaping tablesp. vege-
 table fat
1 onion, chopped
3 large stalks celeriac
4 carrots
1 cup cauliflower
1 cup peas or beans

½ lb. spinach
vegetable stock as required
2 cups flour
6–7 tablesp. butter
salt
9 tablesp. water

Method:
1. Melt fat and sauté onion in it.
2. Prepare vegetables as in Recipe No. 172.
3. Make shortcrust pastry as in Recipe No. 323.
4. Roll out pastry about one-tenth of an inch thick, cut off a piece to make a lid for a baking dish.
5. Fit pastry strips round edge of dish. Put an inverted egg cup in the middle and fill with vegetables either mixed or in layers.
6. Cover with the pastry lid.
7. Press edges together firmly and brush with egg yolk.
8. Bake in a hot oven (400°) for about ½ hr.

177 VEGETABLE TART   177

Ingredients:

2 cups flour	mixed vegetables as liked
6–7 tablesp. vegetable fat	Recipe No. 172
salt	Béchamel Sauce
9 tablesp. water	Recipe No. 299
	grated cheese

Method:
1. Prepare shortcrust pastry as in Recipe No. 323.
2. Line baking pan with pastry and bake the crust.
3. Arrange various mixed vegetables as in Recipe No. 172, or separate vegetables if preferred, on the pastry shell.
4. Cover with a thin Béchamel Sauce, Recipe No. 299.
5. Sprinkle with grated cheese and bake for about 10 min. in a moderate oven.

178 RICE STUFFING FOR VEGETABLES   178

Ingredients:

½ cup rice	3 tablesp. grated cheese
1 cup vegetable stock	chopped herbs
1 egg	3 tablesp. chopped mush-rooms

Method:
1. Boil rice in the stock until soft.
2. Mix all ingredients together and use as required.

179 BREAD STUFFING FOR VEGETABLES   179

Ingredients:

4–5 slices of bread
(½ wholewheat, ½
white if possible)
1 cup milk
1 tablesp. dried mush-
rooms

1 heaping tablesp. vege-
table fat
½ onion, chopped
1½ tablesp. grated cheese
1½ tablesp. chopped herbs
1 egg
½ clove garlic

Method:

1. Soak bread and dried mushrooms for ½ hr. in the milk;
put through a blender.
2. Melt fat and sauté onion in it.
3. Mix all ingredients together and use as required.

Finely chopped fresh mushrooms can be fried with the
onion if liked.

This mixture may be used for small bread dumplings if an
egg or two is added. Use with clear broth, Recipe No. 51 D.

180 SALADS OF COOKED VEGETABLES   180

Ingredients:

Any of the following suitable vegetables:

   carrots   beans
   celeriac   cauliflower
   beetroots   Chinese artichokes

Salad dressing or mayonnaise

Method:

1. Boil vegetables until soft in vegetable stock or salt water.
2. Cut up into cubes or slices.
3. Dress with salad dressing, Recipe No. 8, or with mayonnaise, Recipe No. 318.

Cauliflower can also be covered with a Rémoulade Sauce,
Recipe No. 320, flavored with onion and chopped herbs, either
fresh or dried.

181 POTATO SALAD, I   181

Ingredients:

2 lb. potatoes (approx. 8
medium)
1 cup vegetable stock
4½ tablesp. oil
3 tablesp. lemon juice

3 tablesp. cream
1½ tablesp. chopped onion
salt
nutmeg

Method:
1. Boil potatoes and peel while they are still hot.
2. Slice potatoes and cover with hot vegetable stock.
3. Leave to stand for a short time.
4. Beat oil, lemon juice and cream together and mix with potatoes while still warm.
5. Add seasoning to taste.

182 POTATO SALAD, 2   182

Ingredients:

2 lb. potatoes (approx. 8 medium)
½ cup vegetable stock
2–3 tablesp. lemon juice
1 tablesp. chopped onion

salt
nutmeg
3 tablesp. mayonnaise Recipe No. 318

Method:
1. Boil potatoes and peel while they are still hot.
2. Slice potatoes and cover with hot vegetable stock.
3. Leave to stand for a short time.
4. Mix mayonnaise and flavoring with potatoes and serve.

One medium-sized cucumber may be added to the potatoes in either of the above recipes if desired.

183 D. MIXED VEGETABLE SALAD
(FROM COOKED VEGETABLES)   183 D.

Ingredients:

3–4 different varieties of vegetable such as carrots, celeriac, cauliflower, Chinese artichokes, zucchini, beans, beetroot, potatoes
mayonnaise *or* French dressing

Method:
1. Take the chosen cooked vegetables and dice or slice them.
2. Mix with mayonnaise, Recipe No. 318, or French dressing, Recipe No. 8.

184 RUSSIAN SALAD   184

Ingredients:

4 large carrots	salt
3 large stalks celeriac or celery	4½ tablesp. mayonnaise, Recipe No. 317 or 318
1 cup peas	gherkins, tomatoes, cress to garnish
½ lb. potatoes (2 medium)	
3 tablesp. lemon juice	

Method:

1. Cook carrots, celeriac and peas all separately in a little vegetable stock, with salt, until tender.
2. Cook potatoes in their skins.
3. Leave all vegetables to cool then dice potatoes.
4. Mix in lemon juice and more salt if required.
5. Stir in mayonnaise and garnish.

185 D. NIÇOISE SALAD   185 D.

Ingredients:

5 boiled potatoes	3 hard-boiled eggs
4 tomatoes	4½ tablesp. oil
radishes	3 tablesp. lemon juice
olives	salt
gherkins	cabbage lettuce leaves

Method:

1. Slice vegetables and eggs.
2. Prepare salad dressing as in Recipe No. 8.
3. Mix dressing with vegetables and eggs.
4. Add lettuce leaves to the salad shortly before serving.

186 D. RICE SALAD   186 D.

Ingredients:

1¼ cups rice	2 tomatoes
2½ pt. water	3 gherkins
4½ tablesp. oil	1 tablesp. capers
2 tablesp. lemon juice	chives, parsley or basil
½ tablesp. chopped onion	lettuce leaves optional

Method:

1. Cook rice in the water until soft.
2. Strain through a sieve and rinse well under water.
3. Leave until cold.
4. Mix oil and lemon juice together thoroughly and add, with the onion, to rice.

5. Mix diced tomatoes and gherkins and add with the capers and herbs to other ingredients.

6. Arrange finished salad on lettuce leaves or serve in shells.

187 CELERIAC SALAD WITH MAYONNAISE 187

Ingredients:

1–1¼ lb. celeriac	salt
1½ tablesp. lemon juice	3 tablesp. mayonnaise
6 walnuts	Recipe No. 317
1 apple	3 tablesp. cream

Method:

1. Shred celeriac very finely and mix with lemon juice.

2. Chop walnuts, grate apple, and add to celeriac with salt to taste.

3. Mix carefully with mayonnaise and top with cream.

188 RUSSIAN EGGS 188

Ingredients:

4 hard-boiled eggs	salt
2–3 tablesp. mayonnaise	Marmite or other yeast ex-
Recipe No. 317	tract

Method:

1. Shell eggs and cut in half.

2. Put egg yolks through a fine sieve.

3. Mix yolks with mayonnaise, salt and Marmite, or other yeast extract, and fill the eggs.

Stuffed eggs can be used to garnish salads for special occasions. If liked some of the mixture can be mixed with finely chopped herbs or with tomato purée instead of yeast extract.

189 D. VEGETABLE ASPIC 189 D.

Ingredients:

1 teasp. Agar-Agar*	tomato
2½ pt. vegetable stock	gherkin
lemon juice	pickled cucumber
Marmite or other yeast ex-	cooked cauliflower
tract	cooked peas
salt	cooked beans
hard-boiled egg	

* Agar-Agar is a vegetable gelatine made from seaweed. It can be used for vegetables, desserts, sauces, puddings, etc., and is obtainable in powdered form at health food stores.

Method:

1. Dissolve the Agar-Agar in lukewarm stock, heat slowly, making sure it is completely dissolved.

2. Add lemon juice, Marmite and salt to season.

3. Pour a little aspic into a dish or bowl, previously rinsed out in cold water.

4. Leave to set in a cool place.

5. Garnish with egg and slices of vegetable, pour in a little more aspic and again leave to set.

6. Continue in this manner adding vegetables and aspic alternately until the dish is full.

7. When the aspic has set, turn out and use to garnish salad dishes, or serve with mixed salad as a main dish.

CANAPÉS OR OPEN SANDWICHES

Canapés, or open-type sandwiches, are popular in Switzerland either as an hors d'œuvre or an entrée, or as a warm-weather supper dish. They are excellent also for teas, buffets and cocktail parties. Sandwiches or rolls with similar fillings can also be taken on picnics or for packed lunches. In open-type sandwiches one slice only of bread or biscuit such as Ryvita, etc., is spread with a filling and then decorated. The fillings can be varied almost indefinitely, the fresher and more colorful and attractive the slices look, the more appetizing they will prove. The wholewheat bread used should be at least one day old so that it may be cut into really thin slices.

190 BASIC FILLINGS FOR OPEN SANDWICHES 190

Ingredients:

butter, alone *or*
    5–6 tablesp. curd with
    1½ tablesp. butter
salt or sea salt
Marmite or other yeast extract

2–3 tablesp. cream
chopped chives or other freshly chopped or dried green herbs, caraway seeds or tomato purée
(see also Recipe No. 48 *b*)

Method:

1. Soften the butter.

2. Cream the curd (this can be done more easily if it is first passed through a sieve).

3. Add soft butter to sieved curd and cream well together.

4. Add Marmite and cream.

5. Add salt and herbs.

An alternative is to force cream cheese or any soft cheese through a sieve; add some cream and whip. Flavor as above.

Another method is to grate Swiss Gruyère, English Cheddar or similar type cheese. Mix with cream and allow to stand for ½ hr. Then add herbs and salt, herb-sea-salt or sea salt as above.

GARNISHES

The open sandwiches can be decorated with any of the following: Raw grated carrot or celery, *or* celeriac salad, Recipe No. 187,

> *or* tomatoes, cucumber, radishes, cress, onion rings, gherkins,
>
> *or* capers, olives, walnuts, etc.
>
> *or* chopped egg mixed with mayonnaise,
>
> *or* cress mixed with chopped egg and some mayonnaise or salad dressing,
>
> *or* asparagus tips with mayonnaise, etc.

POTATO DISHES

191 D. POTATOES IN THEIR SKINS   191 D.

Ingredients:

2 lb. potatoes (approx. 8 medium)   salt
                                                  water

Method:

1. Brush any mud off the potatoes and wash well.

2. Steam in a special steamer (or in a wire basket within a saucepan) with salt for 30–40 min., or use a pressure cooker.

192 D. BAKED POTATOES   192 D.

2 lb. potatoes (approx. 8 medium)   3–4 tablesp. oil
                                                  2 tablesp. butter
salt

Method:

1. Brush any mud off the potatoes and wash well.

2. Score skin on upper side three or four times, brush with oil and salt.

3. Bake on a greased baking sheet 30–40 min. in a moderate oven (350°).

4. Put a dab of butter on each potato before serving.

193 D. POTATOES WITH CREAM CHEESE OR CURD   193 D.

Ingredients:
- 2 lb. potatoes (approx. 8 medium)
- salt
- 3 tablesp. oil

Ingredients for Stuffing:
- ½ lb. or 1¾ sticks cream cheese or curd
- ¼ cup milk or cream
- salt
- chives, or caraway, or marjoram, or nasturtium, or other herbs freshly chopped or green dried

Method:
1. Score once across upper side of potatoes, bake in moderate oven (350°) 30–40 min.
2. Mix cream cheese with milk, add herbs and salt to taste.
3. Put into a pastry bag and pipe over the slit in the baked potatoes.

194 D. CARAWAY POTATOES   194 D.

Ingredients:
- 8–10 medium-sized potatoes
- 1 teasp. caraway seeds
- 1 teasp. salt

Method:
1. Brush any mud off the potatoes and wash well.
2. Halve potatoes.
3. Mix caraway and salt, dip the cut side of the potatoes into the mixture.
4. Place on a baking sheet with the cut surface down; brush with oil.
5. Bake in a moderate oven (350°) for ¾ hr.

195 D. POTATOES COOKED IN VEGETABLE STOCK   195 D.

Ingredients:
- 2 lb. potatoes (approx. 8 medium)
- 2½–3 cups vegetable stock
- salt
- 2 tablesp. butter

Method:
1. Wash potatoes, peel and cut into halves or pieces.
2. Cook until tender in stock. Add salt if necessary.
3. Add butter to the cooked potatoes.

196 D. PARSLEY POTATOES   196 D.

Ingredients:

  1¾ lb. potatoes (approx.   water
     7 medium)   3 tablesp. butter
  salt   1½ tablesp. parsley

Method:

  1. Wash and peel potatoes, cut into four lengthwise.
  2. Sprinkle with salt.
  3. Steam potatoes in a wire basket or steamer.
  4. Melt butter and mix with chopped parsley, add to potatoes.

197 CREAM POTATOES, 1   197

Ingredients:

  1¼ lb. potatoes (approx.   2 cups milk
     5 medium)   ½ cup cream
  2½ cups milk or vegeta-   salt
     ble stock   1 bay leaf
  salt   marjoram
  1½ tablesp. vegetable fat
  3 tablesp. flour

Method:

  1. Slice potatoes and cook until tender in milk or stock; add salt.
  2. Prepare Béchamel Sauce, Recipe No. 299, and mix with potatoes.
  3. Season with herbs to taste.

198 D. CREAM POTATOES, 2   198 D.

Ingredients:

  1½ lb. potatoes (approx.   salt
     6 medium)   ½–1 cup cream
  1½ tablesp. vegetable fat parsley
  2½ cups vegetable stock

Method:

  1. Wash and peel potatoes, cut into slices.
  2. Melt fat, sauté potatoes lightly in it.
  3. Add stock, salt, and cook slowly until tender.
  4. Add cream just before serving and sprinkle with parsley.

199 D. POTATOES WITH TOMATOES 199 D.

Ingredients:

1½ tablesp. vegetable fat	1½ cups vegetable stock
1 small onion	salt
1½ lb. potatoes (approx. 6 medium)	2–3 tomatoes
	3–4 tablesp. cream

Method:

1. Melt fat, sauté onion in it.
2. Add peeled, sliced potatoes, vegetable stock and salt, and cook gently.
3. Skin tomatoes, slice and add to potatoes just before they are completely cooked.
4. Add cream just before serving.

200 D. POTATO SNOW 200 D.

(*For Light Diet:* Dabs of fresh butter should be used instead of hot butter.)

Ingredients:

2 lb. potatoes (approx. 8 medium)	salt
water	2 tablesp. melted butter

Method:

1. Wash and peel potatoes, cut into small pieces.
2. Steam or boil in a little water, with salt, until cooked.
3. Force through a sieve or colander on to a warm dish.
4. Pour melted butter over the finished dish.

201 D. MASHED POTATOES 201 D.

Ingredients:

2 lb. potatoes (approx. 8 medium)	1½–2 cups milk
water	nutmeg
salt	3 tablesp. cream, if desired
2–3 tablesp. butter	parsley

Method:

1. Wash and peel potatoes, cut into small pieces.
2. Steam or boil in a little water, with salt, until tender.
3. Melt butter and heat with the milk in a second saucepan.
4. Force hot, cooked potatoes through a sieve or colander (or mash with a wooden spoon) into this saucepan.

5. Mash all together thoroughly, season and add cream.

6. Arrange on a hot dish; make patterns with a knife, dipped in hot water, and garnish with parsley.

202 D. POTATO BALLS   202 D.

(*For Light Diet:* Without fried breadcrumbs.)

Ingredients:

2 lb. potatoes	2–3 tablesp. butter
1 cup milk	1½ tablesp. butter
salt	¾ oz. breadcrumbs
nutmeg	

Method:

1. Prepare potatoes as in Recipe No. 201.

2. Melt butter.

3. Dip small round ladle into hot butter.

4. Scoop out balls of potato and place on a hot dish.

5. Fry breadcrumbs lightly in butter and pour some over each potato ball.

203 POTATO CAKES   203

Ingredients:

1½ lb. potatoes	nutmeg
water	marjoram or basil (fresh or
salt	dried green)
1 egg	flour
4½ tablesp. cheese, if liked	vegetable fat or oil for frying

Method:

1. Wash and peel potatoes.

2. Steam, or boil in the water, with salt till cooked.

3. Force through sieve or mash thoroughly.

4. Mix egg, cheese and seasoning together and add to potatoes.

5. Form mixture into rissoles or cakes and roll in flour.

6. Fry on both sides in a liberal quantity of fat or oil.

If preferred rissoles may be dipped in beaten egg and rolled in breadcrumbs before frying.

204 POTATO PUDDING   204

Ingredients:

1¾ lb. potatoes (approx.)	3 tablesp. butter
water	2 egg whites
salt	¾ oz. breadcrumbs
2 egg yolks	1½ tablesp. butter
4½ tablesp. grated cheese	2 tablesp. butter
nutmeg	¾ oz. breadcrumbs
marjoram	

Method:

1. Wash and peel potatoes, cut into pieces.
2. Steam or boil in a little water, with salt.
3. Force through a sieve or mash thoroughly.
4. Mix with yolks, cheese, butter and herbs to make a damp, but not liquid, paste.
5. Beat egg whites to a stiff froth and fold into potato mixture.
6. Grease pudding mold and coat with breadcrumbs.
7. Fill with mixture, cover with a floured cloth tied firmly.
8. Cook in boiling water 40–50 min., or bake in moderate oven.
9. Turn out pudding and coat with melted butter and breadcrumbs.

205 POTATO RING   205

Ingredients:

The same as in Recipe No. 204.

Method:

Prepare mixture as in Recipe No. 204 up to end of Method 5.
6. Grease ring mold and coat with breadcrumbs.
7. Bake in moderate oven 20–30 min.
8. Turn out. Fill and surround with vegetables.

206 DUCHESS POTATOES   206

Ingredients:

1¼–1½ lb. potatoes	2 tablesp. butter
water	salt
salt	nutmeg
1 egg	1 egg
	1½ tablesp. butter

Method:
1. Cook potatoes as in Recipe No. 204 and put through sieve or mash well.
2. Whisk egg and add with butter, salt and nutmeg to potatoes.
3. Put mixture into a pastry bag and pipe on to a greased baking sheet in a round coil.
4. Brush with beaten egg, dot with butter.
5. Bake in moderate oven until golden brown.

207 POTATO NESTS 207

Ingredients:
The same as for Recipe No. 206.

Method:
1. Prepare potatoes as in Recipe No. 206 and put into a pastry bag.
2. Force out small nests of potato.
3. Fill with cooked vegetables after baking.

208 POTATO NESTS WITH CHEESE STUFFING 208

Ingredients:

Duchess potatoes as in Recipe No. 206	1 egg
	4½ tablesp. cream
10 tablesp. grated cheese	salt

Method:
1. Prepare potatoes as in Recipe No. 206.
2. Put mixture into a pastry bag and press out into small nests.
3. Mix grated cheese, egg, cream and salt and fill nests.
4. Bake in a moderate oven (350°) for about 20 min.

209 POTATO NOODLES 209

Ingredients:

1 lb. potatoes	5 pt. slightly salted vegetable stock
salt water	
1 cup flour	grated cheese
1 egg	breadcrumbs
nutmeg	3 tablesp. butter

Method:
1. Peel potatoes, cook in a little salt water.
2. When cooked force through a sieve or put in a blender.

3. Add flour, egg and nutmeg to make a firm mixture.

4. Roll with a floured hand, on a floured board, into 2-in. sausage-shaped rolls.

5. Choose a large saucepan and bring salted stock to the boil.

6. Add potato rolls and cook gently until they rise to the surface.

7. Take out with a perforated ladle and drain well.

8. Arrange on a hot dish, sprinkle with grated cheese, and pour hot butter and breadcrumbs over.

Serve with Tomato Sauce, Recipe No. 303, if liked.

210 DAUPHIN POTATOES   210

Ingredients:

1¼ cups milk	1 lb. potatoes (approx.)
2 oz. butter or vegetable fat (4 tablesp.)	water for boiling potatoes
	salt
1 cup flour	fat for frying
2 eggs	

Method:

1. Prepare Choux Pastry, Recipe No. 330.
2. Peel potatoes and cook in salt water.
3. Force through a sieve or put into a blender.
4. Mix with pastry and put into a pastry bag without a tip.
5. Heat fat, or oil, in a deep fat frying pan.
6. Squeeze out strips of pastry mixture 1 in. long, straight into the fat.
7. Fry until golden brown.

211 D. BROWNED POTATOES   211 D.

(For Light Diet: Use less fat.)

Ingredients:

8 small potatoes	1½ cups vegetable stock
water	1½ tablesp. vegetable fat (melted) *or* oil.
salt	½ cup cream

Method:

1. Peel potatoes, cut in half and parboil in a little water.
2. Put in a deep roasting pan with the cut surfaces down.
3. Pour vegetable stock and the melted fat over potatoes and braise in moderate oven until the vegetable stock has been absorbed.

4. Pour cream over and continue roasting until the cut surface browns.

5. Arrange on a hot dish with cut sides up, sprinkle with chopped parsley.

212 PRINCESS POTATOES 212

Ingredients:

1¾ lb. potatoes, approx.	½ cup milk ⎫ *or* 1¼ cups
water	¾ cup cream ⎭ milk
salt	nutmeg
3 tablesp. grated cheese	salt
1½ tablesp. vegetable fat	2 tablesp. butter
1 cup milk	
2 eggs	

Method:

1. Cook potatoes, peel and cut into thick slices.
2. Put into a baking dish, sprinkle each layer with grated cheese.
3. Pour hot vegetable fat and 1 cup milk over the potatoes.
4. Bake in hot oven 10–15 min.
5. Whisk eggs and pour over, add milk, and cream if used, add nutmeg and salt.
6. Put dabs of butter on the top and bake for a further 10–15 min.

213 SWISS POTATOES ROESTI 213

Ingredients:

    3 tablesp. vegetable fat
    2 lb. potatoes cooked over-
        night in their skins
    salt

Method:

1. Peel potatoes and grate on a coarse grater.
2. Heat fat in a frying pan, add potatoes and salt.
3. Cover and brown potatoes, turning occasionally.
4. Using a spatula, form into a thick pancake.
5. Allow light brown crust to form on underside.
6. Carefully turn over and slide down to brown other side.
7. Turn on to a hot dish.

If liked, fry chopped onion in butter and add to the potatoes before making the pancake.

214 LYONS POTATOES 214

Ingredients:

1½ tablesp. fat
3 tablesp. oil

2 lb. small potatoes
salt
1 large onion, shredded

Method:
1. Heat fat and oil in a frying pan.
2. Peel potatoes, cut into slices.
3. Cook in the hot fat until half cooked.
4. Add onions, season with salt, and finish cooking.

215 POTATO STICKS OR BALLS 215

Ingredients:

2 lb. potatoes

3 tablesp. vegetable fat *or*
4–6 tablesp. oil

Method:
1. Peel potatoes and cut into small sticks.
2. Dry in a cloth.
3. Heat fat or oil, add potatoes, and salt.
4. Cover with a lid and cook for a short time.
5. Remove lid and allow to brown for about ½ hr.

If large potatoes are used, scoop out little balls and cook as above.

216 HAZELNUT POTATOES 216

Ingredients:

2 lb. potatoes
salt

3 tablesp. vegetable fat
4½ tablesp. breadcrumbs

Method:
1. Peel potatoes, cut into small dice, add salt.
2. Fry in a *covered pan* until soft.
3. Sprinkle with breadcrumbs and continue frying over gentle heat for a short time, without a lid.

217 CASTLE POTATOES 217

2 lb. small potatoes
salt
water

4½ tablesp. vegetable fat *or*
4–6 tablesp. oil

Method:

1. Cut potatoes into quarters lengthwise, round off sharp edges.
2. Cook until semi-soft.
3. Heat vegetable fat, add potatoes, fry slowly in frying pan.
4. Turn carefully several times until a golden brown.

218 FRENCH FRIED POTATOES 218

Ingredients:

2 lb. potatoes   salt
vegetable fat or oil

Method:

1. Cut potatoes into finger-shaped pieces, dry at once in a cloth.
2. Heat fat or oil. Fry potatoes a few at a time.
3. Take out of the fat with perforated spoon, drain on a rack or greaseproof paper, or use a deep fat fryer.
4. Shortly before serving heat up oil again and fry potatoes quickly so that they are crisp outside but remain soft inside.
5. Drain again, sprinkle with salt and serve immediately.

Potato crisps can be done in the same way but should be sliced thinly straight into the smoking fat and fried until golden. Drain and serve hot with salt.

219 POTATO BASKETS 219

(*Small double wire baskets are required to make these baskets.*)

Ingredients:

4 medium-sized potatoes   salt
vegetable fat or oil

Method:

1. Heat the wire baskets in fat.
2. Shred potatoes finely, or cut into matchsticks.
3. Line one basket with potatoes, press the second basket on to them.
4. Fry golden brown in hot fat, or oil, drain.
5. Remove finished baskets very carefully.
6. Keep warm in the oven until required; fill with cooked vegetables.

220 D. POTATO CAKES WITH SPINACH   220 D.

(*For Light Diet:* Without cheese.)

Ingredients:

4 large potatoes
2 cups vegetable stock
salt

¾ lb. spinach (approx. 10 cups)
5–6 tablesp. grated cheese
1½ tablesp. butter

Method:

1. Peel potatoes and cut lentghwise into approx. ½-in. slices.
2. Cook potatoes carefully until tender, place on a greased baking sheet.
3. Prepare spinach as in Recipe No. 99 D.
4. Heap spinach purée on to potato slices.
5. Sprinkle with cheese and put dabs of butter on top.
6. Bake in moderate oven for about 15 min.

221 POTATOES WITH CURLY KALE   221

Ingredients:

1 heaping tablesp. vegetable fat
1 chopped onion
¾ lb. curly kale

1½ lb. potatoes
3 cups vegetable stock
salt
2 tablesp. butter

Method:

1. Melt fat; sauté onion in it.
2. Add chopped kale and sauté.
3. Add diced potatoes and sauté all together.
4. Add stock and salt, cover, and cook for ½–¾ hr.
5. Melt butter and pour over finished vegetables.

222 STUFFED POTATOES   222

Ingredients:

2 lb. potatoes
vegetable stock
salt
Bread Stuffing (Recipe No. 179)

vegetable stock
2 tablesp. butter
cream (if liked)

Method:

1. Choose long potatoes, of the same size if possible, and peel.

2. Cut in half and hollow out a little.

3. Cook in salted stock until half cooked; put in a baking dish.

4. Stuff with bread stuffing and put a dab of butter on each.

5. Pour vegetable stock into the dish until it reaches half-way up each potato.

6. Cover and bake in a moderate oven (350°) for 20–30 min.

7. Pour in cream, if used, just before the dish is ready.

If desired serve with Herb Sauce, Recipe No. 301, or Tomato Sauce, Recipe No. 304.

VEGETABLE DISHES WITH RICE,* CEREALS AND FLOUR

223 D. JAPANESE RICE   223 D.

Ingredients:

1 teasp. vegetable fat	salt
1¼ cups rice	1½ tablesp. butter
2½ cups water	

Method:

1. Melt fat, add rice and sauté.

2. Add water and salt, cover, and cook for about 15 min.

3. Cool rice (which should be separate and grainy).

4. Heat butter, add cooked rice and sauté until really hot.

5. Put dabs of butter on the finished rice before serving.

224 RISOTTO   224

Ingredients:

3 tablesp. vegetable fat	salt
1 chopped onion	rosemary
1¼ cups rice	3 tablesp. grated cheese
2½ pt. vegetable stock or water	1½ tablesp. butter (if liked)

Method:

1. Melt vegetable fat, sauté onion and rice in it until transparent.

2. Add heated stock, salt and rosemary, cook 15–20 min., adding more stock if necessary.

3. Mix in cheese and butter lightly using a fork.

* Whole long grain rice (with silver skin and germ) is used for all savory dishes and whole round grain rice is used for all sweet dishes.

225 SAFFRON OR MARIGOLD RICE   225

Prepare same as Risotto, Recipe No. 224; dissolve ½ teasp. saffron powder in or add 1–2 teasp. marigold petals (fresh or dried) to a little vegetable stock and add to the rice.

226 D. CRÉOLE RICE   226 D.

Ingredients:

3 tablesp. vegetable fat	2½ pt. water or stock
1 onion, chopped	salt
1¼ cups rice	

Method:

As for Recipe No. 224.

Add vegetables to Créole Rice by sautéing 1 cup finely diced vegetables (leeks, celery or celeriac, and carrots), and using 1 cup rice only.

227 D. RICE WITH TOMATOES   227 D.

(*For Light Diet:* Without cheese.)

Ingredients:

1 heaping tablesp. vege- table fat	2 large tomatoes
1 onion, chopped	salt
1 clove garlic	1½–2 cups vegetable stock
1¼ cups rice	1 oz. grated cheese
	1 teasp. butter if liked

Method:

1. Melt fat and sauté onion and garlic in it.
2. Add rice and sauté until it looks transparent.
3. Skin tomatoes, dice and add to the rice.
4. Add salt and vegetable stock; cook for 15–20 min.
5. Mix in the cheese and butter just before serving if liked.

228 RISOTTO WITH PEPPERS   228

Ingredients:

4½ tablesp. oil	2½ cups vegetable stock
1 small onion, chopped	salt
¾ lb. peppers (approx.)	¾ oz. grated cheese
1¼ cups rice	

Method:

1. Cut peppers in half, remove seeds and pith and cut into strips.

2. Heat oil and sauté onion and peppers in it.

3. Add rice and sauté all together.

4. Add stock and salt and cook on the top of the stove or in the oven for 15 min.

5. Sprinkle the finished dish with grated cheese before serving.

Note: If the peppers are bitter, score across the thick parts and soak in cold water for 1 hr. before cooking.

229 D. RICE WITH SQUASH OR ZUCCHINI   229 D.

(*For Light Diet:* Without cheese.)

Ingredients:

1½ tablesp. vegetable fat
½ onion, chopped
1 lb. squash (approx.)

½ cup water or vegetable stock
1¼ cups rice (approx.)
3 tablesp. cheese (if liked)
1½ tablesp. butter

Method:

1. Melt fat and sauté onion in it.

2. Dice squash or zucchini and sauté, with the onion, for 10 min.

3. Add ½ cup of vegetable stock, or water, and the rice and cook gently.

4. Add more stock or water, if necessary, to keep the dish to the consistency of risotto.

5. Add cheese, if used, and butter to the finished dish.

230 D. RICE WITH PEAS   230 D.

(*For Light Diet:* Without cheese.)

Ingredients:

1 heaping tablesp. vegetable fat
½ onion, chopped
3 cups shelled peas
1 cup vegetable stock

Ingredients for Risotto:

1 heaping tablesp. vegetable fat
½ onion, chopped
1½ cups rice (approx.)
3 cups water
3 tablesp. cheese
1½ tablesp. butter

Method:

1. Melt fat and sauté chopped onion in it.

2. Add peas, sauté with onion.

3. Add vegetable stock and cook until tender.

4. Prepare Risotto—see Recipe No. 224.
5. When cooked, add cooked peas to it.
6. Add cheese, if used, and butter to the finished dish.

231 D. RICE WITH SPINACH   231 D.

(*For Light Diet:* Without cheese.)

Ingredients:

1 heaping tablesp. vegetable fat
1 onion, chopped
¾ lb. spinach (approx.)
1¼ cups rice (approx.)

4 cups vegetable stock or water
1½ tablesp. butter
1 oz. cheese, if used

Method:

1. Melt fat and sauté onion in it.
2. Chop spinach and add, with the rice, to the onion and sauté.
3. Add hot stock or water to the other ingredients.
4. Cook for 15–20 min.
5. Add butter and cheese, if used, to the finished dish.

232 RICE SOUFFLÉ WITH TOMATOES   232

Ingredients:

as for Créole Rice,
    Recipe No. 226 D

4–6 tomatoes
3 tablesp. grated cheese
1½ tablesp. butter

Method:

1. Prepare Créole Rice, No. 226 D.
2. Put alternate layers of rice and tomatoes into a well-greased baking dish.
3. Sprinkle with grated cheese and dot with butter.
4. Bake in a moderate oven for about 10 min.

233 TURKISH RICE   233

Ingredients:

as in Recipe No. 224
½ tablesp. vegetable fat
1 cup carrots and celeriac, sliced
½ cup vegetable stock
½ tablesp. vegetable fat
½ onion, chopped

2 cups mushrooms (approx.)
2–3 tablesp. flour
1–1½ cups vegetable stock
1 teasp. lemon juice
salt
1 egg yolk

Method:

1. Prepare rice as in Recipe No. 224.

2. Melt vegetable fat, add carrots and celeriac and ½ cup vegetable stock and cook slightly.

3. Put alternate layers of vegetables and rice in a baking dish.

4. Prepare Mushroom Sauce, Recipe No. 311; pour over rice.

5. Bake in the oven for a short time.

234 D. RICE RING OR PUDDING   234 D.

(*For Light Diet:* With tomatoes as a vegetable, or halved tomatoes, but without Mushroom Sauce.)

Ingredients:

Japanese Rice, Risotto, Saffron or Marigold Rice or Créole Rice, Recipes Nos. 223, 224, 225, 226.

Method:

1. Put the rice into a ring mold, plain mold, or cups rinsed out in cold water. Turn out onto a dish.

2. Finish as follows:

Rice Ring: Fill with tomatoes as a vegetable, or with peas and carrots.

Rice Pudding: With Mushroom Sauce, Recipe No. 311, garnished with tomatoes and slices of hard-boiled egg.

Small Rice Puddings: Garnish with fried halves or small whole tomatoes.

235 RICE RISSOLES OR CROQUETTES   235

Ingredients:

2¼ tablesp. vegetable fat	4½ tablesp. grated cheese
1 small onion, chopped	2 tablesp. butter
1¼ cups rice (approx.)	1 egg
2½ cups vegetable stock	2–3 tablesp. milk
salt	breadcrumbs
	vegetable fat *or* oil

Method:

1. Prepare Risotto, Recipe No. 224.

2. Spread Risotto on a board about ½ in. thick; cool.

3. Cut into rectangles.

4. Whisk egg and milk, dip rice in it, then into breadcrumbs.

5. Fry in a liberal amount of vegetable fat or oil.

236 RICE CAKES WITH SPINACH   236

Ingredients:

2¼ tablesp. vegetable fat	2 eggs
1 small onion, chopped	2 cups raw chopped spinach
1¼ cups rice	4½ tablesp. grated cheese
2½–3 cups vegetable stock	4½ tablesp. flour
	vegetable fat for frying

Method:

1. Prepare Risotto, Recipe No. 224.
2. Whisk eggs and add with the spinach and all other ingredients.
3. Shape into small cakes; dip in flour.
4. Fry in vegetable fat.

237 D. FARINA PUDDING (SAVORY)   237 D.

Ingredients:

4½ oz. farina	salt
3¾ cups milk	1½ tablesp. butter
2½ cups water	

Method:

1. Boil liquid, add farina to it, stirring all the time. Add salt.
2. Cook 15–20 min.
3. Melt butter, pour over finished farina.

238 D. FARINA BALLS   238 D.

Ingredients:

5½ oz. farina	salt
3¾ cups milk	3 tablesp. butter
2½ cups water	1 tablesp. breadcrumbs

Method:

1. Bring milk and water to the boil, add farina, stirring all the time.
2. Add salt and cook for 15–20 min.
3. Dip a small ladle into hot butter then scoop out small balls of farina.
4. Arrange on a hot dish and if liked spread sautéed breadcrumbs over the balls.

Ingredients:

6 oz. farina	½ cup milk
2½ cups milk	½ cup cream
2½ cups water	salt
salt	3 tablesp. grated cheese
nutmeg	1½ tablesp. butter
2 eggs	

Method:

1. Bring milk and water to the boil, add farina, stirring all the time.

2. Add salt and nutmeg and cook for 15–20 min.

3. Spread on a board to a depth of about ½ in. Cool.

4. Cut into small rounds with a pastry cutter.

5. Place any scraps left over from cutting in a greased baking dish, then arrange rounds neatly on top.

6. Beat eggs and mix with milk and cream, pour into dish.

7. Sprinkle with grated cheese and dot with butter.

8. Bake in moderate oven (350°) until firm.

240 FARINA DUMPLINGS   240

Ingredients:

6½ oz. farina	3 tablesp. grated cheese
2½ cups milk	1 egg
2½ cups water	vegetable stock
salt	2 tablesp. butter
	2 tablesp. breadcrumbs

Method:

1. Bring milk and water to the boil, add farina and salt, stirring all the time.

2. Cook for 15–20 min.

3. Mix cheese and egg, and add to the farina.

4. Shape small dumplings with 2 spoons and drop into boiling vegetable stock.

5. Simmer until they rise to the surface.

6. Take out with a perforated ladle, arrange on a hot dish.

7. Melt butter and fry breadcrumbs lightly in it; pour over dumplings.

241 FARINA CAKES   241

Ingredients:

6 oz. farina	salt
2½ cups milk	1–2 eggs
2½ cups water	vegetable fat

Method:
1. Bring milk and water to the boil, add farina and salt, stirring all the time.
2. Cook 15–20 min.
3. Spread on a board to a depth of about ½ in. Cool.
4. Cut into diamond-shaped pieces.
5. Dip into beaten egg and fry both sides in vegetable fat.

242 D. SWEET CORN MASH   242 D.

Ingredients:

1¼ cups milk	1½ cups yellow cornmeal
3¾ cups water	1 heaping tablesp. farina
salt	1 teasp. butter

Method:
1. Bring milk and water to the boil; add salt.
2. Stir cornmeal and farina into the boiling liquid and cook for 5 min., stirring continuously.
3. Cook gently for at least another hour, stirring frequently.
4. Add dabs of butter to the finished dish.

243 D. POLENTA   243 D.

(*For Light Diet:* Without cheese.)

Ingredients:

1½ tablesp. oil	nutmeg
6¼ cups water	1½ tablesp. fresh butter
1½ cups yellow cornmeal	3 tablesp. grated cheese
salt	

Method:
1. Coat saucepan with the oil.
2. Bring water to the boil in the same saucepan.
3. Stir cornmeal, salt and nutmeg into the boiling water and cook fast for 5 min., stirring continuously.
4. Then cook slowly for 1–2 hours.
5. Mix in butter and cheese.

If desired fried onion rings or breadcrumbs and fresh butter may be spread over finished dish.

244 FRIED SWEET CORN   244

Ingredients:

2 cups milk	1 heaping tablesp. farina
3 cups water	salt
1¼ cups yellow cornmeal	3 tablesp. vegetable fat or butter

Method:
1. Bring milk and water to the boil.
2. Stir in cornmeal, farina and salt.
3. Cook for ½ hr., stirring continuously.
4. Spread out on a board, allow to cool.
5. Cut into cubes.
6. Melt fat and fry corn cubes in it.

245 SWEET CORN CAKES, I   245

Ingredients:

1¼ cups milk	1½ heaping tablesp. farina
3¾ cups water	salt
1½ cups yellow cornmeal	1 egg
	3–4½ tablesp. vegetable fat

Method:
1. Prepare Sweet Corn Mash as in Recipe No. 242. Spread out on a board (about ½ in. thick).
2. When cool cut into diamond shapes.
3. Beat egg and dip cakes in it.
4. Heat fat and fry cakes on both sides until golden brown.

246 SWEET CORN CAKES, 2   246

Ingredients:
As in Recipe No. 245.
Thin slices of cheese

Method:
1. Prepare Sweet Corn Cakes as in Recipe No. 245, and place on a well-greased baking sheet.
2. Bake till golden brown in a hot oven (425°).
3. Place a thin slice of cheese on each cake and bake again until cheese has melted.

247 D. MILLOTTO (MADE FROM MILLET)   247 D.

(*For Light Diet:* Without cheese.)

Ingredients:

1 heaping tablesp. vegetable fat	salt
1 onion, chopped	3 tablesp. grated cheese
1¾ cups millet	1½ tablesp. butter
3 cups vegetable stock	½ onion, shredded

Method:

1. Melt fat and sauté onion in it till soft but not brown.
2. Add millet and sauté lightly.
3. Add stock and salt and cook for 20 min.
4. Sprinkle grated cheese and pour butter over finished Millotto.
5. Brown half onion and place on top.

248 D. MILLOTTO (MILLET) WITH VEGETABLES 248 D.

(*For Light Diet:* Without cheese.)

Ingredients:

3 tablesp. vegetable fat	rosemary
½ onion, chopped	3 cups vegetable stock
1 cup diced vegetables	salt
(leeks, celery, carrots)	3 tablesp. cheese, if desired
or carrots and peas	1½ tablesp. fresh butter
1½ cups millet	

Method:

1. Melt fat and sauté onion in it.
2. Add vegetables, millet and rosemary and sauté all together.
3. Add stock and salt and cook for 20 min.
4. Scatter grated cheese and dabs of butter over finished dish.

249 D. BUCKWHEAT 249 D.

Ingredients:

2 cups buckwheat	2 tablesp. butter
4 cups water	cold milk or cream
salt	brown sugar or honey if desired

Method:

1. Soak the buckwheat in the water, with salt, for 24 hours.
2. Cook in well-covered pan for 1 hour.
3. Add butter and serve with cold milk, or cream, and brown sugar, or honey.

250 D. CRUSHED BUCKWHEAT 250 D.

Ingredients:

2 cups buckwheat	salt
4 cups water	cream and brown sugar if desired

Method:
1. Soak buckwheat in water for 24 hours.
2. Drain but keep water.
3. Chop, crush or mix in electric mixer.
4. Bring soaking water to the boil, add salt, and cook buckwheat for ½ hr. in it.
5. Serve with cream and brown sugar.

251 D. WHOLE WHEAT (SAVORY) 251 D.

Ingredients:

1 cup whole wheat berries	salt
4½ tablesp. ground millet	3–4 tablesp. grated cheese
5 cups vegetable stock *or*	1 onion, chopped
milk and water	1½ tablesp. vegetable fat

Method:
1. Wash and dry wheat. Grind coarsely in coffee grinder or electric mixer.
2. Bring liquid to the boil, stir in cereals, cook until tender (30–40 min.).
3. Sprinkle cheese over and add onion lightly sautéed in vegetable fat.

Alternatively the finished pudding may be put in a baking dish, sprinkled with cheese and dotted with butter, then baked for ½ hr.

252 CRUSHED CEREALS* 252

Ingredients:
6 tablesp. crushed cereals (wheat, oats, rye) soaked for 12 hrs. in 9 tablesp. water.
salt

Method:
1. Add 7½ tablesp. water to the soaked cereals, and a little salt.
2. Cook for 10 min. in a saucepan or for ½ hr. in a double boiler.

253 D. WHOLE WHEAT (SWEET) 253 D.

Ingredients:

1 cup whole wheat berries	salt
4½ tablesp. farina or	3 tablesp. sugar *or* honey
ground millet	1 handful raisins, if liked
5 cups milk	1 tablesp. grated nuts

* Available at health food stores.

Method:
1. Prepare as in Recipe No. 251.
2. Bring milk to the boil, stir in cereals, salt, raisins and honey; cook until tender (30–40 min.).
3. Sprinkle grated nuts over the finished pudding if desired.

254 SPAGHETTI, MACARONI, NOODLES 254

(*For Light Diet:* Without cheese but served with Tomato Sauce, Recipe No. 305 D.)

Ingredients:

½ lb. spaghetti, maca- roni, *or* noodles	3¾ pt. water salt

Method:
1. Cook macaroni, spaghetti or noodles in a half-covered saucepan for 15–20 min.
2. Drain through a sieve under running cold water.

Serve in one of the following ways:

Ingredients:	*Method:*
(*a*) 2 tablesp. butter 4½ tablesp. cheese, if liked	Heat butter, add cooked spaghetti, mix well. Sprinkle with cheese.
(*b*) 1½ tablesp. butter 3 tablesp. breadcrumbs	Fry crumbs in butter, pour over cooked spaghetti.
(*c*) Tomato Sauce, Rec. No. 304 1 tablesp. grated cheese	Put spaghetti on a hot dish, sprinkle with cheese and pour sauce over.
(*d*) chopped basil, parsley and a little garlic	Sauté herbs in butter and add to the cooked spaghetti just before serving.

255 D. MACARONI WITH MILK 255 D.

(*For Light Diet:* Without cheese.)

Ingredients:

½ lb. macaroni	1½ cups milk
6¼ pt. water	2 tablesp. butter
salt	3 tablesp. cheese

Method:
1. Boil salted water, add macaroni and cook until nearly tender; drain.
2. Heat milk with butter in it, add macaroni.

3. Boil gently shaking frequently until all the milk has been absorbed and the macaroni is cooked.

4. Sprinkle cheese, if used, over the finished dish before serving.

256 MACARONI SOUFFLÉ   256

Ingredients:

½ lb. macaroni (approx.)	½ cup milk
5 pt. water	1 cup vegetable stock or
salt	water
1½ tablesp. butter	salt
1½ tablesp. vegetable fat	3 tablesp. cream
4½ tablesp. flour	3 tablesp. grated cheese
	1 teasp. butter

Method:

1. Bring water to the boil, add macaroni and salt, boil until cooked.

2. Melt butter, mix with macaroni and put into a baking dish.

3. Prepare Béchamel Sauce, Recipe No. 299.

4. Pour sauce over the macaroni, sprinkle with cheese and dabs of butter.

5. Bake in a moderate oven (350°) for 20 min.

257 MACARONI TIMBALE   257

Ingredients for Pastry:

1¾ cups flour
7 tablesp. butter
6 tablesp. water
salt

Ingredients for Filling:

½ lb. macaroni
water
salt
2 tablesp. butter
3 tablesp. grated cheese
2 eggs
1¼ cups milk

Method:

1. Make Shortcrust Pastry, Recipe No. 323, and leave for at least ½ hr.

2. Roll out four-fifths of the pastry about ½-in. thick.

3. Grease and flour a pudding mold, line this with pastry (it should project about 1 in. over the rim).

4. Prepare filling: boil macaroni for 15–20 min., drain well.

5. Mix butter and grated cheese with the hot macaroni and put into prepared basin.

6. Beat eggs, add to milk, and pour over macaroni.

7. Roll out a lid from the remaining pastry.

8. Turn the projecting pastry over the filling and cover with the lid.

9. Brush with egg yolk.

10. Bake slowly in a moderate oven (350°) for ¾–1 hr.

11. Turn out on to a hot dish and serve with Tomato Sauce, Recipe No. 304.

258 D. HOMEMADE NOODLES   258 D.

Ingredients:

1¾ cups flour	2–3 tablesp. water
(½ should be whole-wheat)	1½ tablesp. oil
2 eggs	salt

Method:

1. Sift flour on to a board, make a well in the center, add other ingredients.

2. Mix well together; there should be no bubbles in the pastry if it is cut through.

3. Leave for ½ hr.

4. Handle only a quarter of the pastry at a time and roll it out as thinly as possible (it should be almost transparent).

5. Put each piece aside as it is finished for about 1 hr.

6. Roll up, cut into fine strips and loosen each carefully with the hands.

7. Dry on a cloth.

If liked, ¼ lb. finely chopped spinach may be added to the other ingredients. Spinach noodles are also available at health food stores.

259 D. NOODLES IN SHELLS   259 D.

(*For Light Diet:* Without cheese.)

Ingredients:

5½ oz. noodles (approx.)	3 tablesp. grated cheese
3¾ pt. water	Tomato Sauce
salt	Recipe No. 305 D
4 shells	1½ tablesp. butter

Method:

1. Cook noodles in boiling salted water.

2. Grease shells and arrange noodles in them.

3. Sprinkle with cheese and pour Tomato Sauce over them.

4. Add dabs of butter and bake for a short time in a moderate oven.

260 D. NOODLES WITH SAGE   260 D.

Ingredients:

½ lb. noodles
6¼ pt. water
salt

2 fresh (or green dried)
sage leaves
2 tablesp. butter

Method:

1. Cook noodles in salted water.
2. Chop sage leaves and heat in melted butter.
3. Add to the noodles and mix well.

261 NOODLES WITH EGG   261

Ingredients:

½ lb. noodles
6¼ pt. water
salt

2 tablesp. butter
2 eggs
½ cup milk or cream

Method:

1. Cook noodles in salted water; drain well.
2. Melt butter and brown noodles slightly in it.
3. Beat eggs and milk, or cream, together and add to the noodles.
4. Fry together until the eggs appear firm and cooked.

262 RAVIOLI   262

Ingredients for Pastry:
1¾ cups flour
1½ tablesp. oil
1 egg
1½ tablesp. water
salt

Ingredients for cooking Ravioli:
5–7 pt. water
salt
2 tablesp. grated cheese
2 tablesp. butter
¼ cup milk if required

Method:

1. Mix all ingredients together to a firm smooth paste.
2. Leave for 15 min.
3. Cut into two pieces and roll each out as thinly as possible.
4. Leave for 1 hr.
5. Put small heaps of the chosen filling (see below) on one piece of dough with a teaspoon, or use a pastry bag (the heaps should be about 1½ in. apart).

6. Put second piece of paste on top and press well together.

7. Cut out small squares or crescent shapes with knife or pastry wheel.

8. Simmer Ravioli in boiling water, a few at a time, until they rise to the surface.

9. Take out with a perforated ladle and arrange alternate layers of Ravioli and cheese on a hot dish.

10. Heat butter (with milk if required) and pour over.

Can also be served with Tomato Sauce, Recipe No. 303.

SIX DIFFERENT TYPES OF FILLINGS

Ingredients:

Method:

(a) ½ tablesp. vegetable fat
3 tablesp. flour
1 cup milk
salt
1 egg
3 oz. grated cheese
nutmeg
chopped basil and pars-
ley

Prepare Béchamel Sauce (Rec. No. 299). Mix egg, cheese, nutmeg and herbs into the sauce.

(b) 3½ oz. grated cheese
1 egg
3–4 tablesp. cream
salt
chopped herbs to taste

Mix all ingredients together to make a thick mixture

(c) ½ tablesp. vegetable fat
¾ lb. chopped spinach
(approx.)
3 tablesp. breadcrumbs
3 tablesp. grated cheese
1 egg

Melt fat and sauté spinach in it. Add cheese, breadcrumbs and egg.

(d) ½ tablesp. vegetable fat
½ onion, chopped
1 clove garlic (if liked)
approx. ½ lb. (9 or 10
cups) chopped spin-
ach
1 tablesp. flour
½ lb. cream cheese
(approx.)

Melt fat, sauté onion, garlic and spinach in it. Mix flour with cream cheese and grated cheese and add to the spinach.

Ingredients:

3–4½ tablesp. grated
cheese
salt

Method:

(e) ½ cup rice
½ lb. spinach (9 or 10
cups)
3 tablesp. grated cheese

Cook rice as for Risotto
(Recipe No. 224). Add
spinach and grated cheese.

(f) 3 tablesp. vegetable fat
or oil
1 onion, chopped
12 tablesp. chopped
scallions
4½ tablesp. chopped
parsley
4 or 5 slices bread
(soaked in water)
1 egg
salt, nutmeg

Sauté onions until golden,
add scallions and parsley
and sauté. Squeeze soaked
bread well and sauté with
herbs until fairly dry. Allow to cool and add egg
and seasoning. Mix well,
and spread on the dough.

Note: If no fresh scallions are available, use 4 tablesp. dried
green onions (reconstituted in a little water or lemon juice)
instead.

263 SPAETZLE (SWABIAN GNOCCHI)   263

Ingredients:

3 cups flour (approx.)
one-third could be
wholewheat
2 eggs
salt
2–2½ cups milk and
water

7½ pt. water
salt
3 tablesp. grated cheese
3 tablesp. butter

Method:

1. Make a well in the center of the flour, add eggs, salt and
water, beat well until bubbles form. Put aside for at least 1 hr.
2. Bring salted water to the boil.
3. Force batter, a small portion at a time, through a sieve
with a large perforation into the boiling water.
4. Simmer until Spaetzle rises to the surface.
5. Take out with a perforated ladle and arrange on dish.
6. Sprinkle with cheese and melted butter.

Cold Spaetzle can be warmed up by heating for a moment in
hot water, or by frying in a frying pan.

Instead of using a sieve, a small wet wooden board may be used. Spread small quantities of batter on to the board and scrape fine strips into the boiling water with a knife.

Spinach can be used in Spaetzle if desired; then use 3 eggs for batter and add ¼ lb. chopped spinach (3 cups) to the batter before cooking.

264 D. SOYA SPAETZLE 264 D.

Ingredients:

2 cups flour (approx.) 2½ cups water
¾ cup soya flour salt
  vegetable stock

Method:
1. Prepare batter as in Recipe No. 263.
2. Cook Spaetzle in vegetable stock and arrange immediately on a hot dish.

265 PANCAKES, 1 265

Ingredients:

1¾ cups flour 2–2½ cups milk
2 eggs and water
  salt
  3 tablesp. vegetable fat

Method:
1. Sift flour and salt into a bowl.
2. Add eggs, milk and water very slowly, beating all the time.
3. Add liquid until the batter is of the consistency of thin cream.
4. Stand aside for at least 1 hr.
5. Heat fat, pour in a small quantity of batter to make a thin pancake.
6. Cook on both sides over good heat until golden brown.

266 PANCAKES, 2 266

Ingredients:

1⅓ cups flour 2 cups milk and water
3–4 eggs salt
  fat for frying

Method:
Cook as for Recipe No. 265.

267 D. SOYA PANCAKES   267 D

Ingredients:

1¼ cup flour	¼ teasp. baking powder
3 heaping tablesp. soya flour	1½ cups water
	1 tablesp. oil
salt	vegetable fat

Method:

1. Put dry ingredients into a bowl, add water very gradually, beating all the time, until smooth.
2. Leave for 1 hr.
3. Melt oil and vegetable fat and cook pancake as in Recipe No. 265.

268 FRENCH OMELETTE   268

Ingredients:

6 eggs	nutmeg
½ cup milk	1½ tablesp. butter for the pan
salt	

Method:

1. Whisk all the ingredients together (or if preferred separate the eggs and add stiffly beaten whites last of all).
2. Melt butter, add mixture and stir lightly with a fork.
3. Turn on to a hot plate when the omelette is firm but not hard.

269 HERB OMELETTE   269

Ingredients and method as in Recipe No. 268, but add 2 tablesp. chopped herbs (chives, parsley, etc.) to the mixture before cooking.

270 FRENCH OMELETTE WITH TOMATOES   270

Ingredients:

6 eggs	1½ tablesp. butter
½ cup milk	2–3 tomatoes
salt	½ tablesp. vegetable fat
nutmeg	½ onion, chopped

Method:

1. Skin and dice tomatoes.
2. Melt vegetable fat, sauté onion first, add tomatoes and sauté until all the juice has been absorbed.
3. Cook omelette as in Recipe No. 268.

4. Make an incision in the finished omelette and pour tomatoes into it.

271 FARMERS' OMELETTE 271

Ingredients:

6 medium-sized potatoes
1½ tablesp. vegetable fat
salt
1½ tablesp. butter
1 tablesp. chopped onion

1 tablesp. chopped mushrooms
parsley, chives, basil
salt
3 eggs
4½ tablesp. cream or milk

Method:

1. Peel potatoes and cut into ½-in cubes.
2. Sauté in vegetable fat in a covered pan, with salt.
3. Melt butter and sauté onion in it, add mushrooms and herbs and cook in their own juice for 10 min.
4. Add potatoes without mixing.
5. Beat eggs with cream and pour over potatoes.
6. Turn over gently until eggs become firm; then fold like an omelette.
7. Arrange on a hot dish.

272 SPINACH OMELETTE 272

Ingredients:

1⅔ cups flour
3 eggs
2 cups milk and water

salt
2 tablesp. vegetable fat
¼ lb. spinach (3 cups)

Method:

1. Mix flour, eggs and salt to a smooth paste with the milk and water.
2. Leave for 1 hr.
3. Melt fat, mix spinach into egg mixture and cook omelette as in Recipe No. 268.

273 PANCAKE WITH SPINACH 273

Ingredients:

1 lb. spinach (approx.)
1½ tablesp. vegetable fat
1 small onion
a little garlic
salt
nutmeg
⅞ cup flour

1 egg
1–1½ cups milk and water
salt
2–3 tablesp. vegetable fat
2 eggs
1½ cups milk

Method:
1. Prepare spinach as in Recipe No. 97.
2. Prepare pancake mixture as in Recipe No. 265.
3. Melt vegetable fat in omelette pan. Pour in enough pancake mixture to cover pan.
4. Spread spinach on finished pancake; roll up and place side by side in a greased baking dish.
5. Whisk 2 eggs into milk, pour over pancake, bake in moderate oven 15–20 min.

274 SPINACH PUDDING   274

Ingredients:

1 heaping tablesp. vegetable fat	salt
	nutmeg
1 onion, chopped	a little lovage (chopped
1 clove garlic	finely)
1 lb. spinach	3 tablesp. grated cheese
4 slices wholewheat bread	2 egg yolks
soaked in	2 egg whites beaten to a stiff
½–1 cup vegetable stock	froth
or milk	Caper Sauce, Rec. No. 302

Method:
1. Melt fat, sauté onion and garlic in it.
2. Chop spinach, add to onion and sauté all together.
3. Squeeze soaked bread and chop finely.
4. Mix all ingredients together thoroughly, folding in stiffly beaten egg whites last of all.
5. Put finished mixture into a greased mold, sprinkle with breadcrumbs.
6. Bake in moderate oven or steam 1–1½ hr.
7. Serve with Caper or Herb Sauce if liked.

275 PARISIAN GNOCCHI   275

Ingredients:

2 cups water	1½ tablesp. vegetable fat
4 tablesp. butter	3 tablesp. flour
1¼ cups flour	1–1½ cups milk and water
2–3 eggs	salt
salt	Marmite or other yeast ex-
nutmeg	tract
4½ tablesp. grated cheese	1 teasp. butter

Method:

1. Prepare Choux Pastry as in Recipe No. 330.
2. Put pastry into a pastry bag without a tip; squeeze out and cut off 1 in. long pieces into boiling vegetable stock.
3. Simmer for a few minutes until gnocchi rises to the surface.
4. Take out with a perforated ladle.
5. Put alternate layers of gnocchi and grated cheese into a greased baking dish.
6. Prepare a thin Béchamel Sauce, Recipe No. 299, and add yeast extract, pour over gnocchi.
7. Add dabs of butter, bake 20–30 min. in moderate oven.

276 VEGETABLE CUTLETS   276

Ingredients:

1¼ cups water	1 cup vegetable stock
4 tablesp. butter	salt
salt	4½ tablesp. grated cheese
1¼ cup flour	1 tablesp. chopped fresh or
3 eggs	dried green herbs
2 cups diced vegetables (carrots, celeriac, peas, leeks)	1 egg breadcrumbs vegetable fat

Method:

1. Prepare Choux Pastry as in Recipe No. 330.
2. Cook diced vegetables gently in the stock until all the liquid has been absorbed. Cool.
3. Mix cheese and herbs with cooked vegetables, salt and pastry.
4. Spread on a board about ½ in. thick; put aside for some hours.
5. Cut out rectangles and shape into cutlets; toss in flour.
6. Dip cutlets in beaten egg, then in breadcrumbs.
7. Melt fat and fry cutlets in a liberal amount of fat.

277 BREAD DUMPLING   277

Ingredients:

6 slices wholewheat bread	1 tablesp. parsley or other chopped herb
1 cup milk	
1 tablesp. mushrooms (fresh or dried)	1–2 eggs salt
1 white roll (medium-sized)	5 pt. vegetable stock for cooking
1 onion	½ onion and butter for the
1 clove garlic	garnish

Method:
1. Soak bread in milk.
2. Put through mincer with the mushrooms, or prepare in blender.
3. Dice the roll and mix with all other ingredients. Add this to first mixture; mix well.
4. Put on a pudding cloth, shape into an elongated dumpling, tie cloth both ends.
5. Simmer in vegetable stock for about 1 hr.
6. Shred onion, fry in butter, spread over sliced dumpling before serving.

278 BREAD AND EGG DISH   278

Ingredients:

½ loaf bread	4 eggs
3 tablesp. vegetable fat	1½–2 cups milk

Method:
1. Slice bread thinly, fry lightly in vegetable fat.
2. Beat eggs and milk and pour over fried bread, stir well and fry until firm.

279 OAT CAKES, FRIED   279

Ingredients:

1 heaping tablesp. vegetable fat	3 tablesp. chopped spinach
1 onion, chopped	1 cup vegetable stock *or* milk
1¼ cup rolled oats	1 egg
1 shredded leek	1½ tablesp. milk
1 piece diced celery	vegetable fat

Method:
1. Melt fat, sauté onion, oats, leek, celery and spinach together.
2. Add stock, or milk, cook until thick.
3. Spread on a board about ½-in. thick; cool.
4. Cut into rectangles.
5. Beat egg and milk, dip cakes into it.
6. Melt fat, fry oat cakes on both sides.

280 WHEAT CAKES, FRIED   280

Ingredients:

1⅓ cups wheat (soaked overnight)

1½ tablesp. vegetable fat

1 onion, chopped

½ cup rice (approx.)

salt

1½ cups vegetable stock

1 cup vegetables (leeks, carrots, celery)

1–2 eggs

herbs (parsley, chives, basil or lovage, fresh or dried green)

breadcrumbs

vegetable fat

Method:

1. Cook wheat for 1–1½ hr. in water previously used for soaking, using a covered saucepan, or for ½ hr. in a pressure cooker.

2. Force through a mincing machine or put in blender.

3. Prepare Risotto as for Recipe No. 224.

4. Mix all ingredients together and cut out into round cakes.

5. Dip cakes into breadcrumbs and fry in a liberal amount of vegetable fat.

281 MUSHROOM CROÛTES   281

Ingredients:

8 slices bread

1 heaping tablesp. vegetable fat

3–4 tomatoes

salt

2–3 eggs, hard-boiled

Mushroom Sauce (Recipe No. 311)

Method:

1. Melt fat and fry bread a golden brown.

2. Cut tomatoes into ½ in. slices, sprinkle with salt, cook for a few minutes.

3. Slice hard-boiled eggs finely.

4. Put two slices of tomato on each piece of fried bread, top with hard-boiled egg.

5. Pour Mushroom Sauce over the prepared slices.

282 CHEESE CROÛTES   282

Ingredients:

8 slices wholewheat bread

½–1 cup milk

1½ tablesp. vegetable fat

4½ tablesp. flour

1 cup milk

½ lb. Swiss cheese

1 egg

Method:
1. Dip slices of bread in milk.
2. Place on well-greased baking sheet.
3. Prepare Béchamel Sauce, Recipe No. 299, and allow to cool.
4. Grate cheese and mix with sauce. Stir in an egg.
5. Spread on the slices of bread and bake in hot oven for about 10 min.

283 CHEESE SOUFFLÉ   283

Ingredients:

3–4 tablesp. butter	4–5 egg yolks
⅞ cup flour	4½ oz. grated cheese
3 cups milk	4–5 egg whites beaten to a
salt	stiff froth
nutmeg	

Method:
1. Prepare Béchamel Sauce, Recipe No. 299.
2. Beat yolks and mix with sauce, add grated cheese.
3. Beat egg whites to a stiff froth; fold into mixture.
4. Put into a greased baking dish, cover with greased paper.
5. Steam over boiling water for 30–40 min.
6. Put into a moderate oven, still over boiling water, for a further 20 min.

284 CREAM PATTIES   284

Ingredients for Pastry:
 1¾ cups flour
 6–7 tablesp. butter
 6–9 tablesp. water
 salt

Ingredients for Filling:
 1 cup milk
 1 cup cream
 2 eggs
 1 teasp. cornstarch or flour
 salt

Method:
1. Prepare Shortcrust Pastry as in Recipe No. 323.
2. Roll out about ⅛ in. thick, cut out rounds, and line greased individual tart pans.
3. Prepare filling, mixing all ingredients together thoroughly.
4. Pour into pastry cases, bake in moderate oven (350°) for about 20 min.

285 CHEESE PATTIES   285

Ingredients for Pastry:
- 1¾ cups flour
- 6–7 tablesp. butter
- 6 tablesp. water
- salt

Ingredients for Filling:
- 1 cup milk
- ½ cup cream
- 2 eggs or 1 whole egg and 1 egg yolk
- 6 tablesp. grated cheese
- 1 teasp. flour or cornstarch

Method:
1. Prepare pastry as in Recipe No. 323.
2. Roll out pastry about ⅛ in. thick and cut into rounds.
3. Line greased individual tart pans.
4. Whisk all ingredients for the filling together.
5. Pour into pastry cases.
6. Bake in moderate oven (350°) for 20 min.

286 CHEESE TART   286

Ingredients for Pastry:
- 1¾ cups flour
- 4–6 tablesp. butter
- 6 tablesp. vegetable fat
- 6 tablesp. water
- salt

Ingredients for Filling:
- 1 large or 2 small eggs
- 1 cup milk
- 1 cup cream or 2 cups milk
- 1 oz. flour or cornstarch
- 5–6 oz. grated cheese
- nutmeg

Method:
1. Prepare Shortcrust Pastry as in Recipe No. 323.
2. Roll out and line large round pie pan.
3. Whisk all the ingredients for the filling together.
4. Pour into pastry case.
5. Bake in moderate oven (350°) for 30 min.

287 CREAM CHEESE SAVORY TART   287

Ingredients for Pastry:
- 1¾ cups flour
- 6–7 tablesp. butter
- 6 tablesp. water
- salt

Ingredients for Filling:
- ½ lb. cream cheese
- 3 tablesp. flour
- 2 eggs
- 1 cup milk
- 3 tablesp. cream, if desired
- salt
- chives

Method:
1. Prepare Shortcrust Pastry as in Recipe No. 323.
2. Roll out ¼ in. thick and line large round pie pan.
3. Whisk all the ingredients for the filling together.
4. Pour into pastry case.
5. Bake in moderate oven (350°) for about 30 min.

288 ONION TART   288

Ingredients for Pastry:
1¾ cups flour
4–6 tablesp. butter
1½ tablesp. vegetable fat
6 tablesp. water
salt

Ingredients for Filling:
1½ tablesp. vegetable fat
1 lb. onions, shredded
  (approx.)
¼ cup flour
1 cup milk
½ cup cream
1 large or 2 small eggs
salt

Method:
1. Prepare Shortcrust Pastry as in Recipe No. 323.
2. Roll out and line large round pie pan.
3. Melt fat and sauté onions till glassy.
4. Sprinkle flour over them and stir well.
5. Whisk the milk, cream and eggs together; mix with onions and salt.
6. Pour over pastry and bake in moderate oven (350°) for 30 min.

289 SPINACH TART   289

Ingredients for Pastry:
1¾ cups flour
4–6 tablesp. butter
1½ tablesp. vegetable fat
6 tablesp. water
salt

Ingredients for Filling:
1 lb. spinach
½ tablesp. vegetable fat
½ onion, chopped
1 teasp. flour
½ cup milk or vegetable
  stock

Ingredients for Coating:
1 egg
½ cup milk
3 tablesp. cream
salt

Method:
1. Prepare Shortcrust Pastry as in Recipe No. 323.
2. Roll out and line large round pie pan.
3. Prepare spinach as in Recipe No. 99.
4. Spread on pastry.
5. Beat egg, milk and cream and salt and pour over spinach.
6. Bake 15–20 min. in moderate oven (350°).

290 TURNOVERS   290

Ingredients for pastry:

1¾ cups flour	6 tablesp. water
7 tablesp. butter	salt
½ tablesp. vegetable fat	

Method:
1. Prepare Shortcrust Pastry as in Recipe No. 323.
2. Roll out and cut out rounds about 4 in. in diameter.
3. Put chosen filling in center of each; brush edges with water or white of egg.
4. Fold over and press edges together firmly. Brush over with egg yolk.
5. Bake in a hot oven (400°) for ¼ hr.

(*a*) *Rice Filling:*
Ingredients:
1½ tablesp. vegetable fat
1 small onion, chopped
½ cup rice
1 cup vegetable stock
salt
1½ tablesp. grated cheese
½ teasp. butter

Method:
Prepare as for Risotto (Recipe No. 224), then allow to cool before using.

(*b*) *Cheese Filling,* 1:
Ingredients:
5 oz. grated cheese
1 egg
9–12 tablesp. cream or milk
salt
nutmeg

Method:
Mix all ingredients together to form a thick mixture.

(c) *Cheese Filling, 2:*
   Ingredients:
   ½ tablesp. vegetable fat
   3 tablesp. flour
   ½ cup milk
   3–4 oz. grated cheese
   1 egg

Method:
Make a sauce with the fat, flour and milk. Cool. Mix the cheese and well-beaten egg into it.

(d) *Vegetable Filling: Ingredients:*
   1½ tablesp. vegetable fat
   1 tablesp. onion, chopped
   1½ cups diced vegetables (carrots, celery leeks, peas)
   1–1½ cups vegetable stock
   salt
   1 tablesp. chopped spinach and various herbs

Method:
Melt fat and sauté onion lightly in it. Add vegetables, stock and seasoning and cook till the liquid has all been absorbed.

(e) *Sauerkraut Filling:*
   Ingredients:
   ½ lb. sauerkraut

Method:
Prepare sauerkraut as in Recipe No. 161, using slightly less stock.

291 CARAWAY FINGERS (WITH CHEESE)   291

Ingredients:
⅞ cup flour
1½ tablesp. butter
1½ oz. grated cheese

3–4 tablesp. water
egg yolk
caraway seeds

Method:
1. Prepare Shortcrust Pastry as in Recipe No. 323, adding cheese.
2. Roll out pastry ⅛ in. thick. Cut into fingers about 2½ in. long and ½ in. wide.
3. Brush with egg yolk, sprinkle with caraway seeds.
4. Bake in moderate oven (350°) about 10 min.

292 FLEURONS 292

Ingredients:

7 oz. Puff Pastry Recipe No. 325   1 egg yolk

Method:

1. Roll out pastry ⅛ in. thick, cut out small crescents.
2. Brush the top only with egg yolk.
3. Bake 5–10 min. in a hot oven (450°).

293 INDIVIDUAL VOL-AU-VENTS 293

Ingredients:
    about 14 oz. finished Puff
        Pastry, Recipe No. 325

Ingredients for Filling:
    mixed vegetables
    Mushroom Sauce, Recipe
        No. 311

Method:

1. Roll out pastry ½ in. thick, cut out rounds 4 in. in diameter.
2. Place half the rounds on a greased baking sheet.
3. Cut out small lids from the remaining rounds, using a smaller cutter, and put on baking sheet.
4. Brush edges of rounds with water or egg white, place pastry rings on them.
5. Brush rings and lids with egg yolk (care must be taken to avoid egg running down cut sides or pastry will not rise).
6. Bake in hot oven (425°) 15–20 min.
7. Fill finished vol-au-vent cases with mixed vegetables, serve with Mushroom Sauce, Recipe No. 311.

294 VOL-AU-VENT 294

Ingredients:
    about 12 oz. Puff Pastry
        Recipe No. 325

Ingredients for Filling:
    mixed vegetables
    Mushroom Sauce, Recipe
        No. 311

Method:

1. Roll out pastry about ¼ in. thick and cut out a round about 8 in. in diameter.
2. Place on baking sheet.
3. Put a plate about 6 in. in diameter on pastry and mark around it, cutting halfway through pastry.
4. Brush pastry with egg yolk without touching incision.
5. Bake in hot oven (425°) for about 15–20 min.
6. Cut out raised center to use as a lid.
7. Fill pie with mixed vegetables and serve with Mushroom Sauce, Recipe No. 311.

295 STUFFED ROLLS 295

Ingredients:
1¼ cups water
4 tablesp. butter
1¼ cup flour
3 eggs
salt

Ingredients for Stuffing:
½ lb. cream cheese
9 tablesp. milk or cream
4½ tablesp. grated cheese
1 tablesp. chopped herbs
salt
Marmite or yeast extract

Method:
1. Prepare Choux Pastry as for Recipe No. 330.
2. Shape into small but longish rolls; place on baking sheet.
3. Bake in moderate oven (350°) for about 15 min.
4. Beat cream cheese until it is of a soft creamy consistency.
5. Add other ingredients and beat well together.
6. Cut rolls in half lengthways; pipe or fill with stuffing.

296 CHEESE AND TOMATO TARTLETS 296

Ingredients:
Shortcrust Pastry Recipe
No. 323

Ingredients for Filling:
¼ lb. Swiss or Cheshire
cheese
3 tomatoes
3 eggs, hard-boiled
2 gherkins
salt
3–4 tablesp. mayonnaise,
Recipe No. 318

Method:
1. Roll out pastry and line individual tart pans.
2. Bake the crusts.
3. Dice cheese and mix with tomatoes, eggs, gherkins and
salt.
4. Fold in mayonnaise.
5. Arrange on tartlets and serve immediately.

297 PUFFS (FOR VEGETABLES) 297

Ingredients:
2¼ cups water
4 tablesp. butter
1¼ cup flour
3 eggs
salt
vegetable fat or oil

Method:
1. Prepare Choux Pastry as in Recipe No. 330.
2. Shape into small balls with a spoon.
3. Drop into moderately hot fat or oil and fry slowly.

298 PIZZA NAPOLITANA 298

Ingredients:
Yeast Pastry
Recipe No. 326
6 ripe tomatoes, skinned
¼ lb. Swiss or Cheddar
cheese

Ingredients for Filling:
thyme or rosemary (fresh
or dried green)
vegetable oil

Method:
1. Prepare Yeast Pastry, Recipe No. 326.
2. Roll out about one-fifth of an inch thick and cut into rounds 5 in. in diameter.
3. Put on a baking sheet and leave to rise in a warm place.
4. Brush each round with a little oil and put some slices of tomato on each.
5. Top with a slice of cheese and some herbs and brush on with a little oil.
6. Bake in moderate oven (400°) 10–20 min.

SAUCES

299 BÉCHAMEL SAUCE 299

Ingredients:
1½ tablesp. vegetable fat
4½ tablesp. flour
1 cup milk

1 cup vegetable stock or
water
salt
nutmeg

Method:
1. Melt fat, sift in flour and sauté.
2. Add the liquid slowly, stirring all the time.
3. Cook for 20 min.

300 BUTTER SAUCE 300

Ingredients:
1½ tablesp. butter
4½ tablesp. flour
2 cups vegetable stock or
water

salt
Marmite or other yeast extract
3 tablesp. cream if desired

Method:
1. Make sauce as in Recipe No. 299.
2. Add Marmite and cream if desired.

301 HERB SAUCE 301

Ingredients:

As for Butter Sauce, Recipe No. 300.

Chopped fresh or dried green herbs (e.g. parsley, lovage, chervil, basil, tarragon, lemon balm, etc.).

egg yolk if desired.

Method:

1. Make Butter Sauce as in Recipe No. 300.
2. Add chopped herbs.
3. Thicken with egg yolk if desired.

302 CAPER SAUCE 302

Ingredients:

As for Butter Sauce
Recipe No. 300

1 tablesp. capers
1 egg yolk
3 tablesp. cream

Method:

1. Make Butter Sauce as in Recipe No. 300.
2. Add capers to finished sauce.
3. Beat yolk and add with the cream.

303 TOMATO SAUCE, I 303

Ingredients:

1 heaping tablesp. vegetable fat
1 onion
1 clove of garlic
½ cup of diced carrots, celery and leeks
2 tomatoes (approx.)
1½ tablesp. flour

½ tablesp. tomato purée
2½ cups vegetable stock or water
¼ bay leaf
rosemary, thyme, or basil
a little hot butter
pinch of sugar

Method:

1. Cut up vegetables.
2. Melt fat and sauté onions and garlic in it.
3. Add vegetables and sauté in the fat.
4. Cut up tomatoes and add.
5. Cook slowly in a covered pan until the liquid has been absorbed.
6. Sprinkle the flour over vegetables.
7. Add purée, stock and herbs and cook for ½ hr.
8. Put through a sieve.
9. Add butter and sugar to improve the flavor.

304 TOMATO SAUCE, 2   304

Ingredients:

1 heaping tablesp. vegetable fat
1 onion, chopped
1 lb. (4) ripe tomatoes
salt
¼ bay leaf

rosemary, basil or thyme
1 teasp. cornstarch
¼ cup vegetable stock
3 tablesp. cream
pinch of sugar if desired

Method:

1. Melt fat and sauté onion in it.
2. Cut tomatoes and sauté with the onion.
3. Cover and cook until tender.
4. Put through a sieve.
5. Add herbs.
6. Mix cornstarch with stock and cook for a few min. with the tomato purée.
7. Add cream and sugar if liked.

305 D. TOMATO SAUCE, 3   305 D.

Ingredients:

1 lb. tomatoes
salt

rosemary, basil or thyme
3 tablesp. cream or a little butter

Method:

1. Cut tomatoes in pieces, cook till tender with salt and herbs.
2. Sieve.
3. Add cream or butter.

306 D. TOMATO SAUCE, 4   306 D.

Ingredients:

1 heaping tablesp. vegetable fat
1 small onion, chopped

1 lb. tomatoes, skinned
salt
basil, rosemary or thyme

Method:

1. Melt fat and sauté onion in it.
2. Dice tomatoes and add to the onion with salt and herbs.
3. Cook till tender.

307 CHEESE SAUCE 307

Ingredients:

1½ cups milk	salt
¼ cup cream	nutmeg
1½ tablesp. flour	1 egg yolk
2 oz. grated cheese	

Method:

1. Mix milk and cream with flour and bring to the boil.
2. Add cheese and seasoning to sauce.
3. Beat the egg yolk and pour the sauce over it.

308 ONION SAUCE 308

Ingredients:

1 heaping tablesp. vegetable fat	salt
2 onions, shredded	powdered caraway seed (if liked)
4½ tablesp. flour	basil
2 cups vegetable stock	1 teasp. butter

Method:

1. Melt fat and sauté onion till golden brown.
2. Mix in flour and cook till golden brown.
3. Add stock and seasonings and cook for 20 min.
4. Sieve, if desired.
5. Stir in butter to improve flavor.

309 HORSERADISH SAUCE 309

Ingredients:

Butter Sauce, Recipe No. 300	1–1½ oz. horseradish

Method:

1. Prepare Butter Sauce, Recipe No. 300.
2. Grate horseradish into the sauce.
3. Cook for 5 min.

310 BROWN SAUCE 310

Ingredients:

1 heaping tablesp. vegetable fat	nutmeg
4½ tablesp. flour	pinch of ground cloves
2 cups vegetable stock	1 teasp. lemon juice
salt	3 tablesp. cream, if liked

Method:

1. Melt fat, stir in flour and cook till chestnut brown. Cool.
2. Add stock, seasoning and lemon juice and cook for 20 min.
3. Stir in cream if desired.

311 MUSHROOM SAUCE   311

Ingredients:

1 heaping tablesp. vegetable fat	1–1½ cups vegetable stock
1 onion, chopped	salt
¾ lb. mushrooms	1 teasp. lemon juice
2–3 tablesp. flour	4½ tablesp. cream
	1 egg yolk

Method:

1. Melt fat and sauté onion in it.
2. Add mushrooms, thinly sliced.
3. Sauté together, cover and cook for ¼ hr.
4. Sprinkle flour over.
5. Add stock, salt and lemon juice and cook for 10 min.
6. Add cream and egg yolk to improve the flavor of the sauce.

312 GREEN PEPPER SAUCE   312

Ingredients:

1 heaping tablesp. vegetable fat	4½ tablesp. flour
1 onion, chopped	2 cups vegetable stock
½ green pepper, shredded finely	salt
	¼ bay leaf, if liked
	3 tablesp. cream, if liked

Method:

1. Melt fat, sauté onion and green pepper in it.
2. Sprinkle flour over.
3. Add stock, salt and bay leaf and cook for 20 min.
4. Add cream to enrich sauce.

313 PIQUANT SAUCE   313

Ingredients:

As for Green Pepper Sauce, Recipe No. 312	1 teasp. capers
1 gherkin, chopped	3 tablesp. diced tomatoes
1 teasp. olives, chopped	1 tablesp. lemon juice
	tarragon
	3 tablesp. cream, if desired

Method:
1. Make as for Green Pepper Sauce, Recipe No. 312.
2. Add other ingredients to the sauce. The cream, if used, should be added just before serving.

314 SAUCE HOLLANDAISE, 1   314

Ingredients:

4½ tablesp. water
1½ tablesp. lemon juice
1 sprig fresh tarragon *or*
    1 teasp. dried green tar-
    ragon
1 small onion

½ bay leaf
1 clove
½ cup vegetable stock
1 tablesp. cornstarch
2 egg yolks
4 tablesp. butter

Method:
1. Boil the water, lemon juice, onion and herbs together until half the liquid has evaporated; strain.
2. Blend cornstarch with the vegetable stock; bring to the boil stirring all the time.
3. Beat egg yolks with the first liquid, in a double saucepan over boiling water until creamy.
4. Cook until the sauce thickens; remove from heat.
5. Add small pieces of butter gradually.
6. Add vegetable stock and cornstarch very carefully stirring all the time.
7. Keep hot over boiling water but do not allow to cook any more.

The vegetable stock and cornstarch may be omitted, in which case double the quantity of all the other ingredients.

315 SAUCE HOLLANDAISE, 2   315

Ingredients:

1½ tablesp. butter
4½ tablesp. flour
2 cups vegetable stock
salt

1 sprig fresh tarragon *or* 1
    teasp. dried green tarra-
    gon
1½ tablesp. butter
1 egg yolk
1½ tablesp. cream
1½ tablesp. lemon juice

Method:
1. Make Butter Sauce as in Recipe No. 300, ading tarragon. Remove sprig after cooking.
2. Add 1½ tablesp. butter, stirring all the time.
3. Add egg, cream and lemon juice just before serving.

316 MOUSSELINE SAUCE   316

Ingredients:

As for Recipe No. 314   ¼ cup cream

Method:

1. Prepare Hollandaise Sauce as in Recipe No. 314.
2. Add stiffly-beaten cream just before serving.

317 MAYONNAISE, 1   317

Ingredients:

1 egg yolk   salt
1½ tablesp. lemon juice   Marmite or other yeast ex-
1 cup oil   tract

Method:

1. Whisk egg yolk with a few drops of lemon juice.
2. Add oil drop by drop whisking constantly.
3. Add a little more lemon juice if the mayonnaise becomes too thick.
4. Season last of all.

Note: The oil should be at room temperature before it is used, not allowed to become too hot or too cold.

318 MAYONNAISE, 2   318

Ingredients:

1 egg yolk   Marmite or other yeast ex-
1½ tablesp. lemon juice   tract
½–¾ cup oil   ½ cup vegetable stock or
salt   water
                              1 tablesp. flour

Method:

1. Prepare mayonnaise as in Recipe No. 317.
2. Blend flour with stock or water, bring to the boil. Cool.
3. Add this thick sauce gradually to the finished mayonnaise.

319 D. MAYONNAISE WITHOUT ANIMAL PROTEIN   319 D.

Ingredients:

3 level tablesp. soya flour   1½ tablesp. lemon juice
9 tablesp. water   Marmite or other yeast ex-
salt   tract
1 cup olive oil   tarragon, chervil or marjo-
                                 ram

Method:
1. Blend flour and water, and whisk until smooth.
2. Add olive oil and lemon juice alternately, whisking all the time.
3. Add herbs and yeast extract to season.

320 REMOULADE SAUCE   320

Ingredients:

mayonnaise, as in Recipe
   Nos. 317, 318 or 319
1 hard-boiled egg, chopped
1 tablesp. chopped gher-
   kins

a few capers
1 teasp. chopped parsley,
   and other herbs if desired
diced tomatoes to garnish

Method:
Mix ingredients with mayonnaise and garnish with tomatoes.

321 D. REMOULADE SAUCE WITHOUT ANIMAL PROTEIN 321 D.

Ingredients:

mayonnaise, as in Recipe
   No. 319 D
1 tablesp. gherkins,
   chopped

a few capers
1 teasp. chopped parsley,
   and other herbs if desired
diced tomatoes to garnish

Method:
1. Mix gherkins, capers and parsley with mayonnaise.
2. Garnish with tomatoes.

322 D. VINAIGRETTE   322 D.

(*For Light Diet:* Without egg, and use sunflower oil only.)

Ingredients:

3 tablesp. olive oil
3 tablesp. peanut oil or
   sunflower oil
4 tablesp. lemon juice
3 tablesp. water or vege-
   table stock

salt
½ onion, chopped
1 hard-boiled egg, chopped
1–2 chopped gherkins, parsley or chives
1½ tablesp. diced tomatoes

Method:
Whisk all the ingredients together.

BATTER AND PASTRY MIXTURES

323 SHORTCRUST PASTRY 323

Ingredients:
6–7 tablesp. butter   salt
1¾ cups flour*   6 tablesp. water

Method:
1. Cut butter into small pieces, rub lightly into flour.
2. Dissolve salt in water.
3. Add to flour and knead lightly until smooth.
4. Leave in a cool place for ½ hr.

324 SHORTCRUST PASTRY (SWEET) 324

Ingredients:
6–7 tablesp. butter   1½ tablesp. sugar
1¾ cups flour   1 egg
salt

Method:
1. Add butter in small pieces to the flour, well sifted with the salt.
2. Rub in lightly.
3. Add sugar and egg, knead lightly until smooth.
4. Leave in a cool place for ½ hr.

325 PUFF PASTRY 325

Ingredients:
4 cups flour (approx.)   1–1½ cups water
11 tablesp. butter (1 stick,   salt
    3 tablesp.)   1 stick, 3 tablesp. butter

Method:
1. Sift flour.
2. Add 11 tablesp. butter, cut into small pieces, and rub in lightly but thoroughly.
3. Dissolve salt in the water, add to the paste and knead until smooth.
4. Roll out into an oblong 6–8 in. wide.
5. Dab half the oblong with the rest of the butter; cut into very small pieces.

---

* When flour is mentioned in the following pastry recipes, regular wholewheat flour or wholewheat pastry flour is intended.

6. Fold the other half of the pastry over the buttered half and press down well.

7. Roll out the pastry in the other direction to another oblong shape.

8. Fold into three, wrap in a damp cloth, and leave in a cool place for 2 hr.

Repeat steps 7 and 8 two or three times more before using the pastry.

326 YEAST PASTRY (for fruit, cheese and onion tarts)   326

Ingredients:

1⅓ cups flour	salt
2 tablesp. butter	⅓ oz. yeast
	6 tablesp. milk

Method:

1. Sift flour and salt into a bowl, make a well in the center and put in a warm place.

2. Cut the butter into small pieces and dot on the flour.

3. Mix the yeast with 2 tablesp. of milk, pour into the well and mix with a little flour to make a thick paste.

4. Cover bowl with a cloth and put in a warm place till the dough doubles its size.

5. Add the rest of the milk and knead into the dough.

6. Beat dough until smooth.

7. Roll out and line pie pan.

Note: For a cheese tart, leave pastry to rise before adding the filling. For fruit and onion tarts, add filling and then leave to rise.

327 YEAST PASTRY (for use with sweet fillings)   327

Ingredients:

(*These should all be kept in a warm place before the pastry is made.*)

1½ cups wholewheat pastry flour	⅓ oz. yeast
3 tablesp. butter	6–7 tablesp. milk
1½ oz. sugar	1 egg
salt	peel of one lemon, grated (if liked)

Method:

1. Working in a warm place, sift flour into a bowl and make a well in the center.

2. Put dabs of butter, sugar and salt round the edge.

3. Mix yeast with a little of the milk; pour into the well.

4. Mix to a thick paste with a little flour.

5. Sprinkle with a little sugar, cover with a cloth and leave to rise, in a warm place.

6. When the dough has doubled its size, add the egg, the rest of the milk and grated peel, if used.

7. Knead to a dough and beat well until smooth.

328 BATTER, 1 (FOR VEGETABLE FRITTERS)   328

Ingredients:

6 tablesp. flour	1 egg yolk
salt	1 egg white
9 tablesp. water	

Method:

1. Sift the flour and salt into a bowl.

2. Mix to a smooth paste with the water and egg yolk and leave to stand for at least ½ hr.

3. Fold in the egg white, beaten to a stiff froth, just before using the batter.

329 BATTER, 2   329

Ingredients:

6 tablesp. flour	3 tablesp. apple juice
7½ tablesp. water	1 egg white
salt	

Method:

1. Sift the flour with the salt.

2. Mix to a smooth paste with water and apple juice and leave to stand for at least ½ hr.

3. Fold in the egg white, beaten to a stiff froth, just before using the batter.

330 CHOUX PASTRY, 1   330

Ingredients:

1 cup milk	1⅓ cups flour
1 cup water	3 eggs
4 tablesp. butter	nutmeg
salt	

Method:

1. Heat the milk, water, butter and salt together.

2. Bring to the boil then remove from the heat.

3. Sift the flour onto a piece of paper, then add it all at once to the milk.

4. Beat well over heat until the mixture leaves the sides of the pan.

5. Allow to cool a little; beat in the eggs one at a time; add nutmeg if desired.

331 CHOUX PASTRY, 2   331

Ingredients:

1¼ cups water	1 cup, 1 oz. flour
3 tablesp. butter	3 eggs
salt	1½ tablesp. sugar

Method:

1. Heat water, butter and salt together.
2. Bring to the boil and remove from heat.
3. Sift the flour onto a piece of paper then add it all at once to the boiling water.
4. Beat well over heat until the paste leaves the sides of the pan.
5. Allow to cool a little, beat in eggs one at a time together with the sugar.

DESSERTS AND CAKES

332 D. FRUIT IN SUGAR SYRUP   332 D.

Ingredients:

2–4 oz. sugar (preferably brown)	Approx. 2 lb. apricots *or* peaches
2 cups water *or* 1 cup water, and 1 cup grape juice	damsons plums greengages

Method:

1. Dissolve sugar in water and bring to the boil.
2. Halve chosen fruit and remove stones.
3. Cook in the syrup until tender. Cool.
4. Arrange attractively in a dish.

333 D. STRAWBERRIES WITH LEMON JUICE   333 D.

Ingredients:

1½ lb. hulled strawberries (approx. 2 pt.)	1 lemon
	3–4½ tablesp. sugar

Method:

1. Halve large strawberries, add sugar and lemon juice.

334 D. FRUIT SALAD

Ingredients:

3½ oz. sugar (preferably brown)
½ cup water or grape juice
2–3 tablesp. lemon juice

Approx. 1½ lb. apricots, *or* peaches
melon
apples
pears
red cherries
any variety of berry

Method:

1. Prepare a selection of fruit according to the season.
2. Dissolve sugar in the water, then bring to the boil.
3. Add fruit juices.
4. Slice fruit finely and add to the cooled syrup.

335 D. STUFFED MELON

Ingredients:

2 small melons   Fruit Salad, Recipe No. 334 D.

Method:

1. Halve melons and remove seeds.
2. Fill with the Fruit Salad.

336 D. FRUIT JELLY

(*For Light Diet:* Without cream.)

Ingredients:

1½ cups water, apple or grape juice
3 oz. sugar
2 small teasp. Agar-Agar

3½ cups fresh fruit juice of grapefruit, orange, berries
whipped cream (if liked)

Method:

1. Whisk water, apple or grape juice with the sugar and heat slowly with Agar-Agar until completely dissolved.
2. Mix in fresh fruit juice and pour at once into glasses or small dishes.
3. Decorate with whipped cream if used.

337 D. APPLE PURÉE

Ingredients:

2 lb. apples (approx. 6 or 7)
1 cup apple juice or water

3–4 oz. brown or granulated sugar
cinnamon or lemon peel
1 tablesp. sugar (to enrich)

Method:
1. Wipe apples, remove stalks and calyxes.
2. Cut into pieces, cook in water or apple juice until tender.
3. Rub through a sieve or prepare in blender.
4. Mix in sugar, cinnamon or peel.
5. If liked, sprinkle 1 tablesp. sugar over finished apple and brown.

338 APPLE PURÉE WITH MERINGUE 338

Ingredients:

ingredients as in Recipe No. 337	2–3 egg whites
	⅓–½ cup sugar

Method:
1. Prepare purée as in Recipe No. 337, put into a baking dish.
2. Beat egg whites to a very stiff froth; fold in sugar.
3. Decorate, using a pastry bag, or spread lightly over the purée, and cook in a moderate oven until lightly brown.

339 D. STEWED APPLES 339 D.

Ingredients:

2 lb. apples (approx.)	⅓–½ cup sugar
1–1½ cups water or apple juice	grated peel of 1 lemon *or* a little cinnamon

Method:
1. Peel apples, remove cores and slice.
2. Bring liquid to the boil.
3. Add sugar, fruit and lemon peel or cinnamon.
4. Cook until tender.

340 D. APPLE HALVES 340 D.

Ingredients:

2 lb. apples (approx.)	1 stick cinnamon
2½ cups water or apple juice	quince, raspberry or redcurrant jelly
5½ oz. sugar	

Method:
1. Peel apples, cut in half, and remove cores.
2. Bring liquid to the boil, flavor with sugar and cinnamon, and add the apples, a portion at a time, and cook until tender.
3. Remove with perforated ladle, put on a dish with cut surface uppermost.
4. Fill with the chosen jelly.

341 D. BLUEBERRY SWEET 341 D.

Ingredients:

2 lb. blueberries (approx.)

7 oz. brown *or* granulated sugar

1 cup water

1 tablesp. flour

3 tablesp. water

2 tablesp. butter

bread cubes

Method:

1. Wash fruit and remove any unsound berries.
2. Cook 5–10 min. in water with sugar.
3. Blend flour with water, add to blueberries and bring to the boil.
4. Put into serving dish or individual glasses.
5. Fry bread cubes in butter and use as a garnish.

342 D. STEWED RHUBARB 342 D.

Ingredients:

2 lb. rhubarb (approx.)

5–7 oz. brown *or* granulated sugar

½ cup water

½ tablesp. cornstarch

Method:

1. Wash rhubarb, cut into small pieces.
2. Cook in water, with sugar, until tender.
3. Remove with perforated ladle and put into a serving dish.
4. Boil juice to thicken, or mix ½ tablesp. cornstarch with water, add to the juice and bring to the boil.
5. Pour over rhubarb.

343 D. STRAWBERRIES AND CREAM 343 D.

Ingredients:

1 lb. strawberries (about 1½ pt.)

3½ oz. sugar

1 cup cream

Method:

1. Hull strawberries, clean and put through sieve or prepare in blender.
2. Add sugar, mix carefully and put into dish or individual glasses.
3. Garnish with whole berries.

Other fruit may be prepared in the same manner, and could be served with cream, junket or yogurt.

344 FRUIT DISH (individual)   344

Ingredients:

½ lb. fruit (approx.)   ¼ portion Sponge
1 cup water   Recipe No. 409
3–4 tablesp. sugar   ½ portion Vanilla Cream
                      Recipe No. 350
                      ½ cup cream

Method:

1. Cook fruit, with sugar, in water until tender.
2. Cut sponge into rounds, divide among 4 glasses.
3. Add cut-up fruit and a little juice.
4. Pour Vanilla Cream over and garnish with whipped cream if liked.

Suitable fruit to use: Pears, apricots, peaches and berries.

345 SURPRISE FRUIT DISH   345

Ingredients:

ingredients as for Recipe   ½ cup cream
   No. 334   4 meringue shells

Method:

1. Prepare Fruit Salad as in Recipe No. 334, put into individual glasses.
2. Garnish with whipped cream and meringues.

346 D. STUFFED APPLES   346 D.

Ingredients:

4 large or 8 small apples   grated peel of 1 lemon
6 tablesp. grated filberts   ½ tablesp. butter
3 tablesp. currants   1½ tablesp. sugar
6 tablesp. cream   ½–1 cup apple juice
4½ tablesp. sugar

Method:

1. Wipe fruit, core and make an incision round the apple skin.
2. Mix nuts, currants, cream, sugar and lemon.
3. Put apples into a baking dish and fill centers with mixture.
4. Put dabs of butter on to the fruit, sprinkle with sugar.
5. Pour in apple juice to a depth of about ½ in., bake 20–30 min.

347 CARAMEL PEARS   347

Ingredients:

2 lb. pears	2 teasp. cornstarch
7 oz. sugar	¼ cup milk
2½–3¾ cups boiling water	½–1 cup cream

Method:

1. Peel pears, cut in half and remove cores.
2. Dissolve sugar over low heat then cook gently until golden brown; add boiling water.
3. Cook pears in sugar and water until tender.
4. Lift out fruit with perforated ladle and arrange in a glass dish, about 2½ cups liquid should remain).
5. Mix cornstarch with milk, add to the boiling juice, bring again to the boil.
6. Pour hot sauce over cream, stirring well, then pour over pears.

348 VIENNESE PEARS   348

Ingredients:

2 lb. pears (approx.)	½ portion Vanilla Cream Recipe No. 350
1–1½ cups water	3 tablesp. sugar
3½ oz. sugar	1½ oz. whole filberts
lemon peel	

Method:

1. Peel pears, cut in half and remove cores.
2. Bring water, sugar and lemon peel to the boil, cook pears in liquid until tender.
3. Arrange pears on a flat dish, pour Vanilla Cream over them.
4. Melt 2 tablesp. sugar over gentle heat, cook until chestnut brown.
5. Add filberts to sugar and cook for a short time.
6. Pour on to greased baking sheet.
7. When cool, grate nuts in a nut-mill and sprinkle over pears.

349 APPLE PORCUPINES WITH VANILLA CREAM 349

Ingredients:

2 lb. apples (approx.)	1½–3 tablesp. sugar
2½ cups water or apple juice	1 teasp. cornstarch
5½ oz. sugar	1 egg
1½ cups milk	½ cup cream
½ vanilla bean *or* ½ teasp. vanilla extract	1½ oz. almonds

Method:

1. Prepare apples as in Recipe No. 340, omitting jelly.
2. Prepare Vanilla Cream, Recipe No. 350.
3. Beat cream until it is thick; fold into cold Vanilla Cream.
4. Blanch almonds in boiling water; cut into thin strips; roast in oven.
5. Heap apple halves, cut surface downwards on a flat dish; stick in almond strips to represent porcupine quills.
6. Pour Vanilla Cream over.

350 VANILLA CREAM (CUSTARD) 350

Ingredients:

3¾ cups milk	1 tablesp. cornstarch
1 vanilla bean *or* 1 teasp. vanilla extract	4½ tablesp. milk
	3 eggs
	2–4 oz. sugar

Method:

1. Bring milk to the boil with the vanilla in it.
2. Mix cornstarch with cold milk, add to the boiling milk, and bring again to the boil.
3. Beat eggs and sugar together; add some of the hot milk, stirring all the time.
4. Pour back into pan, stir well, bring again to near boiling point.

351 FILBERT WHIP 351

Ingredients:

2 oz. filberts	1 tablesp. cornstarch
3 oz. sugar	2 eggs
3¾ cups milk	2 oz. sugar
1 vanilla bean *or* 1 teasp. vanilla extract	

Method:
1. Roast nuts lightly in the oven until the skins rub off easily.
2. Cook sugar over low heat until golden brown.
3. Add nuts to sugar and mix well; put on a baking sheet.
4. Leave until set.
5. Grate in a nut-mill or coarse grater.
6. Prepare Vanilla Cream, Recipe No. 350, using the same saucepan as used for browning the sugar.
7. Mix 2 oz. sugar and the ground nuts with Vanilla Cream while it is still hot.

352 BAVARIAN FILBERT WHIP   352

Ingredients:

½ portion Filbert Whip,   ½ cup water
   Recipe No. 351   1 cup cream
1 small teasp. Agar-Agar*

Method:
1. Whisk Agar-Agar into the water and heat over low heat until it is completely dissolved (do not allow to boil).
2. Mix with cold Filbert Whip.
3. Whip cream until stiff, mix half into Filbert Whip and pour into mold, previously rinsed in cold water.
4. Leave in a cool place for some hours until set.
5. Turn out and garnish with remaining whipped cream.

353 STRAWBERRY OR RASPBERRY WHIP   353

Ingredients:

¾ lb. berries (approx.)   1 egg
1¼ cups milk   3–4½ tablesp. sugar
1 teasp. cornstarch   ½–1 cup cream
1½ tablesp. milk

Method:
1. Clean and hull berries.
2. Put through blender or force through sieve.
3. Make as Vanilla Cream, Recipe No. 350, and cool.
4. Mix with berries.
5. Whip cream and fold into fruit or use as a garnish.

* See p. 41 and footnote p. 118.

354 APPLE WHIP 354

Ingredients:

1¼ cups milk
½ vanilla bean *or*
½ teasp. vanilla extract
1 teasp. cornstarch
1½ tablesp. milk
1 egg

1½ tablesp. sugar
1 lb. apples (approx. 3 medium)
¼ cup water or apple juice
2 tablesp. sugar
grated lemon peel
½–1 cup cream

Method:

1. Prepare Vanilla Cream, Recipe No. 350.
2. Prepare thick Apple Purée, Recipe No. 337 D.
3. Mix purée with Vanilla Cream.
4. Whip cream until stiff, fold into Apple Purée or use as a garnish.

355 RHUBARB WHIP 355

Ingredients:

1 lb. rhubarb
3–3½ oz. sugar
water
1¼ cups milk
½ vanilla bean *or*
½ teasp. vanilla extract

1 teasp. cornstarch
1½ tablesp. milk
1 egg
1½ tablesp. sugar
½–1 cup cream

Method:

1. Wash rhubarb and dice.
2. Cook until tender, with sugar.
3. Put through blender or force through sieve.
4. Prepare Vanilla Cream, Recipe No. 350, and cool.
5. Mix with rhubarb.
6. Whip cream until stiff; fold into rhubarb or use as a garnish.

356 APRICOT WHIP 356

Ingredients:

As for Rhubarb Whip (Recipe No. 355) substituting apricots for rhubarb and adding 1 teasp. lemon juice.

Method:

The same as for Recipe No. 355.

357 LEMON WHIP 357

Ingredients:

3¾ cups milk	3 eggs
1–2 lemons	3½–5½ oz. sugar
1 tablesp. cornstarch	½–1 cup cream
4½ tablesp. milk	

Method:

1. Peel lemons very thinly, and squeeze juice.
2. Bring peel to the boil in the milk.
3. Mix cornstarch with cold milk.
4. Add to boiling peel and milk, and bring again to the boil.
5. Whisk eggs and sugar, add a little of the boiling mixture, stir well.
6. Pour back into the saucepan, stirring constantly and bring again to near boiling point.
7. Cool, then strain.
8. Add a few spoonfuls lemon juice and mix with whipped cream.

358 LEMON WHIP (UNCOOKED) 358

Ingredients:

1 piece lemon peel	2 eggs
¾ cup water	7½–9 tablesp. sugar
1 small teasp. Agar-Agar*	½–1 cup cream
½ cup lemon juice	

Method:

1. Whisk peel, water and agar-agar well together.
2. Heat slowly over gentle heat until the agar-agar is completely dissolved (do not allow to boil).
3. Stir in lemon juice.
4. Beat eggs and sugar together until creamy; add to fruit cream.
5. Whip cream until stiff; fold in carefully; pour into serving dish.
6. Leave to stand about 1 hr.

359 ORANGE WHIP 359

Ingredients:

As for Lemon Whip (Recipe No. 357), substituting oranges for lemons.

Method:

The same as for Recipe No. 357.

* See p. 41 and footnote p. 118.

360 ORANGE WHIP (UNCOOKED) 360

Ingredients:

1 piece orange peel	1 teasp. lemon juice
¾ cup water	7½–9 tablesp. sugar
1 small teasp. Agar-Agar*	2 eggs
½ cup orange juice	½–1 cup cream

Method:

Prepare as for Lemon Whip (cold), Recipe No. 358.

361 D. ORANGE SHAPES 361 D.

Ingredients:

1½ cups orange juice	1½ tablesp. sugar
1 small teasp. Agar-Agar*	1 extra cup orange juice

Method:

1. Whisk agar-agar into orange juice; add sugar.
2. Heat slowly over gentle heat until agar-agar is completely dissolved (do not allow to boil).
3. Add the other cup of orange juice.
4. Pour into individual molds previously rinsed out in cold water.
5. Leave in a cool place to set.

362 CHAUDEAU 362

Ingredients:

2 eggs	¾ cup apple or grape juice
2 oz. sugar	1½ tablesp. lemon juice

Method:

1. Mix all ingredients together thoroughly.
2. Put into a double boiler over lukewarm water.
3. Beat well until creamy.

Note: If Chaudeau appears too thick, add more juice.

363 CUSTARD FILLING FOR ALL TARTS OR TARTLETS 363

Ingredients:

2½ cups milk	3 tablesp. vanilla sugar or
½ cup flour	plain sugar and vanilla
2 eggs	extract
	2 tablesp. butter

* See p. 41 and footnote p. 118.

Method:
1. Mix flour with milk, bring to the boil, stirring constantly; cook for a few more minutes.
2. Beat eggs, mix with sugar and vanilla sugar.
3. Add to flour and milk, bring to just under boiling point.
4. Mix butter into cooked custard.

364 BANANA CREAM   364

Ingredients:

1–2 bananas	1½ tablesp. sugar
3–4 tablesp. cream	a dash of lemon juice
	8 oz. whipped cream

Method:
1. Prepare bananas in blender or force through sieve.
2. Mix with 3–4 tablesp. cream.
3. Add lemon juice and sugar and fold in whipped cream.
4. Put in a pastry bag and use to fill tartlets or garnish other sweet dishes.

365 SWEET CHESTNUT PURÉE WITH CREAM   365

Ingredients:

2 lb. chestnuts	3½–5½ oz. sugar
2 cups milk	½ cup water
1 vanilla bean *or*	1–1½ cup cream
1 teasp. vanilla extract	

Method:
1. Make a diagonal cross on the flat side of the chestnuts; bake in oven until shells split.
2. Remove shells and skin from chestnuts.
3. Cover chestnuts with milk, add vanilla and cook until tender.
4. While still hot force through a sieve.
5. Dissolve sugar in water and cook until syrupy.
6. Mix with chestnut purée; the mixture should be fairly moist.
7. Press through a ricer or suitable sieve to form 'vermicelli' on a serving dish.
8. Whip cream until stiff; garnish purée with it.

366 VANILLA SAUCE

366

Ingredients:

1½ cups milk
½ vanilla bean *or*
½ teasp. vanilla extract

1½ tablesp. sugar
½ teasp. cornstarch
1 egg
½ cup cream if desired

Method:

1. Prepare as a thin Vanilla Cream as in Recipe No. 350.
2. Whip cream if used; mix with sauce.

367 D. ALMOND MILK SAUCE

367 D.

Ingredients:

2 cups milk
2 oz. almonds
1½ oz. sugar

1 tablesp. cornstarch
3 tablesp. water

Method:

1. Peel almonds and put through nut-mill or coarse grater.
2. Add almonds and sugar to milk and bring to the boil.
3. Mix cornstarch with water, then add to the boiling milk, stirring all the time.
4. Put into blender, or force through sieve several times.

368 D. 'RED WINE' SAUCE

368 D.

Ingredients:

1 cup water
lemon or orange peel
1 stick cinnamon

1 clove
2–2½ oz. sugar
1 cup red grape juice
about 1 tablesp. almonds

Method:

1. Boil the water, peel, cinnamon, clove and sugar together for a few minutes.
2. Strain, add grape juice, heat but do not boil again.
3. Peel almonds, cut into long strips and add to sauce.

369 ROSE HIP SAUCE

369

Ingredients:

2½ oz. rose hip purée
1 cup water or grape juice

2½ oz. sugar
lemon juice, if liked

Method:
    1. Bring purée, water and sugar to the boil.
    2. Add lemon juice if used.

Note: Rose Hip Purée is necessary in order to make Rose Hip Purée. As no Rose Hip Purée is available at present, directions are given below for preserving rose hips as purée, made either from fresh or from dried hips.

Preparing Fresh Rose Hips for Purée:

Ingredients:
2½ lb. rose hips   3¾ cups water

Method:
    1. Pick only ripe rose hips, vivid red and slightly soft, after frost has touched them.
    2. Select whole, undamaged hips.
    3. Top and tail (using scissors if soft).
    4. Wash quickly and drain in colander (not aluminum).
    5. Boil the water in stainless steel or undamaged enamel saucepan.
    6. Add the hips and bring again to the boil.
    7. Simmer with the lid on until the hips are soft (about 15 min.).
    8. Rub through a fine hair or stainless steel sieve, using a wooden spoon, masher or pestle.

Do not over-boil or the color and flavor will be spoiled, but the hips must be soft enough to sieve.

369*b* ROSE HIP PURÉE (*from fresh hips*)   369*b*

Ingredients:
1 lb. sugar per 1 lb. mashed sieved hips
castor sugar for covering jars

Method:
    9. Beat hips and sugar for about 20 min., using a wooden spoon.
    10. Bring to boil, then cook gently for 10 min.
    11. Fill well-cleaned, dry and hot earthenware or glass jars.
    12. Allow purée to cool.
    13. Cover with waxed paper, soaked in alcohol.
    14. Cover waxed paper with about half an inch of castor sugar.
    15. Cover with cellophane to make jars airtight.

Note: This purée will keep for one year if carefully prepared and stored in a dark, cool and airy place, but its vitamin content will decrease with keeping.

369c DRYING ROSE HIPS FOR PURÉE   369c

Purée can also be made from dried hips. If fresh hips are carefully dried immediately after picking and stored well, they will retain their vitamin content for a longer period than cooked purée in jars. They can then be used for making purée and for other purposes when convenient.

Dehydration:
1. Cut in half lengthwise.
2. Spread on clean surface near a fire or in an airing cupboard.
3. Avoid too much heat, otherwise hips will become brown and lose aroma.
4. Hips should be brittle and distinctly red when dry.
5. Shake hips in a sieve (preferably out of doors) to remove hairs.
6. Store in earthenware or cardboard containers or in a tin lined with paper, in a dry place.

369d COOKED ROSE HIP PURÉE   369d

Ingredients:

4 oz. dried hips	1¾ cups boiling water
	2 oz. sugar

Method:
1. Put hips into boiling water and bring quickly to the boil.
2. Simmer for 15 min.
3. Rub through a hair or stainless steel sieve.
4. Boil the sugar with 1–2 tablesp. water until it forms a thread.
5. Mix this syrup with 5 oz. mashed hips and boil for 10 min.

370 PUNCH (NON-ALCOHOLIC)   370

Ingredients:

1¾ cups water	1¾ cups red grape juice
1 quarter lemon	1½ tablesp. lemon juice
¼ stick cinnamon	6 tablesp. sugar
1 clove	4½ tablesp. fruit syrup
1¾ cups apple juice	slices of lemon

Method:

1. Boil water, lemon and spices for 5 min. Strain.
2. Add apple and grape juice.
3. Heat again, add lemon juice, sugar and syrup.
4. Serve as hot as possible, decorated with lemon slices.

371 D. FARINA SHAPE

371 D.

Ingredients:

1⅓ cups farina	1 egg
3¾ pt. milk	grated peel of 1 lemon
salt	1½ oz. almonds
3–4 tablesp. sugar	

Method:

1. Cook farina as in Recipe No. 237, add sugar last of all.
2. Beat egg.
3. Mix with cooked farina; add peel and grated almonds.
4. Fill mold, previously rinsed in cold water.
5. Cool, turn out when set.

372 D. RICE RING WITH STEWED FRUIT

372 D.

Ingredients:

2 cups rice	salt
3 cups water	2½ cups hot milk
grated peel of 1 lemon	4½ tablesp. sugar
	2 tablesp. butter

Method:

1. Bring water to the boil, add rice, lemon and salt. Cook 15 min.
2. Add milk and sugar, cook until rice is tender.
3. Add butter and mix well.
4. Rinse ring mold in cold water, pour in rice and cool.
5. Turn out when set and fill with stewed fruit.

373 D. RICE AND LEMON PUDDING

373 D.

Ingredients:

4½ cups water	5½ oz. sugar
juice of 1 lemon	salt
chopped lemon peel	1 cup rice
	1 cup cream

Method:
1. Bring water to the boil with lemon juice, peel, sugar and salt.
2. Add rice, cook for ½ hr., cool.
3. Whip cream, mix with rice, fill mold, previously rinsed in cold water.
4. Put in a cool place to set.

374 RICE PUDDING WITH PINEAPPLE   374

Ingredients:

1 cup rice	3 tablesp. sugar
1½ cups water	½ cup water
salt	1 small teasp. agar-agar*
1 vanilla bean *or*	2 slices pineapple
1 teasp. vanilla extract	1 cup cream
3 cups hot milk	

Method:
1. Bring water to the boil, add rice, salt, vanilla, and cook for 10 minutes.
2. Add milk, cook until thick, add sugar.
3. Mix agar-agar with water, heat slowly over low heat until agar-agar is completely dissolved (do not allow to boil).
4. Add to cool rice.
5. Dice pineapple and whip cream.
6. Add pineapple and half the cream to the rice mixture and fill mold, previously rinsed in cold water.
7. Leave to set, turn out, garnish with remaining cream and a few pineapple cubes.
8. Serve with pineapple juice.

375 MILK RICE PUDDING   375

Ingredients:

1 cup rice	2½ cups water
3 cups milk	pinch of salt

Method:
1. Cook all ingredients together slowly for 30–40 min.

Can be served with sugar and ground cinnamon or with stewed fruit.

* See p. 41 and footnote p. 118.

376 D. ALMOND FLAMMERI

Ingredients:

5 cups milk	salt
grated peel of 1 lemon	3 oz. almonds
3½ oz. cornstarch	4½ tablesp. sugar
1¼ cups milk	2 eggs
	raspberry syrup

Method:

1. Bring 5 cups milk, with grated lemon peel, to the boil.
2. Mix cornstarch with 1¼ cups milk, add salt and add both to the boiling milk and lemon.
3. Cook for 5 min.
4. Peel and grate almonds and add with sugar to the cornstarch mixture.
5. Beat the eggs and fold into the mixture.
6. Rinse a mold in cold water and pour pudding into it.
7. Put in a cool place to set, turn out and serve with raspberry or other fruit syrup.

377 ALMOND PUDDING

377

Ingredients:

4 tablesp. butter	1½ tablesp. butter
3½ oz. sugar	milk
3 egg yolks	3 egg whites
¾ cup almonds	1½ oz. raisins
6 slices bread	cinnamon

Method:

1. Beat butter and sugar until creamy, add egg yolks.
2. Peel almonds, roast lightly then grate, add to mixture.
3. Cut thin slices of bread.
4. Crisp bread in hot butter, then soak in a little milk and add to the mixture.
5. Beat egg whites to a stiff froth, mix carefully with remaining ingredients. Fold carefully into mixture.
6. Put into a mold and steam over boiling water for 1 hr.
7. Serve with fruit or 'Red Wine' Sauce, Recipe No. 368 D.

378 RED FRUIT SHAPE (Rote Gruetze)

378

Ingredients:

2 cups red currants, or black currants	1 cup raspberries or strawberries
1 cup apple juice, grape juice or water	5 oz. farina
3–5 oz. sugar	1 tablesp. cornstarch
	Vanilla Sauce, Rec. No. 350

Method:

1. Cook currants in juice or water.
2. Put through sieve or blender.
3. Add sugar and berries and cook without breaking.
4. Stir in farina; cook for 10 min.
5. Mix cornstarch with cold water, add and bring again to the boil.
6. Rinse mold in cold water; pour mixture into it.
7. Leave in a cool place to set.
8. Turn out and serve with Vanilla Sauce, Recipe No. 350, or cream.

If no berries available, use 3 cups currants.

379 CHERRY PUDDING   379

Ingredients:

8 slices wholewheat bread	¾ cup shelled filberts, finely chopped
1 cup hot milk	
5 tablesp. butter	3½ 1 lb. cans black cherries, pitted
3½ oz. sugar	
grated peel of 1 lemon	cinnamon
3 egg yolks	3 egg whites, beaten
	confectioner's sugar

Method:

1. Prepare as for Fresh Cherry Cake, Recipe No. 413.
2. Instead of baking in the oven, put into a pudding mold and steam for 1 hr.
3. Serve with Vanilla Sauce, Recipe No. 350.

380 SANS SOUCI APPLE PUDDING   380

Ingredients:

2 tablesp. butter	¾ cup milk
currants	4 tablesp. cornstarch
approx. 2 medium apples (½ lb.)	1 tablesp. butter
	2 egg yolks
3 oz. sugar	3 egg whites, stiffly beaten
1½ tablesp. butter	
pinch cinnamon	

Method:

1. Grease plain pudding mold with 2 tablesp. butter; line with currants.
2. Peel apples and cut into dice.
3. Stew apples in their own juice with sugar, butter and cinnamon (apples should be tender, but retain their shape).

4. Mix cornstarch with cold milk and butter, then cook for a few min., stirring constantly.

5. Add egg yolks and lastly the egg whites alternately with apple.

6. Fill pudding mold and steam for 1 hr.

381 D. BAKED APPLE SWEET WITH TAPIOCA 381 D.

Ingredients:

3–4 tablesp. tapioca
9–12 tablesp. water
6 apples, peeled
2 oz. sugar

apple peels and cores
1 cup apple or grape juice *or* water
2 oz. sugar
1½ tablesp. butter

Method:

1. Soak tapioca for 3 hr.

2. Slice apples, put in buttered baking dish alternately with tapioca.

3. Cook peels and cores in the apple or grape juice for 10 min.

4. Strain, add sugar and pour over mixture.

5. Put dabs of butter on mixture and bake 40–50 min.

382 BAKED CHERRY SWEET 382

Ingredients:

10 oz. cherries, pitted
2½ oz. sugar
2 rusks (if liked)
2 tablesp. butter
6 tablesp. wholewheat flour

1 cup milk
salt
2 oz. brown sugar
2 eggs

Method:

1. Pit cherries, sprinkle with sugar and put in a baking dish.

2. Crush rusks (if used) and mix with cherries.

3. Melt butter and cook flour in it.

4. Add hot milk and salt and cook until thick.

5. Add sugar, then the eggs, one at a time, beating well.

6. Pour over cherries, steam for 20 min. over boiling water.

7. Bake for a further 20 min. in a moderate oven (350°).

Other fruit which may be cooked in this way includes apricots, peaches or any mixture of similar fruit.

383 BAKED LEMON SWEET   383

Ingredients:

5 tablesp. butter	3 eggs
1¼ cup flour	grated lemon peel
2 cups milk	3 tablesp. lemon juice
5½ oz. sugar	

Method:

1. Melt butter, cook flour in it.
2. Add milk and cook until thick.
3. Add sugar, mix in eggs one at a time, add flavoring, beat well.
4. Pour into a greased baking dish, steam for 20 min. over boiling water.
5. Bake for a further 20 min. in a moderate oven.

384 CREAM CHEESE SOUFFLÉ   384

Ingredients:

3 tablesp. butter	2 eggs
6 tablesp. flour	2½ oz. sugar
salt	1½ oz. raisins
1½ cups milk	grated lemon peel
1 lb. cream cheese	6 tablesp. cream

Method:

1. Melt butter, cook flour in it. Add salt.
2. Add hot milk and cook for a few min.
3. Mix in cheese and eggs, one at a time, then add other ingredients.
4. Grease a deep baking dish and pour mixture into it.
5. Bake in moderate oven for 30–40 min.

385 ALMOND SLICES WITH FRUIT SAUCE   385

Ingredients for the Slices:	*Ingredients for Fruit Sauce:*
2 egg whites	½ lb. apricots (canned or
¼ lb. peeled almonds	stewed)
2¾ oz. sugar	1½–3 tablesp. cream
8 thin slices white bread	

Method:

1. Beat egg whites to a stiff froth.
2. Grate almonds and fold into egg whites; add sugar.
3. Spread fairly thickly on the slices of bread.
4. Place on a greased baking sheet, bake in moderate oven until lightly browned.

5. Put apricots through a sieve or reduce to pulp in an electric blender.

6. If too thick, thin with a little juice.

7. Add cream, if liked, and serve with almond slices.

386 RHUBARB SLICES 386

Ingredients:

8 slices wholewheat or white bread	5½ oz. sugar
	½ cup cream
3 tablesp. butter	vanilla sugar *or* extract
1¼ lb. rhubarb	

Method:

1. Fry bread on both sides in the butter until golden yellow.

2. Stew rhubarb in its own juice and sugar; cool.

3. Arrange rhubarb on the slices.

4. Beat cream until stiff, mix in vanilla shortly before serving and use to garnish the slices.

387 APPLE SLICES 387

Ingredients:

approx. ⅓ of Puff Pastry, Recipe No. 325	3 tablesp. sugar
	1 egg yolk
4 medium-sized apples	apricot jam

Method:

1. Roll out pastry to a thickness of about ¼ in.

2. Cut out rectangles about 3 in. by 4 in., and put on a baking sheet.

3. Peel apples, slice thinly and put on pastry so that they overlap (leaving about ½ in. clear round edge).

4. Sprinkle with sugar and brush this edge with egg yolk without touching outsides.

5. Bake in hot oven (400°) 10–15 min.

6. Pour a layer of jam over the hot slices.

388 PINEAPPLE SLICES 388

Ingredients:

2 small eggs	6 tablesp. flour
4½ tablesp. sugar	¼ teasp. baking powder
salt	1 tablesp. butter
grated peel of 1 lemon	4–6 slices pineapple and some juice
½ tablesp. water	
	½–1 cup cream

Method:

1. Prepare sponge as in Recipe No. 409.
2. Bake in a rectangular cake pan. Cool.
3. Cut into slices about 2½ in. by 4 in.
4. Sprinkle slices with pineapple juice, and put overlapping pieces of pineapple on each.
5. Garnish with whipped cream.

389 BANANA SLICES 389

Ingredients:

As in Recipe No. 388	6 tablesp. currant, rasp-
2 bananas instead of	berry *or*
pineapple	quince jam or jelly, diluted

Method:

1. Prepare as for Pineapple Slices.
2. Slice bananas, place on sponge.
3. Brush with jelly and garnish with cream.

390 APPLE TART 390

Ingredients:

1¾ cups flour	6 tablesp. water
6–7 tablesp. butter	6–7 medium-sized apples
salt	Coating as below

Method:

1. Prepare Shortcrust Pastry as in Recipe No. 323. Roll out and line pie plate.
2. Peel, core and slice apples and put in circles on the pastry. Finish with the chosen coating.

Coating, 1

Ingredients:

2 tablesp. sugar	1½ tablesp. butter
cinnamon	

Method:

1. Sprinkle sugar and cinnamon over the apples.
2. Dot with butter and bake in moderate oven (400°).

Coating, 2

Ingredients:

1 egg	1 teasp. cornstarch
½ cup milk	1½–3 tablesp. sugar
½ cup cream	

Method:

1. Whisk egg, milk, cream, cornstarch and sugar together and pour over the tart when it is half cooked.
2. Bake until the pastry is cooked and the custard set.

Coating, 3

Ingredients:

1¼ cups apple juice	3 tablesp. sugar
½ teasp. Agar-Agar*	

Method:

1. Make required apple juice by cooking peel and cores of apples for 10 min. and straining.
2. Dissolve agar-agar in the liquid, heat together but do not boil. Sweeten with the sugar.
3. Cool, but before it sets, pour over the tart after it is baked.

Coating, 4

1 cup sour cream	1½ tablesp. sugar
1 egg	½ tablesp. melted butter
2 teasp. flour	

Method:

1. Whisk egg, flour and sugar together.
2. Stir lightly into the cream.
3. Add melted (not hot) butter.

If liked, sprinkle sugar and cinnamon over the apples before pouring on the coating. Bake in a moderate oven.

391 GRAPE TART 391

Ingredients:

As for Apple Tart (Recipe No. 390), substituting grapes for apples.

Method:

Prepare as for Apple Tart, Recipe No. 390.

* See p. 41 and footnote p. 118.

392 APRICOT TART
392

Ingredients:

Shortcrust Pastry as in Recipe No. 323 or 324	1½ lb. apricots
2 tablesp. grated filberts or almonds *or* breadcrumbs	4½ tablesp. sugar

Method:

1. Line a pie plate with shortcrust.
2. Sprinkle nuts or breadcrumbs on to it.
3. Halve apricots, place on the pastry just overlapping.
4. Sprinkle with sugar and bake for 10–15 min.

If desired sprinkle hot tart with more sugar, or with the following mixture:

Alternative Filling:

Ingredients:

1 egg	1 teasp. cornstarch
½ cup milk	3 tablesp. sugar
½ cup cream	

Method:

Whisk together, pour over tart and bake until set.

393 PLUM OR DAMSON TART
393

Ingredients:

As for Recipe No. 392, substituting plums or damsons for apricots.

Method:

Prepare as for Apricot Tart, Recipe No. 392.

394 RHUBARB TART
394

Ingredients:

As for Recipe No. 392, substituting rhubarb for apricots.

Method:

Prepare as for Apricot Tart, Recipe No. 392.

395 MORELLA TART
395

Ingredients:

As for Recipe No. 392, substituting cherries for apricots.

Method:

Prepare as for Apricot Tart, Recipe No. 392.

396 STRAWBERRY TART 396

Ingredients:

1¾ cups flour	1 lb. strawberries or rasp-
5–7 tablesp. butter	berries (about 1½ pt.)
1½ tablesp. sugar	4½ tablesp. sugar
1 egg	½–1 cup cream *or* 2–3 egg
salt	whites
	3½ oz. sugar

Method:

1. Prepare sweet shortcrust pastry as in Recipe No. 324. Put aside for a short time.
2. Roll out and line pie plate.
3. Bake pastry case in moderate oven (400°) 20 min.
4. Arrange prepared berries on the cold pastry case.
5. Garnish with whipped cream, if used, *or*
6. Beat egg whites until stiff, mix carefully with sugar, swirl over berries or use a pastry bag.
7. Brown lightly in the oven for a few min.

397 CREAM CHEESE (CURD) TART 397

Ingredients:

1¾ cups flour	2 egg yolks
5–7 tablesp. butter	3 oz. sugar
salt	1½ oz. almonds, grated
6 tablesp. water	1½ oz. raisins
¾ lb. cream cheese	⅓ oz. cornstarch
6 tablesp. cream	peel of 1 lemon, grated
	2 egg whites

Method:

1. Prepare shortcrust pastry as in Recipe No. 323.
2. Roll out ¼ in. thick and line a pie plate.
3. Mix all other ingredients, spread on the pastry and bake (350°) 30 min.

398 EASTER TART 398

Ingredients:

Shortcrust Pastry	1½ oz. sugar
Recipe No. 323	2 eggs
2–2½ cups milk	lemon peel, grated
½ cup farina *or*	1½ oz. sultanas
½ cup rice	1½ oz. filberts, grated
salt	1½ tablesp. sugar
3 tablesp. butter	

Method:
1. Roll out pastry and line pie plate.
2. Cook the farina or rice in milk till really thick; add salt.
3. Cream butter and sugar together until fluffy.
4. Add eggs and lemon peel and beat well.
5. Add to the farina or rice and mix in the sultanas and filberts. Cool.
6. Spread on the pastry and bake for 30–40 min. (400°).
7. Sprinkle with 1 tablesp. sugar.

399 APPLE STRUDEL   399

Ingredients:

1¾ cups flour	6–7 oz. sugar
1½ tablesp. oil	2 oz. breadcrumbs, lightly fried
1 egg	
6–7½ tablesp. warm water	3 oz. raisins or sultanas
salt	3 oz. almonds or filberts, grated
2–2½ lb. apples (6–8 medium)	4–5 tablesp. melted butter
1½ tablesp. melted butter	confectioner's sugar

Method:
1. Mix flour, oil, egg, 1½ tablesp. butter, water and salt to a smooth paste.
2. Knead well for ¼ hr.
3. Cover with a damp cloth and leave for at least ½ hr.
4. Peel and core apples, and slice thinly.
5. Spread a large cloth on a table and sprinkle with flour.
6. Roll out the pastry on it very thinly.
7. Pull it out over the back of your hands until it is transparent.
8. Brush pastry with 5 tablesp. melted butter and sprinkle with fried breadcrumbs.
9. Arrange apple slices on it then cover with raisins, nuts and sugar.
10. Lift up the cloth on one side and roll up pastry to form a roll.
11. Brush roll with butter.
12. Bake in a hot oven (425°) for 30–40 min.
13. Sprinkle with confectioner's sugar.

Note: Prepared and rolled-out Apple Strudel pastry is available: it needs only to be filled and baked.

400 APPLES EN ROBE DE CHAMBRE   400

Ingredients:

1¾ cups flour	salt
5–7 tablesp. butter	4–6 apples
1½ tablesp. sugar	6 tablesp. sugar and cinna-
1 egg	mon mixed
	1 egg yolk

Method:

1. Make shortcrust pastry as in Recipe No. 324.
2. Roll out ½ in. thick and cut into 4–5 in. squares.
3. Peel and core apples and arrange on pastry.
4. Sprinkle with sugar and cinnamon.
5. Fold four corners to the center.
6. Cut out small fancy pastry shapes and put on top.
7. Brush with egg yolk and bake in hot oven (425°) for 30–45 min.

Apples may also be stuffed with currants.

401 APPLE CHARLOTTE   401

Ingredients:

6–8 apples	3 tablesp. raisins
½ tablesp. butter	2 tablesp. filberts, ground
3 tablesp. sugar	½ loaf bread
cinnamon	4–5 tablesp. melted butter
	3–4½ tablesp. sugar

Method:

1. Peel and core apples, slice thinly.
2. Cook slowly in their own juice with the ½ tablesp. butter until soft.
3. Add sugar, cinnamon, raisins and filberts.
4. Cut bread into slices about ¼ in. thick.
5. Dip one side of bread into melted butter and then into sugar.
6. Line first bottom and then sides of a deep casserole or a charlotte mold with the slices, which must be touching.
7. Fill the dish with the apple mixture and cover with pieces of bread left over.
8. Bake in a moderate oven (400°) for 40–60 min. until golden brown.
9. Turn out. Invert on a serving dish.

Custard Filling, Recipe No. 363, may be spread (about ½ in. thick) over the baked Apple Charlotte, sprinkled with sugar and then browned under a broiler.

Charlotte may also be served with Vanilla Sauce, Recipe No. 366.

402 PEACH CHARLOTTE 402

Ingredients:
As for Recipe No. 401, substituting peaches for apples.

Method:
Prepare as for Apple Charlotte, Recipe No. 401.

403 APPLE PIE 403

Ingredients:

1⅓ cups flour	7 medium-sized apples
5 tablesp. butter	4–6 tablesp. sugar
1 egg	cinnamon
1½ tablesp. sugar	2 tablesp. raisins or sultanas
salt	1½ tablesp. melted butter
	egg yolk

Method:
1. Prepare pastry as for Recipe No. 324. Leave for ½ hr.
2. Peel, core and slice apples thinly.
3. Mix with sugar, cinnamon, raisins and melted butter.
4. Put mixture into a pie pan.
5. Roll out pastry to about ⅛ in. thick and cut out a lid for the dish from it.
6. Line upper edge of the dish with the remnants of pastry.
7. Put a cup upside down in the dish and put on the pastry lid.
8. Press edges firmly and brush with egg yolk.
9. Bake (400°) for ½ hr.

404 APPLE FRITTERS 404

Ingredients:

6 tablesp. flour	1 egg white
7½ tablesp. water	6 apples
3 tablesp. apple juice	vegetable fat
salt	sugar and cinnamon mixed

Method:

1. Mix flour to a smooth batter with the water and apple juice.
2. Add salt and stiffly beaten egg white.
3. Peel and core the apples and cut slices about ½ in. thick.
4. Dip in batter.
5. Fry in deep vegetable fat until golden brown.
6. Dip finished fritters in sugar and cinnamon.

405 SAVARIN   405

Ingredients:

1½ cups flour
½ cake yeast
½ cup milk
salt
1 egg
1½ tablesp. sugar
3–4 tablesp. butter
stewed fruit
cream

Ingredients for Punch Sauce:

½ cup water
lemon and orange peel
2 cloves
1 cup white grape juice
    or apple juice
6 tablesp. sugar
1½ tablesp. fruit syrup,
    if liked

Method:

1. Prepare Yeast Pastry as in Recipe No. 327.
2. Put into a well-buttered ring mold and leave to rise.
3. Bake in a hot oven (425°) 20–30 min.
4. Turn out, serve with Punch Sauce made as follows:
5. Bring water, peel and cloves to the boil and allow to draw for ¼ hr.
6. Strain and add juice and sugar.
7. Pour hot sauce over finished Savarin.
8. Fill the center with stewed fruit, and garnish with whipped cream.

If preferred use Chaudeau, Recipe No. 362, instead of Punch Sauce.

406 SPLITS   406

Ingredients:

1¼ cups water
3 tablesp. butter
1¼ cup flour
3 eggs
¾ oz. sugar

salt
Cream, *or*
    Banana Cream, Rec. No.
    364 *or* Custard Filling,
    Rec. No. 363
confectioner's sugar

Method:

1. Prepare Choux Pastry as in Recipe No. 331.
2. Scoop out small heaps (size of small apples) or force through pastry bag and place on buttered baking sheet.
3. Bake in moderate oven 20–30 min. (400°).
4. Leave to dry for a short time.
5. Fill with whipped cream, Banana Cream, Recipe No. 364, or Custard Filling, Recipe No. 363.
6. Sprinkle with confectioner's sugar.

407 PUFFS 407

Ingredients:

1¼ cups water	¾ oz. sugar
3 tablesp. butter	vegetable fat
1¼ cup flour	sugar and cinnamon mixed
salt	'Red Wine' Sauce,
3 eggs	Recipe No. 368 D.

Method:

1. Prepare Choux Pastry as in Recipe No. 331.
2. Scoop out small balls with a spoon.
3. Fry slowly in moderately hot vegetable fat.
4. Dip finished puffs in sugar and cinnamon and serve with 'Red Wine' Sauce.

408 CREAM CHEESE (CURD) TURNOVERS 408

Ingredients:	*Ingredients for Filling:*
1½ cups flour	6 oz. cream cheese curd
3 tablesp. butter	3 tablesp. cream
⅓ oz. yeast	1 egg
6–7½ tablesp. milk	1½ oz. sugar
salt	1 tablesp. grated almonds
1 egg	1 tablesp. raisins
1½ oz. sugar	1 teasp. cornstarch
peel of 1 lemon (grated)	peel of ½ lemon (grated)
vegetable fat or oil for deep frying	
sugar and cinnamon, mixed	

Method:

1. Prepare Yeast Pastry as in Recipe No. 327. Roll out ¼ in. thick.

2. Cut out rounds 4 in. in diameter.

3. Mix other ingredients together and put a small heap on each pastry round.

4. Brush edges with water and turn over, pressing edges well together.

5. Deep fry turnovers in moderately hot vegetable fat.

6. Dip turnovers in sugar and cinnamon mixture.

409 SPONGE (FOR FRUIT CAKES, SLICES, ETC.)   409

Ingredients:

3 eggs	1½ tablesp. water
8–9 tablesp. sugar	¾ cup flour
salt	½ teasp. baking powder
grated peel of 1 lemon	2 tablesp. melted butter

Method:

1. Line bottom of round layer cake pan with waxed paper.

2. Mix sugar and eggs, add salt, peel and water.

3. Whisk until creamy in a bowl over lukewarm water (or in a double boiler).

4. Fold flour into mixture alternately with baking powder and melted butter.

5. Pour mixture into cake pan.

6. Bake in moderate oven (350°) for 15–20 min.

410 FRUIT SPONGE   410

Ingredients:

6 tablesp. butter	3 egg whites
3 egg yolks	1 teasp. baking powder
3½ oz. sugar	1½ lb. apricots, peaches or apples
grated peel of 1 lemon	
1¼ cup flour	3–4 tablesp. sugar
	1 tablesp. confectioner's sugar

Method:

1. Beat butter until creamy.

2. Add yolks, sugar and peel, beat again until soft and creamy.

3. Whisk egg whites to a stiff froth; fold into the mixture alternately with the flour and baking powder.

4. Line bottom of round layer cake pan with waxed paper and cover with mixture.

5. Halve or slice the chosen fruit and put on top of the sponge.

6. Sprinkle 2–3 oz. sugar on top and bake for ¾ hr. in moderate oven (350°).

7. Sprinkle confectioner's sugar over finished dish before serving.

411 STRAWBERRY CREAM CAKE   411

Ingredients:

½ quantity of Sponge Mixture Recipe No. 409
1 lb. hulled strawberries (about 1½ pt.)
4½ tablesp. sugar
1 cup cream

Method:

1. Put the sponge mixture into a greased and lined layer cake pan and bake slowly for 20 min.

2. Arrange strawberries on the sponge, sprinkle with sugar.

3. Whip cream and use to garnish fruit, or spread half the cream over sponge before adding strawberries.

If liked the strawberries can be coated with diluted strawberry jam.

412 CHESTNUT CREAM CAKE   412

Ingredients:

½ quantity Sponge Mixture Recipe No. 409
6 tablesp. Apple Purée, Recipe No. 337
½ portion Sweet Chestnut Purée, Recipe No. 365
1 cup cream

Method:

1. Put sponge mixture into greased and lined layer cake pan and cook slowly for 20 min.

2. Spread apple purée over sponge.

3. Cover with Chestnut Vermicelli and garnish with stiffly whipped cream.

413 FRESH CHERRY CAKE   413

Ingredients:

8 slices wholewheat bread
1 cup hot milk
5 tablesp. butter
3½ oz. sugar
grated peel of 1 lemon
3 egg yolks
¾ cup shelled filberts, finely chopped
3½ cans (17 oz. each) of pitted bing cherries, drained
cinnamon
3 egg whites, beaten
confectioner's sugar

Method:

1. Soak slices of bread in the hot milk; put through a blender.

2. Beat butter and sugar together until creamy, add peel and yolks, one at a time.

3. Mix in the rest of the ingredients lightly, put into a greased baking pan, 8″x8″x2″.

4. Bake in moderate oven (350°) for about 1 hr.

5. Sprinkle confectioner's sugar over the finished cake.

414 CARROT CAKE 414

Ingredients:

5 egg yolks
7 oz. white or brown sugar
grated peel of 1 lemon
4 large carrots, grated or chopped in blender (equals 1¾ cups)
1½ cups almonds, grated (equals 2 cups grated)
1 teasp. cinnamon
½ teasp. powdered clove
5 oz. wholewheat flour
5 egg whites
confectioner's sugar

Method:

1. Beat yolks and sugar until creamy.

2. Fold in all the other ingredients, adding the stiffly beaten egg whites last.

3. Put into a greased loaf pan (9x9x1½ in.) and bake for approximately 50 minutes in a moderate oven (350°).

4. Sprinkle confectioner's sugar over the finished cake.

415 DUTCH CURRANT BREAD 415

Ingredients:

4 cups wholewheat flour
7 tablesp. butter
salt
6 tablesp. sugar (if liked)
1 oz. compressed yeast
¼ cup lukewarm milk
½ lb. currants
6 oz. seedless raisins
3 tablesp. flour
2 oz. candied peel (lemon)
2½ cups milk (warmed)
2 eggs

Method:

1. Sift flour into a warm bowl, make a well in the center.

2. Put dabs of butter all around flour.

3. Add salt, and sugar if liked, in the same way.

4. Dissolve yeast in 2 oz. milk, pour into well, mix to a thin paste with a little flour. Allow to work.

5. Mix flour with yeast, using the milk for mixing and knead until smooth.

6. Put bowl in a warm place and leave to rise until dough has doubled its bulk.

7. Wash and dry fruit and sprinkle with flour, add to the dough with the eggs.

8. Put into a loaf pan and leave in a warm place to rise again.

9. Bake for 1 hr. in a hot oven (400°).

10. Serve with butter, nut butter or honey for breakfast or supper.

416 MIXED FRUIT CAKE
416

Ingredients:

2 sticks butter	3½ oz. pitted prunes
8 oz. sugar	1 oz. candied peel (orange)
5 eggs	1½ oz. walnuts
grated peel of 1 lemon	salt
1½ tablesp. lemon juice	2 cups wholewheat flour
½ lb. raisins	1 teasp. baking powder

Method:

1. Heat butter until creamy, add sugar, eggs, peel and lemon juice and beat well.

2. Cut prunes and candied peel into small pieces, mix all fruit with flour.

3. Mix all ingredients together thoroughly.

4. Line a loaf pan with waxed paper, put in cake mixture.

5. Bake in a slow oven (200°–250°) for 3 hr. approximately.

417 D. SOYA CAKE (WITHOUT EGGS)
417 D.

Ingredients:

2 sticks butter	6 tablesp. soya flour
5 oz. sugar	1¾ cups wholewheat flour
grated orange peel	1½ cups grated filberts
salt	½ tablesp. baking powder
7½ tablesp. water	4 tablesp. chopped walnuts
9 tablesp. Rose Hip Purée, Recipe No. 369	6 tablesp. currants or raisins

Method:

1. Beat butter until creamy, add sugar and beat again.

2. Add orange peel and salt.

3. Wash and dry fruit and toss in flour.

4. Mix all ingredients together thoroughly, except 2 tablesp. Rose Hip Purée. Reserve these for filling.

5. Grease cake pan, put in half the mixture, spread with this Rose Hip Purée.

6. Cover with second half of mixture.

7. Bake in moderate oven (350°) for 1–1½ hr.

If liked, instead of 2 tablesp. Rose Hip Purée use ⅛ teasp. powdered clove and a pinch of cinnamon and mix with the cake mixture just before baking.

418 ROLLED OAT BISCUITS 418

Ingredients:

1¾ cups rolled oats	vanilla extract
7 tablesp. butter	⅞ cup flour
1 egg	egg yolk
9 oz. sugar	

Method:

1. Melt butter and sauté oats in it.

2. Beat egg, add sugar, vanilla and flour and add to the oats.

3. Knead all together until smooth and pliable.

4. Roll out dough ⅛ in. thick.

5. Cut into rounds.

6. Brush with egg yolk.

7. Bake in moderate oven (350°) until golden brown.

419 SWABIAN BISCUITS 419

Ingredients:

1 stick, 3 tablesp. butter	1–2 eggs
9 oz. brown sugar	juice and grated peel of 1
¾ cup roasted and grated filberts	lemon
	pinch of cinnamon
3 cups, 2 tablesp. whole-wheat flour	pinch of salt
	egg yolk

1. Beat butter until creamy, add sugar and beat again.

2. Add all other ingredients, except final egg yolk, and knead until smooth.

3. Leave in a cool place for 1 hr.

4. Roll out dough ⅛ in. thick.

5. Cut into fancy shapes and brush with egg yolk.

6. Bake in moderate oven (350°) until golden brown.

WHOLEWHEAT BREAD

FOR HOME-BAKING

If wholewheat bread is not obtainable at the bakers, or is of a poor quality, excellent wholewheat bread can be baked at home in an ordinary oven. Though more work may be involved, we can make certain that home-made bread contains absolutely fresh coarsely ground whole grains, and that the full value of this is retained. It is advisable to buy compost-grown wheat grains, flour and other cereals from health food stores.*

It is wiser to make bread in small quantities until experience in bread-making has been gained. When using whole wheat, pick over and remove any hard grains, bits of wood or small stones which may be found. The wheat should then be coarsely ground in a small cereal grinder or in a coffee grinder set to coarse grinding.

The oil suggested in the following recipe is added to the bread to prevent it crumbling so easily, to make a loaf of better consistency which is easier to cut, and to give a pleasant flavor.

420   420

Ingredients for 1 loaf weighing 3 lb. approx:

8 cups coarsely ground wholewheat flour *or* crushed whole wheat	2½ cups water
	1 level tablesp. salt (sea salt)
	1½ tablesp. oil
½ oz. yeast	

Method:

1. Put coarsely ground flour into a bowl, make a well in the center.
2. Dissolve the yeast in a little lukewarm water until it is of a pouring consistency.
3. Pour into the well and mix with a little of the flour to 'set the sponge.'
4. Sprinkle a little more flour over the surface to prevent a crust forming.
5. Cover the bowl and stand it in a warm place until the dough doubles its bulk. (1–3 hr., depending on the temperature).
6. Dissolve salt in lukewarm water, add oil and mix with the dough.
7. Knead thoroughly for 15–20 min. until the dough becomes pliable.

* See p. 10.

8. Beat dough 20 times by holding it in both hands high above the head and then knocking it against the table.

9. Stand the bowl in a warm place for another 30 min.

10. Shape into a longish loaf and put into a buttered or oiled loaf pan sprinkled with flour.

11. Fill only two-thirds of the pan and press well against the sides.

12. Allow to rise for 10–15 min.

13. Put into a pre-heated oven (400°) for about 2 hr.

Note: The baking time and temperature vary from oven to oven, and can only be ascertained with experience. The correct time is 2 hr., a shorter length of time tends to make the crust too thick and the crumb doughy, too long baking gives a dry bread.

This bread should not be eaten until the day after it is baked; it can be kept for at least a week if kept in a cool (not cold) place.

421 BREAD ROLLS   421

Ingredients:

The same as for Wholewheat Bread only instead of 2½ cups water and 1½ tablesp. oil, use 1¼ cups water, 1¼ cups milk, and 2 tablesp. butter.

Method:

1. Prepare dough as for bread.

2. Form into balls (using about 3 oz. of the dough for each).

3. Flatten a little and allow to rise for a short time.

4. Put into a moderate oven (400°) for 10 min.

5. Reduce heat to 350° and bake for another 10–15 min.

2. CULINARY HERBS AND HERB TEAS

When Dr. Bircher-Benner discovered the curative action of raw vegetable foods fifty years ago, he was faced with the task of adapting such an unusual diet to the palates and digestive organs of his patients, and of preparing it in an appetizing way. This led to the rediscovery of the culinary herbs in all their richness and variety, to the investigation of their inherent possibilities and the fresh application of the forgotten knowledge of bygone days. Culinary herbs not only cannot do any harm; they even, in many respects, add to the therapeutic effect of the diet by means of definite curative action. The use of culinary herbs was then also extended to normal diets.

There is a whole range of wonderful culinary herbs at the housewife's disposal, with which she can prove her 'artistry' by emphasizing, enriching and modifying the natural taste of food, without overpowering it in any way. As a general rule, the average modern cook knows little of this art. It is a matter of developing the instinct for that subtle addition of seasoning which provides a satisfying, harmonious taste; of testing the affinities between different flavors, and at the same time providing as much variety as possible. Culinary herbs stimulate a jaded appetite and also help to reduce an exaggerated craving for food to normal requirements. They facilitate, to an unbelievable degree, the often necessary task of decreasing the daily intake of common salt from the frequently exaggerated quantities to the wholesome quantity of 5 gm. per day at the most; and this in a pleasant way, acceptable to the patient.

Usually, far too much salt is used and in addition hot spices, such as the peppers, mustard, curry powder, excessive quantities of paprika, or even the pungent, artificial seasonings of unknown composition sold on the market, some of which have no flavor of their own but act as stimulants to our taste buds, e.g. monosodium glutamate. These frequently overpower the inherent flavor of the various foods, blunt the palate, overstimulate the digestive organs and overload the eliminative system. The instincts which influence the selection of foods will gradually deteriorate and often reject the natural for the artificial and refuse friut and vegetables in favor of an excessive amount of meat or alcohol. They may even refuse to function altogether, thus resulting in a poor appetite which has to be titillated by exotic 'luxuries'.

When, as a result, the liver, the kidneys and the digestive organs finally cease to do their work properly, the sufferer is forced to keep to a diet. Such a diet must of necessity be a so-called protective diet, unseasoned and unattractive, even at times completely salt-free, and therefore often the despair of the patient because many cooks can think only in terms of salt and hot spices. A recent technical publication complains of the unimaginative use of flavoring in most clinics and hospitals, which makes the diet so monotonous.

For many people, therefore, any special diet has become synonymous with dull and tasteless food. And yet a special diet —even a salt-free, protective one—can be made so palatable, so varied and well-flavored, that it can be followed for weeks and months without difficulty. The chief means of attaining this is by the skilled use of culinary herbs.

Botanically, the culinary herbs belong to the following plant families: The *umbelliferae,* such as caraway, fennel, dill, chervil, parsley, lovage, etc.; the *liliaceae,* such as onion, garlic, chives, leeks, etc.; the *labiatae,* such as summer savory, marjoram, mint, peppermint, rosemary, thyme (the labiates have a strong aroma, and are specially suitable as seasonings); the *compositae,* such as tarragon; the *cruciferae,* such as horseradish. As a rule, the leaves and stalks are used and sometimes the roots and fruit. The pharmacologically effective substances in culinary herbs are: volatile oils, tannins, bitter principles, secretins, balsams, resins, mucilages, glucosides and organic vegetable acids.

The volatile oils are very important substances contained in culinary herbs, being present in proportions of a few per cent to fractions of one per cent. In the small doses in which they are eaten in dishes flavored with such herbs, these oils stimulate secretion in the mouth and the stomach, activate peristalsis, reduce processes of fermentation and decomposition, thus reducing flatulence, and have an anti-spasmodic and pain-relieving (anodyne) action. In general, these oils stimulate, aid digestion and act as gastric tonics. Certain oils help to dilate cramped blood vessels (vasodilators) so that, for example, in cases of inadequate output, an increased discharge of urine may result.

Tannins are present in various culinary herbs and have an astringent anti-inflammatory action on the gastro-intestinal system, inhibiting fermentation and decomposition.

The bitter principles stimulate the secretion of digestive juices and are frequently employed in cases of general digestive debility. They have a tonic effect on the smooth muscles of the gastro-intestinal system and thus have a stimulating action on the appetite. Well-known bitter principles are to be found in wormwood, centaury, gentian, and of the culinary herbs in anise, fennel, marjoram and rosemary.

The *secretins* are substances that enhance the external secretion of the pancreas, and are found especially in cabbage, onions, nettles, peas, soya beans, wheat and rice.

Organic acids may stimulate the appetite, have an antibiotic action and are valuable in the digestion of fats.

If at all possible, culinary herbs should be used in their fresh state, a small herb garden being kept for this purpose, or at any rate, a few window boxes with marjoram, basil and others. Some culinary herbs can also be gathered wild in hedges and at the edge of woods. A greengrocer should moreover be found who supplies herbs fresh—a regularly expressed demand will help to achieve this—and in as great a variety as possible. If they are unobtainable freshly grown, or in winter, they can be used in the dried form, obtainable at supermarkets, good-class grocers and health food stores. When buying dried herbs, it is preferable to choose those which retain their natural, mostly green color, as they will have been dried carefully and have preserved their volatile oils, which are identical with their aroma. But these can only be retained if stored in airtight, sealed glass jars, as the elusive aroma escapes easily or mingles with other herb flavors. All dried herbs have to be kept in the dark, to retain aroma and color.

The following are among the most important culinary herbs:

BASIL (*Ocimum basilicum*)

An herb with a strong flavor, slightly bitter if used in excess. Wonderful aromatic scent, belonging to the best and most delicate of the culinary herbs.

Use: With salads, raw vegetables, herb sauces, cream cheese with herbs, sauerkraut, rissoles, cucumber, pumpkin, zucchini, all bean and tomato dishes, sauces and soups.

Cultivation: There are two kinds, one with large leaves, one with small. Can be grown as an annual in the garden in a warm, protected place, or cultivated in a window box. Grows 10–12 in. tall. Leaves can be picked from July–November.

SUMMER SAVORY (*Satureia hortensis*)

Strong flavor and wonderful scent.

Use: With green beans, fresh, frozen or canned, fried potatoes, raw vegetables, sauerkraut. Use sparingly. Can best be mixed with thyme. Choose only the youngest shoots to eat raw.

Cultivation: Grows as an annual 10–12 in. high in a sunny place in the garden. Can also be cultivated in a window box.

BORAGE (*Borago officinalis*)

Imparts a pleasantly refreshing cucumber-like flavor, slightly salty.

Use: With lettuce and all leafy salads, and especially with cucumber or potato salad and in all summer drinks and cups. Only use fresh, small young leaves and blossoms, since it is quite tasteless when dried in the ordinary way. These young leaves should be finely chopped or crushed and added in small quantities. The blossoms, which are mostly blue but sometimes pink, are also edible and are attractive when used to decorate raw salads, particularly cucumber, carrot or fennel salad. Suitable for mixtures of fresh herbs.

Cultivation: It is an annual, easily grown and seeds itself, therefore needs little care. Grows 12–28 in. high. Can be cultivated in a window box.

NETTLES (*Urtica dioica and urens*)

The young leaves of the stinging nettle, found everywhere, have special curative values. They are hematinic (increasing the hemoglobin of the blood) and have a high content of silicic acid.

Use: Take only the young, fresh, tender leaves, which can be found on every plant at different times of the season. They can be used for salads and cooked in the same way as spinach. Can also be employed as a flavoring herb in vegetable juices, with spinach and soups.

DILL (*Anethum graveolens*)

An herb of peculiarly pleasant, refreshing fragrance.

Use: With cucumber and potato salad, finely chopped. Mixed with butter it makes an excellent sandwich spread. Do not cook. It can be used with practically every type of dish, and is also good as an addition to other herbs. Use the feathery leaves. They lose much of their aroma when domestically dried but the flat seeds retain it. The latter can be used in the same way as caraway seeds, for instance, with potatoes. Use leaves fresh from June–November; at other times use green dried dill or seeds.

Cultivation: Dill is an annual and needs little care in a garden; seeds itself. Can also be cultivated in a window box.

TARRAGON (*Artemisia dracunculus*)

A very aromatic herb, especially popular in French cooking.

Use: With salads and raw vegetables, potatoes, herb mixtures and sauces. Better aroma when fresh than dried domestically.

Cultivation: Hardy perennial, 12–20 in. tall. Gather leaves before flowers appear (May–June). Grow from cuttings and plant in dry, sunny spot.

FENNEL (*Foeniculum vulgare*) AND SWEET or FLORENCE FENNEL (FINOCCHIO) (*Foeniculum dulce*)

Sweet Fennel is cultivated principally as a piquant-tasting vegetable.

Use: To give aroma to raw juices and salads. The feathery shoots (similar to dill), leaves and seeds, can also be used as a seasoning, for fennel sauce for instance, chopped finely. Young shoots of sweet fennel can be cooked as a vegetable (see Recipes Nos. 108 and 109).

Cultivation: The ordinary garden fennel will also grow as a perennial up to 2–4 ft. high. Never grow fennel and dill near to each other.

CHERVIL (*Anthriscus cerefolium*)
Pleasant-tasting, spicy, slightly sweet spring herb.
Use: Gather the leaves before the flowers open. Use freshly chopped with salads, raw vegetables, chervil soup, herb soups, sauces, spinach and herb sandwiches.
Cultivation: Grown as a summer annual. To ensure a regular supply throughout the summer begin sowing March–April as it seeds quickly and can only be used before the flowers appear. Can also be planted in a window box.

LOVAGE (*Levisticum officinale*)
Very powerful herb, therefore use sparingly and with care.
Use: Raw with salads and raw vegetables. Improves cooked vegetables, soups and stews, but do not use too often. Characteristic flavor.
Cultivation: Perennial; grows up to 6 ft. high. Plant in good soil in damp place. One plant is sufficient for one family for the whole year.

MARJORAM (*Origanum* [Wild or Pot] and *Marjorana hortensis*)
Has a strongly aromatic scent and taste. One of the best culinary herbs.
Use: With salads, raw vegetables, herb sauces, soups and rissoles. Must be used with care, since it easily overpowers the natural tastes of foods. Loses scarcely any of its aroma when dried.
Cultivation: Grows 12–15 in. high as an annual; has a strongly aromatic scent and taste. Needs sunny position in garden. Can also be cultivated in a window box.

LEMON BALM (*Melissa officinalis*)
The leaves impart a delicate, lemon-like scent and slightly bitter flavor.
Use: With salads, especially lettuce, raw vegetables and various cooked foods.
Cultivation: A perennial; needs little care and seeds itself.

PARSLEY (*Petroselinum sativum or crispum*)
Pleasant, strongly aromatic scent and flavor. There are varieties with curly leaves and with plain leaves, and Hamburg Parsley with thick roots. The last is used as an aromatic vegetable alone, or as an excellent seasoning with other vegetables, particularly in soups.

Use: Leaves with all herb mixtures, salads, soups, vegetables, potatoes and sauces. Grated roots and leaves with raw salads.

Cultivation: Biennial, needs good soil. The roots can be harvested in the second year before the plant flowers.

MINT (SPEARMINT) (*Mentha spicata*) or PEPPERMINT (*Mentha piperita*)

The different varieties of mint are used for many flavoring purposes and sprigs of fresh mint also make a refreshing summer tea. Peppermint is not only used as an excellent hot beverage (see Herbal Teas, pp. 219–20), but also as a strong, pleasantly piquant herb for seasoning. The first taste is mildly burning, followed by a cooling, agreeable one. Leaves of the curly mint (*Metha crispa*) can be used in the same way.

Use of mint: With salads, herb sandwiches, peas, new potatoes, spinach.

Use of peppermint: Fresh leaves with all dishes mentioned above, dried leaves for peppermint tea.

SALAD BURNET (*Poterium sanguisorba*)

Herb with cucumber-like flavor, with round, pinnate leaves.

Use: With salads, herb mixtures, soups, vegetables, especially in combination with parsley and lovage.

Cultivation: Grows 12–20 in. high. Plant in sunny position or can be cultivated in a window box.

ROSEMARY (*Rosmarinus officinalis*)

Penetrating, somewhat camphorous scent, and spicy, bitter taste. Shrub with thick, needle-shaped leaves.

Use: With risotto, baked potatoes, vegetable broth and raw vegetable juice. Powdered rosemary can be used in small quantities in salads and cooked vegetables. Use sparingly.

Cultivation: Perennial but not hardy. Grows up to 6 ft. high. Can be brought into the house in winter and planted out in summer.

SAGE (*Salvia officinalis*)

Herb with bitter, astringent taste and camphorous smell.

Use: With spinach, soup, pancakes and rissoles. Also sage fritters in batter.

Cultivation: Grows as a small shrub up to 28 in. high. Hardy perennial and is easy to grow. Can be cultivated in a window box.

CHIVES (*Allium schoenoprasum*)

A useful herb for those who do not like strong onion flavors.

Use: With salads and raw vegetables, soups, potatoes, vegetables, sauces, pancakes, cream cheese, bread and butter. Can be used frequently and in large quantities.

Cultivation: Hardy perennial. Clumps should be divided in the second year. The flowering stems should be removed because only the leaves are wanted. Can also be cultivated in a window box. Not suitable for domestic drying.

THYME (*Thymus vulgaris*)

Strong, aromatic fragrance with a camphorous flavor. A low, plant-like shrub, cultivated in gardens. Wild thyme can be used in similar ways.

Use: With salads, raw and cooked vegetables, soups (bean soup), stuffings. Excellent when mixed with marjoram. Use in moderation.

Cultivation: Perennial, cultivated in garden or in a pot. Needs a dry, sunny position.

CARAWAY (*Carum carvi*)

Seeds, leaves and roots. Grows up to 3 ft., 4 in. high, with tap root.

Use: Young leaves and roots, in the same way as seeds, with salads, vegetables, herb soups, potatoes, special caraway dishes, all cabbage dishes. Specially good with Browned Wholewheat Soup (Recipe No. 78), long radishes and sauerkraut.

Note: In Switzerland caraway seeds are exclusively used for savory dishes and are considered a good aid to the digestion of, for example, cabbage dishes, because of their antiflatulent properties.

ANISE SEEDS (*Pimpinella anisum*)

Seeds have a pleasant, sweetish, spicy taste.

Use: With salads, carrots, bread, biscuits, plum and pear preserves.

ONION (*Allium cepa*)

The onion can be used—finely chopped—in a number of ways with salads, vegetables, potatoes, soups, sauces or as a vegetable. When fried they are a good basis for many vegetable dishes, etc., also vegetable broth. Chopped onions, mixed with tomatoes, bread and oil, make a tasty stuffing.

The chopped green of the onion, especially of the scallion, makes an excellent flavoring and can be used fried as a basis for many dishes and soups.

HORSERADISH (*Cochlearia armoracia*)

Raw horseradish root can be grated and added sparingly to salad dressings and other sauces or be made into sandwich spreads. If other herbs are used at the same time, horseradish enhances the taste of the mixture.

GARLIC (*Allium sativum*)

The strong smell moderates if parsley or grated apples are served at the same time. Can be used to rub round the salad bowl; excellent for seasoning many vegetable dishes, such as spinach and particularly bean dishes. Use sparingly.

No exact directions can be given as to the quantities of culinary herbs to be used. A sense of taste for herbal flavorings will gradually develop and improve with experience. The use of herbs, in fact, provides an excellent opportunity for developing a sensitive and discriminating palate.

HERB TEAS

We have tested, approved and frequently served the following kinds of Herb Tea at our Clinic.

Use approximately 1 teasp. of dried herbs per cup unless stated otherwise.

422 BITTER TEA   422

Wormwood (*Artemisia absinthium*)⎫
Centaury (*Centaurium umbellatum*) ⎬in equal parts
Blessed Thistle (*Cnicus benedictus*)⎭

Pour boiling water over herbs, allow to steep for 5 min. Strain. In the case of a poor appetite: drink 2–3 tablesp. of this tea half an hour before meals; mild cholagogue, i.e. increases flow of bile. For people with delicate constitutions use centaury only.

423 SEED TEA (carminative, i.e. anti-flatulent)   423

Caraway (*Carum Carvi*)   ⎫
Fennel (*Foeniculum vulgare*)   ⎬in equal parts
Anise (*Pimpinella anisum*)   ⎭

Pour boiling water over seeds, allow to steep for 20 min. Strain. In the case of flatulence: drink 1 cupful after meals.

424 CHAMOMILE TEA (*Matricaria chamomilla*)   424

Pour boiling water over dried flowerheads; allow to steep for 3–5 minutes. Strain.

In the case of colic drink as an infusion: has a cleansing and soothing action on the gastro-intestinal tract; as mouthwash after extraction, etc.; also used for enemas and lavages.

425 PEPPERMINT TEA (*Mentha piperita*)   425

Pour boiling water over dried leaves; allow to steep for 3–5 minutes. Strain.
Sedative, cholagogue, i.e. increases flow of bile.

426 VERBENA TEA (*Verbena officinalis*)   426

LEMON VERBENA TEA (*Lippia citriodora*)

Pour boiling water over dried herb; allow to steep for 3–5 min. Strain.
Sedative, mucolytic, choleratic. Very popular in France, where it is drunk like ordinary tea.

427 LINSEED TEA   427

1 tablesp. linseed to 2½ cups water.
Boil 7–10 min., allow to draw for a few minutes. Strain. Mucolytic, mildly purgative.

428 LADY'S MANTLE (*Alchemilla vulgaris*)   428

Pour boiling water over dried or fresh herb, allow to steep for 10 min. Strain.

429 SOLIDAGO (GOLDEN ROD) (*Solidago virgaurea*).   429

Either dry the upper part of the herb in flower and break apart, or buy the tea ready prepared. Boil for 1 minute, allow to steep 10 min. Strain. Use in cases of dropsy, inflammation of bladder and kidneys. Diuretic. 2–3 cups daily.

430 HORSETAIL TEA (*Equisetum arvense*)   430

Soak 1 teasp. per cup for several hours; then boil the herb in the soaking water for 10–15 minutes and allow to steep for another 10–15 minutes. Strain.
Rich in silicic acid, diuretic. Can also be used to bathe rims of eyelids in cases of irritation.

431 ROSE HIP TEA (*Rosa canina, etc.*)   431

Soak 2–3 tablesp. rose hips (pods and seeds in balanced proportion) in 3¾ pt. water for 12 hr. Simmer 30–40 min. Strain.
Mildly stimulates the flow of bile, diuretic.

Note: All the above teas should preferably be drunk without sugar, or sweetened only with honey or brown sugar.

SOPORIFIC TEAS
(for inducing good sleep)

432 LEMON PEEL TEA (peel of 1 lemon for 2 cups of tea)　432

Wash and dry the lemon well. Pare outer yellow skin with potato peeler. Pour boiling water over this, allow to steep for 5 minutes. Strain. Add a little honey or brown sugar. Drink before going to sleep.

433 RED BERGAMOT (Gold Melissa) *Monarda didyma*　433

Pour boiling water over herb, allow to steep for 5 min. Strain. Sweeten with brown sugar or honey if desired. Drink before going to sleep.

434 ORANGE BLOSSOM　434

Boil 2–3 blossoms for 2–3 min. in 2 cups of water. Allow to steep for a few min. Strain. Sweeten with brown sugar or honey. Drink before going to sleep.

3. NORMAL BIRCHER-BENNER DIET: FULL DIET

FOR THE HEALTHY

The Bircher-Benner diet was intended by its originator for two purposes. First, to provide wholesome and protective nourishment for normal healthy people, to build up strong children full of vitality, and to retain energy and active functioning of all faculties until old age. Secondly, to use it for therapeutic purposes, in cases of general debility or convalescence, and for the treatment of special diseases and conditions—in fact, as a diet-therapy.

For the normal diet for healthy people menus for varying economic and social conditions are given below. For each month sixteen EVERYDAY MENUS for the main meal such as are served in our Clinic on the 'full diet,' are printed opposite six ECONOMICAL MENUS for the main meal (preferably the midday meal). These last comprise six well-thought-out combinations of quickly prepared and thoroughly satisfying dishes, containing the desired equal proportion of raw and cooked foods, the latter mostly in the form of a main or casserole dish. Then follow four FESTIVE MENUS for each month for Sundays and special occasions, such as we at the Clinic serve at these times.

In addition to the everyday menus given in this section, a number of menus for LIGHT DIETS are included in Part III. Fruit, raw vegetables and wholewheat bread are served as in 'full diet' menus, but soup, vegetables, potatoes and cereal dishes are prepared in a slightly different way.

PLAN FOR A DAY'S MENU

We give here a brief summary of the menus for the two light meals of the day, breakfast and supper, supposing that the main meal can be taken at midday, which is always preferable from a dietetic point of view. If, however, the main meal has to be taken in the evening then lunch must be light. In any case, young children and old people should preferably have their light meal in the evening, possibly containing the second Muesli. The structure of these two light meals remains basically the same, though inside this framework variations, sometimes of a seasonal nature, are suggested.

Breakfast

1. Bircher Muesli (see Recipe Nos. 1 D–7 D).
2. Wholewheat bread and butter. (Nut butter is a good and easily digested substitute for those who do not like, or should not have, butter.)

    Instead of Muesli and bread and butter, fruit and a whole-grain cereal with cream or yogurt may be given.
3. Nuts, ground or whole.
4. Weak tea or Herb Tea (rose hip, mint, or peppermint, Melissa, blackberry leaf, etc., see p. 220), sweetened with brown sugar or honey.

    Or milk (if possible, unpasteurized tuberculin tested milk).

Those in good health who cannot do without coffee should take a good coffee substitute, e.g., malt, fig or dandelion coffee, together with milk.

Evening Meal

It is advisable to have this meal early in the evening, if possible between 6:30 and 7:30 P.M., so that the digestive processes do not disturb the first important hours of sleep. For the same reason this meal is kept a simple one. Those who have a hard day's work behind them should eat something like the following for the last meal of the day:

1. Bircher Muesli *or* fruit with yogurt.
2. Cooked dish, such as: Potato dish with cheese salad, *or* a nourishing soup made according to one of our recipes, Nos. 60–96.
   Risotto of natural rice, No. 224, *or*
   Salad Niçoise, No. 185, with wholewheat bread and butter.
3. As a beverage we at the Clinic give an Herb Tea or rose hip tea, or a vegetable broth.

If, however, a delicate constitution or impaired functions have to be considered, then it is advisable to eat the same combination of dishes as for breakfast; perhaps adding a little soft or cream cheese. Dried fruit (if not treated with sulphur) and salads are also recommended. Honey or rose hip syrup or purée are valuable supplements to wholewheat bread.

The fundamental rule we so often stress applies here: begin every meal with raw food.

BEVERAGES

Hardly any thirst is felt if the meal begins with raw fruit, and little salt and no strong seasonings are used. Never drink without being thirsty! One glass or cup of some liquid sipped slowly is ample for each meal, and even this is not always necessary. In addition to freshly expressed fruit and vegetable juices and Herb Teas (see pp. 58–9, 214–5) we serve apple juice preserved by a cold process, and for festive occasions red and white grape juice. Black currant juice or syrup is specially rich in Vitamin C. Blueberry juice, made of fresh or dried berries, has a disinfectant effect on the intestines and is therefore valuable in cases of stomach upsets. Certain mineral waters and sea water (if available in bottled form) are also useful beverages.

4. MENUS FOR MANY OCCASIONS

JANUARY

Note: For Raw Salad recipes, see Nos. 8–39.

Everyday Menus	*Economical Menus*

FRUIT

RAW SALAD:
   cauliflower, tomatoes, lettuce

COOKED DISHES:
   Clear broth No. 50 D, with diced egg No. 57
   Leeks as a vegetable No. 166.
   Rice cakes Nos. 235, 236.

FRUIT

RAW SALAD:
   tomatoes, lettuce or watercress

COOKED DISHES:
   Rice with spinach No. 231 D.

FRUIT

RAW SALAD:
   black radishes, white cabbage, endives

COOKED DISHES:
   Chicory No. 103 D, potato balls No. 202 D

DESSERT:
   Apple tart No. 390

FRUIT

RAW SALAD:
   carrots, sauerkraut or white cabbage

COOKED DISHES:
   Minestrone No. 96, whole-wheat bread and cheese

FRUIT

RAW SALAD:
   celery, spinach, lettuce

COOKED DISHES:
   Spring soup No. 86 D, curly kale No. 158, spaghetti No. 254, with tomato sauce No. 303

FRUIT

RAW SALAD:
   beetroot, lettuce or watercress

COOKED DISHES:
   Potatoes and cream cheese No. 193 D.

FRUIT

RAW SALAD:
   chicory, tomatoes, carrots, lettuce

FRUIT

RAW SALAD:
   celery or celeriac, endives

Everyday Menus

COOKED DISHES:
Cauliflower soup No. 84,
dried beans No. 120, po-
tato salad Nos. 181, 182

FRUIT
RAW SALAD:
salsify, savoy, lettuce or
watercress
COOKED DISHES:
Mixed vegetables (carrots,
tomatoes, Brussels
sprouts, cauliflower)
No. 172, with wheat
cakes No. 280 and cran-
berries
DESSERT:
Cold banana sweet No. 364

FRUIT
RAW SALAD:
beetroot, sauerkraut or
white cabbage, endives
COOKED DISHES:
Rice soup No. 61 D to 64 D
Chinese artichokes with
sauce No. 173
Filbert potatoes No. 216

FRUIT
RAW SALAD:
black radishes, red cab-
bage, lettuce or water-
cress
COOKED DISHES:
Minestra No. 95 D,
spinach No. 97 to 100 D
Tomatoes No. 129 D with
noodles No. 254

Economical Menus

COOKED DISHES:
Fried potatoes No. 213 and
cream cheese No. 48b

FRUIT
RAW SALAD:
salsify, lettuce, cream
cheese with ryvita or
wholewheat rolls
COOKED DISHES:
Oat groats soup No. 71 D

FRUIT
RAW SALAD:
fennel, chicory or seakale
COOKED DISHES:
Macaroni au gratin No.
254(c)
DESSERT:
Apple whip No. 354

Everyday Menus	*Festive Menus for Special Occasions*

FRUIT
RAW SALAD:
  fennel, tomato, lettuce or
    watercress
COOKED DISHES:
  Browned wholewheat soup
    No. 78
  Stuffed cabbage leaves No.
    159
  Potatoes in cream sauce
    No. 198 D

FRUIT
RAW SALAD:
  beetroot, cauliflower, let-
    tuce or watercress
COOKED DISHES:
  Salsify or scorzonera with
    sauce No. 173
  Fried potatoes No. 213
DESSERT:
  Filbert whip No. 351

FRUIT
RAW SALAD:
  carrots decorated with
    finely chopped leeks,
    black radishes, lettuce
    or watercress
COOKED DISHES:
  Spinach soup No. 82 D
  Endives as a vegetable No.
    102 D
  Risotto No. 224

FRUIT
RAW SALAD:
  salsify, endives, lettuce or
    watercress
COOKED DISHES:
  Leek soup No. 87, carrots
    Nos. 111D–113
  Bread dumplings No. 277

FRUIT
RAW SALAD:
  beetroot, lettuce or water-
    cress
COOKED DISHES:
  Stuffed rolls No. 295
  chicory No. 103 D
  Lyons potatoes No. 214
DESSERT:
  Lemon whip Nos. 357, 358

FRUIT
RAW SALAD:
  carrots, sauerkraut or
    white cabbage, lettuce or
    watercress
COOKED DISHES:
  Cheese and tomato tartlets
    No. 296
  Endives as a vegetable No.
    102
  Potato snow No. 200 D
DESSERT:
  Apple purée with meringue
    No. 338

Everyday Menus	*Festive Menus for Special Occasions*

FRUIT
RAW SALAD:
  black radishes, cress, let-
  tuce or watercress
COOKED DISHES:
  Spinach Nos. 97–100 D
  Potatoes with cream
    cheese No. 193 D
DESSERT:
  Apple purée with caramel
    sugar No. 337 D

FRUIT
RAW SALAD:
  beetroot, spinach, endives
COOKED DISHES:
  Celeriac soup No. 83 D
  Sauerkraut or white cab-
    bage No. 161
  Spaetzle No. 263

FRUIT
RAW SALAD:
  cauliflower, cress, endives
COOKED DISHES:
  Spinach No. 97 to 100 D
    garnished with potatoes
    No. 192 D
  Macaroni timbale No. 257
    with tomato sauce Nos.
    303–306 D.
DESSERT:
  Almond flammeri No. 376
    D with raspberry syrup

FRUIT
RAW SALAD:
  fennel or celery garnished
    with carrots, lettuce
COOKED DISHES:
  Chopped cabbage No. 157
  French fried potatoes No.
    218
DESSERT:
  Almond slices No. 385
    with apricot sauce

FRUIT
RAW SALAD:
  tomatoes, savoy, lettuce

FRUIT
RAW SALAD:
  celery or celeriac, toma-
    toes, lettuce or water-
    cress

Everyday Menus

COOKED DISHES:
Clear broth No. 51 D with
caraway fingers No. 291
Brussels sprouts No. 155
Chestnuts No. 168

FRUIT
RAW SALAD:
salsify, chicory, lettuce or
watercress
COOKED DISHES:
Clear rice soup No. 61 D
carrots No. 112
Spinach omelette No. 272

Festive Menus for Special Occasions

COOKED DISHES:
Vol-au-vent No. 293 with
dumplings No. 52
Mushrooms and mush-
room sauce No. 311
Brussels sprouts No. 155
Duchess potatoes No. 206
DESSERT:
Bavarian orange whip No.
360

FEBRUARY

Everyday Menus

FRUIT
RAW SALAD:
celery or celeriac, toma-
toes, lettuce or water-
cress
COOKED DISHES:
Potato and leek soup No.
90
Red cabbage with apples
No. 162
Farina gnocchi No. 239

FRUIT
RAW SALAD:
beetroot, cress, lettuce or
watercress
COOKED DISHES:
Spinach Nos. 97–100 D
Potatoes with cream
cheese No. 193 D.
DESSERT:
Apple strudel No. 399

Economical Menus

FRUIT
RAW SALAD:
carrots, spinach or Brus-
sels sprouts
COOKED DISHES:
Tapioca soup No. 60 D
Spaghetti with tomato
sauce No. 254 (c)

FRUIT
RAW SALAD:
cauliflower, lettuce
COOKED DISHES:
Millotto No. 247 D
DESSERT:
Apple purée No. 338

Everyday Menus

FRUIT
RAW SALAD:
  cauliflower, carrots, en-
    dives
COOKED DISHES:
  Barley soup No. 72 D
  Salsify in sauce No. 124 D
  Lyons potatoes No. 214

FRUIT
RAW SALAD:
  black radishes or carrots or
    turnips, chicory, lettuce
    or watercress
COOKED DISHES:
  Oatmeal soup No. 69 D
  Brussels sprouts No. 155
  Potato cakes No. 203

FRUIT
RAW SALAD:
  tomatoes, fennel or chic-
    ory, lettuce
COOKED DISHES:
  Celeriac slices No. 123
  Japanese rice No. 223 D
DESSERT:
  Hot almond pudding No.
    377 with wine sauce No.
    368 D

FRUIT
RAW SALAD:
  celery or celeriac, spinach
    lettuce or watercress
COOKED DISHES:
  Golden cubes No. 59, soup
    No. 51
  Tomatoes as a vegetable
    No. 129 D
  Millotto No. 247 D.

Economical Menus

FRUIT
RAW SALAD:
  tomatoes, lettuce or water-
    cress
COOKED DISHES:
  Clear vegetable broth No.
    51 D
  Potato cakes (rissoles)
    No. 203

FRUIT
RAW SALAD:
  celery or celeriac, endives
COOKED DISHES:
  Cauliflower with Béchamel
    sauce No. 173
  Caraway potatoes No.
    194 D

FRUIT
RAW SALAD:
  beetroot, sauerkraut or
    white cabbage, lettuce
    or watercress
COOKED DISHES:
  Bread soup No. 76
DESSERT:
  Caramel No. 347

FRUIT
RAW SALAD:
  savoy, fennel or celery
COOKED DISHES:
  Risotto No. 224 and baked
    tomatoes with parsley
    and onions No. 130 D.

Everyday Menus	*Festive Menus for Special Occasions*

FRUIT
RAW SALAD:
    carrots, chicory, endives
COOKED DISHES:
    Vegetable rice soup No. 63 D
    Cauliflower au gratin No. 173
    French fried potatoes No. 218

FRUIT
RAW SALAD:
    salsify, red cabbage, lettuce or watercress
COOKED DISHES:
    Spinach Nos. 97–100 D
    Rice creole No. 226 D
DESSERT:
    Savarin with fruit salad No. 405

FRUIT
RAW SALAD:
    tomatoes, endives, chicory
COOKED DISHES:
    Cheese patties No. 285
    Fennel or celery au gratin No. 173
    Mashed potatoes No. 201 D
DESSERT:
    Apple pudding No. 380

FRUIT
RAW SALAD:
    black radishes or carrots, cress, lettuce or watercress
COOKED DISHES:
    Carrot soup No. 81 D
    Celery No. 107 D or 110 D
    Sweet corn cakes Nos. 245–6

FRUIT
RAW SALAD:
    celery or celeriac, tomatoes, lettuce or watercress
COOKED DISHES:
    Barley soup No. 72 D
    Fennel or chicory No. 108 D and 103 D
    Potato balls No. 202 D

FRUIT
RAW SALAD:
    black radishes or carrots, beetroot, lettuce or watercress
COOKED DISHES:
    Vegetable cutlets No. 276
    Salsify in sauce No. 124 D
    Filbert potatoes No. 216
DESSERT:
    Rice pudding with pineapple No. 374

Everyday Menus	*Festive Menus for Special Occasions*

FRUIT

RAW SALAD:
  cauliflower, endives, lettuce or watercress

COOKED DISHES:
  Chopped savoy No. 157
  Farmer's omelette No. 271

DESSERT:
  Apples en robe de chambre No 400

FRUIT

RAW SALAD:
  beetroot, sauerkraut or white cabbage
  lettuce or watercress

COOKED DISHES:
  Minestra No. 95 D
  Spinach pudding No. 274 with caper sauce No. 302
  Potatoes cooked in vegetable stock No. 195 D

FRUIT

RAW SALAD:
  carrots, fennel or chicory, lettuce or watercress

COOKED DISHES:
  Tomato soup No. 79 or 80 D
  Salsify in sauce No. 124 D
  Caraway potatoes No. 194 D

FRUIT

RAW SALAD:
  black radishes or carrots, cress, lettuce or watercress

FRUIT

RAW SALAD:
  celery or celeriac, chicory, endives

COOKED DISHES:
  Omelettes with spinach No. 272
  Brussels sprouts No. 155 with potatoes cooked in vegetable stock No. 195 D

DESSERT:
  Caramel pears No. 347

Everyday Menus	*Festive Menus for Special Occasions*

COOKED DISHES:
Lettuce as a vegetable No.
101 D
Risotto No. 244
DESSERT:
Apple fritters No. 404

FRUIT
RAW SALAD:
salsify, red cabbage,
lettuce or watercress
COOKED DISHES:
Tapioca soup No. 60 D
Dried beans No. 120
Potato salad Nos. 181, 182

FRUIT
RAW SALAD:
salsify, spinach, lettuce
COOKED DISHES:
Turkish rice No. 233
Cauliflower No. 153
Castle potatoes No. 217
DESSERT:
Apricots with cream

MARCH

Everyday Menus	*Economical Menus*

FRUIT
RAW SALAD:
beetroot, sauerkraut or
white cabbage, lettuce
COOKED DISHES:
Potato soup No. 89 D
Spinach Nos. 97–100 D
Onion tart No. 288

FRUIT
RAW SALAD:
chicory or celery, toma-
toes, lettuce, or water-
cress mixed
COOKED DISHES:
Rice pudding and stewed
damsons or rhubarb No.
372 D

FRUIT
RAW SALAD:
salsify, fennel or chicory,
lettuce
COOKED DISHES:
Chicory, No. 103 D
Risotto No. 224 with to-
mato sauce Nos. 303–
306 D

FRUIT
RAW SALAD:
carrots, dandelion or
watercress
COOKED DISHES:
Beetroot as a vegetable
No 126 D
Fried potatoes No. 213

FRUIT
RAW SALAD:
celery or celeriac, chicory,
carrots, lettuce

FRUIT
RAW SALAD:
lettuce or watercress

Everyday Menus

COOKED DISHES:
Farina soup No. 74 D
Potatoes in their skins No.
191 with cheese and let-
tuce

FRUIT
RAW SALAD:
carrots, cress, lettuce
COOKED DISHES:
Clear soup No. 51 D with
pancake strips No. 55
Brussels sprouts No. 155
Potato cakes No. 203

FRUIT
RAW SALAD:
stuffed tomatoes with
white cabbage and let-
tuce
COOKED DISHES:
Carrots Nos. 111 D–113
Cheese patties No. 285
DESSERT:
Orange whip Nos. 359–
360

FRUIT
RAW SALAD:
cauliflower, spinach, en-
dives
COOKED DISHES:
Oatmeal soup No. 69 D
Chopped cabbage No. 157
Spaghetti with tomato
sauce No. 254 (c)

FRUIT
RAW SALAD:
black radishes or carrots,
lettuce, tomatoes
COOKED DISHES:
Browned wholewheat soup
No. 78
Lettuce as a vegetable No.
101 D
Filbert potatoes No. 216

Economical Menus

COOKED DISHES:
Potato salad Nos. 181, 182
Cooked carrots No. 111 D–
113, garnished with
boiled eggs
Swiss or Cheddar cheese
wholewheat bread
FRUIT
RAW SALAD:
black radishes or carrots
or turnips, lettuce
COOKED DISHES:
Vegetable soup or Mine-
strone No. 96
Farina pudding No. 237 D

FRUIT
RAW SALAD:
celery or celeriac, endives
COOKED DISHES:
Cheese tart No. 286

FRUIT
RAW SALAD:
beetroot, sauerkraut or
white cabbage
COOKED DISHES:
Purée of split peas gar-
nished with diced to-
matoes No. 169

Everyday Menus	*Festive Menus for Special Occasions*

FRUIT
RAW SALAD:
  salsify, lettuce
COOKED DISHES:
  Stuffed beetroot No. 127
    and herb sauce No. 301
  Potatoes cooked in vege-
    table broth No. 195 D
DESSERT:
  Pineapple slices No. 388

FRUIT
RAW SALAD:
  radishes, cauliflower, en-
    dives
COOKED DISHES:
  Mushroom croûtes No. 281
  Lettuce as a vegetable No.
    101 D
  Noodles Nos. 254, 259,
    260
DESSERT:
  Raspberry sweet (frozen
    raspberries) No. 353

FRUIT
RAW SALAD:
  tomatoes, celery or chic-
    ory, lettuce
COOKED DISHES:
  Bread dumpling soup Nos.
    51 D, 179
  Cabbage No. 156
  Mashed potatoes No.
    201 D

FRUIT
RAW SALAD:
  salsify or carrot, dandelion
    or watercress, lettuce
COOKED DISHES:
  Spring soup No. 86 D
  Lettuce as a vegetable
    No. 101 D
  Sweet corn cakes with
    cheese Nos. 245, 246

FRUIT
RAW SALAD:
  salsify or carrots, spinach,
    lettuce or watercress
COOKED DISHES:
  Cheese soufflé No. 283
  Carrots in a sauce
    Nos. 112, 113
  Potato snow No. 200 D
DESSERT:
  Apple halves with jelly
    No. 340 D and vanilla
    sauce No. 366

FRUIT
RAW SALAD:
  celery or celeriac, cress,
    lettuce

Everyday Menus	*Festive Menus for Special Occasions*

COOKED DISHES:
  Salsify with sauce No.
   124 D
  Lyons potatoes No. 214
DESSERT:
  Chestnut cream cake No.
   412

FRUIT
RAW SALAD:
  black radishes, carrots or
   turnips, tomatoes, en-
   dives
COOKED DISHES:
  Vegetable soup (sieved)
   No. 96
  Cauliflower au gratin No.
   173
  Caraway potatoes No.
   194 D

FRUIT
RAW SALAD:
  kohlrabi or turnips,
   chicory, diced tomatoes,
   lettuce
COOKED DISHES:
  Carrot soup No. 81 D
  Fennel Nos. 108 D, 109 or
   celery No. 107 D or leeks
   No. 166
  Noodles No. 254

FRUIT
RAW SALAD:
  beetroot, sauerkraut or
   white cabbage, endives
COOKED DISHES:
  Turkish rice No. 233
  Spinach Nos. 97–100 D
   with French fried pota-
   toes No. 218
DESSERT:
  Fruit salad and cream No.
   334 D

FRUIT
RAW SALAD:
  cauliflower, chicory
COOKED DISHES:
  Globe artichokes No. 148
   D or celery No. 107 D or
   celeriac with sauce Hol-
   landaise No. 123 or au
   gratin No. 173
  Princess potatoes No 212
   with raw lettuce
DESSERT:
  Red currant jelly No. 336 D

Everyday Menus

FRUIT
RAW SALAD:
  salsify or beetroot, cress,
  lettuce
COOKED DISHES:
  Rice soup Nos. 61 D–64 D
  Spinach Nos. 97–100 D
  Omelette No. 268

Festive Menus for Special Occasions

FRUIT
RAW SALAD:
  lettuce garnished with to-
  matoes
COOKED DISHES:
  Globe artichokes with
  sauce Hollandaise No.
  148 D
  Rice ring No. 234 D with
  tomatoes as a vegetable
  No. 129 D
DESSERT:
  Fruit and cream dish No.
  344

APRIL

Everyday Menus

FRUIT
RAW SALAD:
  celeriac or chicory, cress,
  lettuce
COOKED DISHES:
  Farina soup No. 74 D
  Spinach Nos. 97 D–100 D
  garnished with
  caraway fingers No. 291
  Potatoes cooked in vegetable stock No. 195 D

FRUIT
RAW SALAD:
  beetroot, sauerkraut or
  white cabbage, lettuce
COOKED DISHES:
  Carrots with pearl onions
  in No. 117
  Risotto No. 224
  Cream cheese turnovers
  No. 408
FRUIT
RAW SALAD:
  radishes, fennel or chicory,
  endives

Economical Menus

FRUIT
RAW SALAD:
  carrots and fennel or
  chicory mixed
COOKED DISHES:
  Minestrone No. 96
  Cheese, wholewheat bread
  and lettuce

FRUIT
RAW SALAD:
  beetroot, lettuce
COOKED DISHES:
  Clear broth No. 51 D
  Caraway potatoes No. 194
  D or baked potatoes No.
  192 D and cream cheese
  No. 48*b*

FRUIT
RAW SALAD:
  tomatoes and dandelion or
  cabbage

Everyday Menus

COOKED DISHES:
Cheese soup No. 77
Lettuce as a vegetable No.
101 D
Potato cakes No. 203

FRUIT
RAW SALAD:
carrots, cauliflower, let-
tuce
COOKED DISHES:
Vegetable soup No. 96
Spinach beet stalks No.
105 D, 106 with
Remoulade sauce No.
320
Browned potatoes No.
211 D

FRUIT
RAW SALAD:
fennel or chicory, red or
white cabbage, lettuce
COOKED DISHES:
Mixed vegetable platter
(lettuce as a vegetable
No. 101 D, cauliflower
No. 153, carrots Nos.
111 D–113, tomatoes
No. 129 D)
Rolled oat cakes No. 279
DESSERT:
Apple whip No. 354

FRUIT
RAW SALAD:
carrots, spring cabbage,
lettuce
COOKED DISHES:
Clear broth No. 51 D with
dumplings No. 52
Fennel Nos. 108 D, 109 or
chicory No. 103 D or
celery No. 107 D

Economical Menus

COOKED DISHES:
Browned wholewheat soup
No. 78
Spinach Nos. 97–100 D
with potatoes cooked in
vegetable stock No.
195 D

FRUIT
RAW SALAD:
black radishes, carrots or
turnips, lettuce
COOKED DISHES:
Sauerkraut or cooked cab-
bage No. 161
Bread dumpling No. 277

FRUIT
RAW SALAD:
celeriac or chicory, lettuce
COOKED DISHES:
Polenta with cheese No.
243 D
Carrots Nos. 111 D–113

FRUIT
RAW SALAD:
turnips, tomatoes
COOKED DISHES:
Barley soup No. 72 D
Fried potatoes No. 213 or
218 and lettuce as a
vegetable No. 101 D

Everyday Menus	*Festive Menus for Special Occasions*

FRUIT

RAW SALAD:
  tomatoes, dandelion, lettuce

COOKED DISHES:
  Barley soup No. 72 D
  Red cabbage No. 162 or white cabbage No. 156
  Mashed potato balls No. 202 D

FRUIT

RAW SALAD:
  salsify or carrots, spinach, lettuce

COOKED DISHES:
  Celeriac as a vegetable No. 121
  Spinach noodles with tomato sauce No. 258 D

DESSERT:
  Filbert whip No. 351

FRUIT

RAW SALAD:
  beetroot, cress, lettuce

COOKED DISHES:
  Macaroni timbale with tomato sauce No. 257
  Spinach Nos. 97–100 D
  Castle potatoes No. 217

DESSERT:
  Chaudeau and biscuits No. 362

FRUIT

RAW SALAD:
  cabbage, cucumber, lettuce

COOKED DISHES:
  Tomato soup Nos. 79, 80 D
  Lentils No. 170
  Potato salad Nos. 181, 182

FRUIT

RAW SALAD:
  radishes, tomatoes, lettuce

COOKED DISHES:
  Chervil No. 85 D or any herb soup No. 66a D
  Chicory No. 103 D
  Mashed potatoes No. 201 D

FRUIT

RAW SALAD:
  beetroot, tomatoes, lettuce

COOKED DISHES:
  Potato cakes No. 203 with spinach Nos. 97–100 D
  Rice ring No. 234 D with carrots and peas No. 114 D

DESSERT:
  Rhubarb whip with wafers No. 355

Everyday Menus

FRUIT

RAW SALAD:
cauliflower, spinach, lettuce

COOKED DISHES:
Globe artichokes with vinaigrette sauce No. 148 D
Rice ring with tomatoes as a vegetable No. 234 D

DESSERT:
Orange shapes No. 361 D

FRUIT

RAW SALAD:
beetroot, spring cabbage, lettuce

COOKED DISHES:
Spring soup No. 86
Fennel Nos. 108 D, 109 or chicory No. 103 D or celery hearts No. 107 D
Millotto No. 247

FRUIT

RAW SALAD:
cress, tomatoes, radishes or carrots, cooked beetroot

COOKED DISHES:
Vermicelli soup No. 51 D
Various cheeses with potatoes in their jackets No. 192 D

FRUIT

RAW SALAD:
carrots, zucchini, lettuce

COOKED DISHES:
Lettuce as a vegetable No. 101 D
Noodles au gratin No. 254 or 256

DESSERT:
Almond slices with apricot sauce No. 385

Festive Menus for Special Occasions

Easter Menu

FRUIT
Grapefruit

RAW SALAD:
Russian salad, with vegetable aspic, garnished with eggs and tomatoes, lettuce

COOKED DISHES:
Lettuce as a vegetable No. 101 D with browned potatoes No. 211 D

DESSERT:
Strawberries and cream No. 343 D

Everyday Menus

FRUIT
RAW SALAD:
  carrots, cress, lettuce
COOKED DISHES:
  Spring soup No. 86 D
  Peas No. 115 D
  Parisian gnocchi No. 275

Festive Menus for Special Occasions

FRUIT
RAW SALAD:
  radishes, cauliflower, lettuce
COOKED DISHES:
  Cream patties No. 284
  Sugar-peas (edible-podded),
    young peas or any available young vegetable
    No. 118 on fried bread
  Potato snow No. 200 D
DESSERT:
  Pineapple slices No. 388

MAY

Everyday Menus

FRUIT
RAW SALAD:
  radishes, lettuce
COOKED DISHES:
  Spinach soup No. 82 D
  Zucchini with tomatoes
    No. 137
  Risotto No. 224

FRUIT
RAW SALAD:
  radishes, cauliflower, lettuce
COOKED DISHES:
  Sugar-peas (edible-podded
    young peas) No. 118,
    croûtes No. 282
  Potato salad Nos. 181, 182
DESSERT:
  Rhubarb tart No. 394

FRUIT
RAW SALAD:
  beetroot, zucchini, lettuce

Economical Menus

FRUIT
RAW SALAD:
  tomatoes stuffed with celeriac or turnips, lettuce
COOKED DISHES:
  Onion tart No. 288

FRUIT
SALAD:
  Salad Niçoise (radishes,
    tomatoes, lettuce, potatoes, egg) No. 185 D
COOKED DISH:
  Pea soup No. 94

FRUIT
RAW SALAD:
  beetroot, zucchini or tomatoes, lettuce

Everyday Menus

COOKED DISHES:
Broth No. 51 D with caraway fingers No. 291
Cauliflower with sauce No. 153
Potatoes with chives No. 196

FRUIT
RAW SALAD:
carrots, cabbage, lettuce
COOKED DISHES:
Barley soup No. 72 D
Broccoli with sauce as in No. 153
French fried potatoes No. 218

FRUIT
RAW SALAD:
cress garnished with radishes, lettuce
COOKED DISHES:
Stuffed tomatoes Nos. 132, 133 D
Noodles No. 254
Strawberries and cream No. 343 D

FRUIT
RAW SALAD:
beetroot, cauliflower, lettuce
COOKED DISHES:
Potato and leek soup No. 90
Lettuce as a vegetable No. 101 D
Cheese croûtes No. 282

Everyday Menus

FRUIT
RAW SALAD:
radishes, carrots or turnips, tomatoes, lettuce

Economical Menus

COOKED DISHES:
Spring soup No. 86 D
Lyons potatoes No. 214

FRUIT
RAW SALAD:
fennel or chicory, carrots, lettuce
COOKED DISH:
Tomato-rice No. 227 D

FRUIT
RAW SALAD:
tomatoes and lettuce
COOKED DISHES:
Millotto No. 247 or 248 D
DESSERT:
Fruit salad and cream No. 334 D

FRUIT
RAW SALAD:
black radishes, carrots or turnips, lettuce
COOKED DISHES:
Macaroni soufflé No. 256

Festive Menus for Special Occasions

| *Everyday Menus* | *Festive Menus for Special Occasions* |

COOKED DISHES:
  Oat soup No. 69 D
  Cabbage No. 156
  Potatoes and cream cheese
    No. 193 D

FRUIT
RAW SALAD:
  carrots, cress, lettuce
COOKED DISHES:
  Carrots and peas No. 114 D
  Filbert potatoes No. 216
DESSERT:
  Farina pudding with
    strawberry or black cur-
    rant sauce No. 371 D

FRUIT
RAW SALAD:
  zucchini, cucumber, let-
    tuce
COOKED DISHES:
  Tomato soup Nos. 79, 80 D
  Spinach Nos. 97–100 D
  Bread and Egg Dish No.
    278

FRUIT
RAW SALAD:
  radishes, spinach, lettuce
COOKED DISHES:
  Herb soup No. 66 *a* D
  Red or white cabbage No.
    162 or 156
  Spaetzle fried with bread-
    crumbs No. 263

FRUIT
RAW SALAD:
  stuffed tomatoes with
    cauliflower, cress, let-
    tuce
COOKED DISHES:
  Ravioli No. 262 and let-
    tuce
  Peas No. 115 D
  Castle potatoes No. 217
DESSERT:
  Lemon whip and wafers
    Nos. 357 and 358

FRUIT
RAW SALAD:
  beetroot garnished with
    olives, sauerkraut or
    white cabbage, lettuce
COOKED DISHES:
  Asparagus with sauce Hol-
    landaise No. 151 D
  Cauliflower polonaise No.
    153
  Parsley potatoes No. 196 D
DESSERT:
  Apple Strudel No. 399

| *Everyday Menus* | *Festive Menus for Special Occasions* |

FRUIT
RAW SALAD:
  carrots, fennel or chicory,
    lettuce
COOKED DISHES:
  Beans Nos. 119, 120
  Lyons potatoes No. 214
DESSERT:
  Rhubarb whip with wafers
    No. 355

FRUIT
RAW SALAD:
  beetroot, cucumber, let-
    tuce
COOKED DISHES
  Cheese soup No. 77
  Spinach beet stalks No.
    105 D or asparagus with
    remoulade sauce No.
    151 D and No. 320
  Potatoes cooked in vegeta-
    ble stock No. 195 D

FRUIT
RAW SALAD:
  radishes, cauliflower, let-
    tuce
COOKED DISHES:
  Oatmeal or flake soup Nos.
    68 D, 69 D
  Carrots Nos. 111 D, 112
  Spinach pudding No. 274
    with caper sauce No.
    302 or herb sauce No.
    301

FRUIT
RAW SALAD:
  zucchini, chicory, lettuce
COOKED DISHES:
  Celery hearts as a vegeta-
    ble No. 107 D or 173
  Rice with tomatoes No.
    227 D

FRUIT
RAW SALAD:
  salsify or scorzonera, let-
    tuce
COOKED DISHES:
  Vegetables served in shells
    No. 175 D
  Rice ring and tomatoes as
    a vegetable No. 234 D
DESSERT:
  Strawberry whip and wa-
    fers No. 353

243

Everyday Menus

DESSERT:
Almond flammeri No. 376 D

FRUIT
RAW SALAD:
carrots, cucumbers, lettuce
COOKED DISHES:
Clear broth No. 51 D with pancake strips No. 55
Zucchini Nos. 136 D, 137 or eggplant Nos. 145 D–147
Caraway potatoes No. 194 D with herb sauce No. 301

Festive Menus for Special Occasions

FRUIT
RAW SALAD:
radishes, chicory, lettuce Russian salad
COOKED DISHES:
Spinach pudding No. 274 and tomato Nos. 303–316 or herb sauce No. 301
Frozen beans No. 119
DESSERT:
Meringues. See No. 338

JUNE

Everyday Menus

FRUIT
RAW SALAD:
beetroot, squash or zucchini, lettuce, turnip

COOKED DISHES:
Bread soup No. 76
Carrots Nos. 111 D–113
Potato pudding No. 204

FRUIT
RAW SALAD:
carrots, red peppers, lettuce
COOKED DISHES:
Potato soup No. 89 D
Rice cakes with spinach No. 236

FRUIT
RAW SALAD:
cress garnished with radishes, cucumber, lettuce

Economical Menus

FRUIT
RAW SALAD:
Radishes, cress

COOKED DISHES:
Sugar-peas (edible-podded young peas) No. 118
French fried potatoes No. 218

FRUIT
RAW SALAD:
carrots, lettuce, turnips
COOKED DISHES:
Chervil soup No. 85 D
DESSERT:
Lemon soufflé No. 383

FRUIT
RAW SALAD:
Tomatoes and spinach
COOKED DISHES:
Turkish rice No. 233

Everyday Menus   *Economical Menus*

COOKED DISHES:
Peperonata No. 144 D
Spaghetti à la napolitaine
(with tomato sauce) No.
254
DESSERT:
Strawberry slices. See No.
388

FRUIT
RAW SALAD:
tomatoes, cabbage, lettuce
COOKED DISHES:
Spinach soup No. 82 D
Peas No. 115 D
Potatoes cooked in vegeta-
ble stock No. 195 D

FRUIT
RAW SALAD:
new carrots, lettuce
COOKED DISHES:
Cauliflower cheese, No.
173
Oat cakes fried No. 279

FRUIT
RAW SALAD:
beetroot, white cabbage,
lettuce
COOKED DISHES:
Tomato soup with tapioca
No. 79
Sugar-peas (edible-podded
young peas) croûtes No.
118
Millotto No. 247 D

FRUIT
RAW SALAD:
squash or zucchini and
tomatoes or red peppers
mixed, lettuce
COOKED DISHES:
Noodles with cheese No.
254

FRUIT
RAW SALAD:
carrots, lettuce
COOKED DISHES:
Carrots Nos. 111 D–113
Small whole fried potatoes
as in No. 215
DESSERT:
Farina shape No. 371 D

FRUIT
RAW SALAD:
Radishes, cucumber and
cress
COOKED DISHES:
Peas No. 115 D or spinach
beet No. 105 D or spring
cabbage No. 156
Mashed potatoes No. 201 D

Everyday Menus	*Festive Menus for Special Occasions*

FRUIT
RAW SALAD:
carrots, cucumber, lettuce
COOKED DISHES:
Farina soup No. 74
Spinach Nos. 97 D–100 D
Potatoes and cream cheese
No. 193 D

FRUIT
RAW SALAD:
cauliflower, tomatoes
mixed with red peppers,
lettuce
COOKED DISHES:
Chervil soup No. 85 D
Lettuce as a vegetable No.
101 D
Polenta No. 243 D

FRUIT
RAW SALAD:
carrots, squash, lettuce
COOKED DISHES:
Asparagus No. 151 D with
mousseline sauce No.
316
Lettuce as a vegetable No.
101 D
New potatoes, fried whole
No. 215
DESSERT:
Strawberry tart No. 396

FRUIT
RAW SALAD:
radishes or carrots, spin-
ach, lettuce
COOKED DISHES:
Cauliflower au gratin No.
173
Caraway potatoes No.
194 D
DESSERT:
Lemon whip with biscuits,
Nos. 357, 358

FRUIT
RAW SALAD:
beetroot, cucumber, let-
tuce
COOKED DISHES:
Broth No. 51 D with egg
custard No. 57
Beans No. 119
Cheese patties No. 285

FRUIT
RAW SALAD:
tomatoes, cress, lettuce
COOKED DISHES:
Young peas No. 116 D,
fried whole tomatoes
and fleurons No. 292
Saffron rice No. 225
DESSERT:
Raspberry jelly No. 336 D

Everyday Menus	*Festive Menus for Special Occasions*

FRUIT
RAW SALAD:
  tomatoes, spinach, lettuce
COOKED DISHES:
  Cauliflower soup No. 84
  Carrots Nos. 111 D–113
  Spinach spaetzle No. 263

FRUIT
RAW SALAD:
  carrots, zucchini, lettuce
COOKED DISHES:
  Spinach beet stalks in sauce or au gratin No. 105 D or 173
  Millet No. 247 D with young peas No. 116 D
DESSERT:
  Blueberry sweet No. 341 D

FRUIT
RAW SALAD:
  radishes or carrots, spinach, lettuce
COOKED DISHES:
  Cream of oatmeal soup No. 69 D
  Beans No. 119
  Baked potatoes No. 192 D or fried potatoes No. 216

FRUIT
RAW SALAD:
  beetroot, cucumber, turnip, lettuce
COOKED DISHES:
  Vegetable tart No. 177
  Spinach Nos. 97–100 D with potatoes cooked in vegetable stock No. 195 D
DESSERT:
  Strawberry whip No. 353

FRUIT
RAW SALAD:
  cauliflower, cucumber, lettuce, turnips
COOKED DISHES:
  Vegetable broth No. 51 D with diced egg custard No. 57
  Sugar-peas (edible-podded young peas) No. 118, croûtes No. 282
  Risotto No. 224

Everyday Menus	*Festive Menus for Special Occasions*

FRUIT

RAW SALAD:
spinach beet, radishes, beetroots, lettuce

COOKED DISHES:
Mixed vegetable platter (carrots, spinach, beans, cauliflower, tomatoes). See individual recipes.
Wheat cakes No. 280 and cranberries

DESSERT:
Fresh cherry cake No. 413

FRUIT

RAW SALAD:
cauliflower, cucumber, lettuce

COOKED DISHES:
Vegetable cutlets No. 276 and herb sauce No. 301
Carrots Nos. 111 D–113.
Browned potatoes No. 211 D

DESSERT:
Rhubarb slices No. 386

JULY

Everyday Menus	*Economical Menus*

FRUIT

RAW SALAD:
radishes, young carrots or turnips, tomatoes, lettuce

COOKED DISHES:
Broth No. 51 D with cheese dumplings No. 54
Carrots and peas No. 114 D
Fried potatoes No. 213

FRUIT

RAW SALAD:
lettuce, tomatoes, cucumber

COOKED DISHES:
Peperonata No. 144
Risotto No. 224

FRUIT

RAW SALAD:
beetroot, cucumber, lettuce

COOKED DISHES:
Cauliflower cheese No. 173
French fried potatoes No. 218

DESSERT:
Apricots and cream No. 344

FRUIT

RAW SALAD:
cucumber, radishes, lettuce

COOKED DISHES:
Cheese croûtes No. 282

Everyday Menus

FRUIT
RAW SALAD:
  radishes, tomatoes, lettuce
COOKED DISHES:
  Tapioca soup No. 60 D
  Squash (stuffed) No. 138
  Ravioli No. 262

FRUIT
RAW SALAD:
  carrots, cauliflower, lettuce
COOKED DISHES:
  Oat cream soup No. 68 D
  Tomatoes baked No. 130 D
  Japanese rice No. 223 D

FRUIT
RAW SALAD:
  beetroot, squash, lettuce, turnip
COOKED DISHES:
  Lettuce as a vegetable No. 101 D
  Cream patties No. 284
DESSERT:
  Raspberry whip No. 353

FRUIT
RAW SALAD:
  cucumber, cress, lettuce
COOKED DISHES:
  Minestra No. 95 D
  Stuffed red peppers with noodles No. 143
  Potatoes cooked in vegetable stock No. 195 D

Economical Menus

FRUIT
RAW SALAD:
  tomatoes, lettuce, turnips
COOKED DISHES:
  Noodles with tomato sauce No. 254
DESSERT:
  Strawberry or raspberry whip No. 353

FRUIT
RAW SALAD:
  radishes or young carrots, lettuce
COOKED DISHES:
  Tomatoes as a vegetable No. 129 D
  Spinach spaetzle No. 263

FRUIT
RAW SALAD:
  cucumber, lettuce
COOKED DISHES:
  Broad beans as in No. 115 D or green beans No. 119
  Potato pudding No. 204

FRUIT
RAW SALAD:
  carrots, lettuce
COOKED DISHES:
  Beetroot as a vegetable No. 126 D
  Potatoes with cream cheese No. 193 D

| *Everyday Menus* | *Festive Menus for Special Occasions* |

FRUIT
RAW SALAD:
  carrots, red peppers, lettuce
COOKED DISHES:
  Tomato soup Nos. 79, 80 D
  Beans No. 119
  Baked potatoes No. 192 D

FRUIT
RAW SALAD:
  radishes or carrots, spinach, lettuce
COOKED DISHES:
  Eggplant fried in egg and breadcrumbs No. 174
  Millotto No. 248 D
DESSERT:
  Peach tart. As in No. 392

FRUIT
RAW SALAD:
  various raw vegetables arranged with rice salad No. 186 D, served in shells
COOKED DISHES:
  Beans No. 119 with fresh tomato purée
  Potato snow No. 200 D
DESSERT:
  Fresh cherry cake No. 413

FRUIT
RAW SALAD:
  beetroot, cucumber, lettuce
COOKED DISHES:
  Spinach soup No. 82 D
  Kohlrabi No. 163
  Potato cakes No. 203

FRUIT
RAW SALAD:
  tomatoes, fennel, lettuce
COOKED DISHES:
  Broth No. 51 D with caraway fingers No. 291
  Chopped spinach Nos. 97–100 D
  Omelettes Nos. 265, 266

FRUIT
RAW SALAD:
  peppers, cauliflower, lettuce
COOKED DISHES:
  Cheese and tomato tartlets No. 296 or Pizza napolitana No. 298
  Lettuce as a vegetable No. 101 D
  French fried potatoes No. 218
DESSERT:
  Rice pudding with pineapple No. 374

Everyday Menus	*Festive Menus for Special Occasions*

FRUIT
RAW SALAD:
  kohlrabi, cucumber, lettuce, turnip
COOKED DISHES:
  Spinach beet stalks au gratin No. 106
  Polenta No. 243 D
DESSERT:
  Blueberry junket

FRUIT
RAW SALAD:
  cauliflower, cress, lettuce
COOKED DISHES:
  Carrot soup No. 81 D
  Globe artichokes with sauce Hollandaise No. 148 D
  Potatoes cooked in vegetable stock No. 195 D

FRUIT
RAW SALAD:
  beetroot, cucumber, lettuce
COOKED DISHES:
  Broth No. 51 D with diced egg custard No. 57
  Tomatoes as a vegetable No. 129 D with peppers No. 141 D
  Potato noodles No. 209

FRUIT
RAW SALAD:
  radishes or carrots, tomatoes, lettuce
COOKED DISHES:
  Spinach Nos. 95–100 D
  Cheese patties No. 285
DESSERT:
  Red currants and cream No. 344

FRUIT
RAW SALAD:
  kohlrabi or beetroot, lettuce, cucumber
COOKED DISHES:
  Tomatoes with cheese slices No. 131
  Sugar-peas (edible-podded peas) No. 118, croûtes No. 282
  Small fried potatoes No. 215
DESSERT:
  Strawberries and cream No. 343 D

251

Everyday Menus

FRUIT
RAW SALAD:
  carrots, white cabbage, radishes, lettuce
COOKED DISHES:
  Spinach soup No. 82 D
  Cauliflower cheese No. 173
  Potato balls No. 202 D

Festive Menus for Special Occasions

FRUIT
RAW SALAD:
  raw vegetables on Canapés (open sandwiches) spread with cheese and egg, served with lettuce
COOKED DISHES:
  Eggplant au gratin No. 146
  Potatoes cooked in vegetable stock No. 195 D
DESSERT:
  Fruit jelly No. 336 D

AUGUST

Everyday Menus

FRUIT
RAW SALAD:
  beetroot, spinach, lettuce
COOKED DISHES:
  Minestra No. 95
  Spinach beet stalks No. 105 D with tomato sauce No. 303
  Polenta No. 243 D

FRUIT
RAW SALAD:
  radishes or carrots, tomatoes, lettuce
COOKED DISHES:
  Vegetable cutlets No. 276
  Spinach Nos. 97–100 D garnished with potatoes cooked in vegetable stock No. 195 D

FRUIT
RAW SALAD:
  beetroot, cucumber, lettuce

Economical Menus

FRUIT
RAW SALAD:
  carrots, cabbage
COOKED DISHES:
  Polenta with cheese No. 243
DESSERT:
  Raspberries, loganberries or blackberries

FRUIT
RAW SALAD:
  beetroot, tomatoes, lettuce
COOKED DISHES:
  Potato soup No. 89 D or bean soup No. 93
  Stuffed squash No. 138

FRUIT
RAW SALAD:
  Salad Niçoise (radishes, lettuce, beans, tomatoes, egg, olives) No. 185 D

Everyday Menus

COOKED DISHES:
Corn-on-the-cob with butter No. 152
Cauliflower au gratin No. 173
French fried potatoes No. 218

FRUIT
RAW SALAD:
carrots, cucumber, lettuce
COOKED DISHES:
Potato soup No. 89 D
Squash with tomatoes No. 137 D
Cheese croûtes No. 282

FRUIT
RAW SALAD:
cauliflower, spinach, lettuce
COOKED DISHES:
Tomatoes with cheese slices No. 131
Millotto No. 248 D
DESSERT:
Apricot tart No. 392

FRUIT
RAW SALAD:
radishes, squash, lettuce
COOKED DISHES:
Tapioca soup No. 60 D
Carrots and peas No. 114 D
Castle potatoes No. 217

FRUIT
RAW SALAD:
beetroot, tomatoes, lettuce
COOKED DISHES:
Spinach soup No. 82 D
Beans No. 119
Spaghetti à la Napolitaine No. 254

Economical Menus

COOKED DISHES:
Potatoes in their skins No. 191 with various cheeses

FRUIT
RAW SALAD:
beetroot, lettuce
COOKED DISHES:
Minestrone No. 96
DESSERT:
Blackberries or loganberries and cream No. 344

FRUIT
RAW SALAD:
carrots and lettuce
COOKED DISHES:
Sauerkraut or white cabbage No. 160 or 161
Spaetzle No. 263

FRUIT
RAW SALAD:
beetroot and lettuce
COOKED DISHES:
Silver or spinach beet stalks with sauce No. 105 D
French fried potatoes No. 218

Everyday Menus

FRUIT
RAW SALAD:
radishes or carrots, spinach, lettuce
COOKED DISHES:
Chopped cabbage No. 157
Stuffed potatoes No. 222
with herb sauce No. 301
DESSERT:
Damson tart No. 393

FRUIT
RAW SALAD:
carrots, squash, lettuce
COOKED DISHES:
Spring soup No. 86 D
Red peppers stuffed with
tomato-rice No. 142
Potato salad Nos. 181, 182

FRUIT
RAW SALAD:
beetroot, cucumber, lettuce
COOKED DISHES:
Cheese soup No. 77
Spinach Nos. 97–100 D
French fried potatoes No.
218

FRUIT
RAW SALAD:
cauliflower, tomatoes, lettuce
COOKED DISHES:
Beetroot as a vegetable No.
126 D
Potatoes and cream cheese
No. 193 D
DESSERT:
Blackberry jelly No. 336 D

Festive Menus for Special Occasions

FRUIT
RAW SALAD:
Russian salad No. 184 garnished with tomatoes
and cucumber
COOKED DISHES:
Spinach Nos. 97–100 D
French fried potatoes No.
218
DESSERT:
Peaches and cream No.
344

FRUIT
RAW SALAD:
Tomatoes No. 134 garnished with cucumber,
radishes and lettuce
COOKED DISHES:
Carrots and peas No.
114 D
French fried potatoes No.
218
DESSERT:
Filbert whip No. 351 or
352

Everyday Menus

FRUIT
RAW SALAD:
Tomatoes No. 134, cucumber, lettuce
COOKED DISHES:
Barley soup No. 72 D
Cauliflower au gratin No. 173
Potatoes cooked in vegetable stock No. 195 D

FRUIT
RAW SALAD:
peppers, savoy, lettuce
COOKED DISHES:
Clear No. 51 D soup with pancake strips No. 55
Vegetable fritters: squash, tomatoes, beetroot, cauliflower No. 174
Remoulade sauce No. 320
DESSERT:
Peach purée

FRUIT
RAW SALAD:
radishes or carrots, squash, lettuce
COOKED DISHES:
Beans No. 119, risotto No. 224
DESSERT:
Filbert whip with biscuits No. 351 or 352

FRUIT
RAW SALAD:
carrots, celery, peppers, lettuce
COOKED DISHES:
Cream of oatmeal soup No. 69 D
Red cabbage with apples No. 162
Potato snow No. 200 D

Festive Menus for Special Occasions

FRUIT
RAW SALAD:
beetroots, spinach, lettuce
COOKED DISHES:
Corn-on-the-cob with butter No. 152
Squash No. 136 D or 137 D with rice croquettes No. 235
DESSERT:
Blackberry tart. As in No. 392

FRUIT
RAW SALAD:
beetroot, stuffed tomatoes with cucumber, cabbage salad
COOKED DISHES:
Vegetable tart No. 177
Lettuce as a vegetable No. 101 D
French fried potatoes No. 218
DESSERT:
Red currants and cream, biscuits No. 344

SEPTEMBER

Everyday Menus

FRUIT
RAW SALAD:
  cauliflower, cress, lettuce
COOKED DISHES:
  Leek soup No. 87
  Stuffed eggplant No. 147
    and tomato sauce Nos.
    303–306 D
  Potatoes cooked in vegeta-
    ble stock No. 195 D

FRUIT
RAW SALAD:
  celeriac or beetroot, toma-
    toes, lettuce
COOKED DISHES:
  White or red cabbage No.
    162
  French fried potatoes No.
    218
  Apple charlotte No. 401

FRUIT
RAW SALAD:
  carrots, cucumber, lettuce
COOKED DISHES:
  Spring soup No. 86
  Tomatoes as a vegetable
    No. 129 D
  Macaroni timbale No. 257

FRUIT
RAW SALAD:
  radishes or carrots, spin-
    ach, endives
COOKED DISHES:
  Oatmeal soup No. 69 D
  Stuffed cabbage leaves
    No. 159
  Potato salad Nos. 181,
    182

FRUIT
RAW SALAD:
  fennel or chicory, cauli-
    flower, lettuce

Economical Menus

FRUIT
RAW SALAD:
  beetroot, lettuce
COOKED DISHES:
  Stuffed potatoes No. 222
DESSERT:
  Plum or greengage sweet
    as in No. 353

FRUIT
RAW SALAD:
  tomatoes stuffed with car-
    rots, lettuce
COOKED DISHES:
  Cheese soufflé No. 283

FRUIT
RAW SALAD:
  cucumber, endives
COOKED DISHES:
  Stuffed eggplant No. 147
    with tomato sauce Nos.
    303–306 D
DESSERT:
  Blackberries and cream
    No. 344

FRUIT
RAW SALAD:
  carrots, lettuce
COOKED DISHES:
  Barley soup No. 72 D
  Wholewheat bread and
    cheese

FRUIT
RAW SALAD:
  cauliflower, cress

Everyday Menus

COOKED DISHES:
Corn-on-the-cob with butter No. 152
Potato cakes with spinach No. 220 D

DESSERT:
Apricots and cream No. 344

FRUIT
RAW SALAD:
beetroot, squash, lettuce
COOKED DISHES:
Cheese soup No. 77
Spinach Nos. 97–100 D
Bread and egg dish No. 278

Everyday Menus

FRUIT
RAW SALAD:
celery, tomatoes, lettuce
COOKED DISHES:
Broth No. 51 D with diced egg custard No. 57
Spinach beet stalks in sauce No. 105 D
Turkish rice No. 233

FRUIT
RAW SALAD:
cress, cauliflower garnished with radishes, lettuce
COOKED DISHES:
Celeriac slices with sauce Hollandaise No. 123
Potatoes cooked in vegetable stock No. 195 D

DESSERT:
Blackberry jelly No. 336 D

Economical Menus

COOKED DISHES:
Green beans as a vegetable No. 119
Parsley potatoes No. 196 D

FRUIT
RAW SALAD:
tomatoes, white cabbage, lettuce
COOKED DISHES:
Stuffed peppers with noodles No. 143

Festive Menus for Special Occasions

FRUIT
RAW SALAD:
celery or celeriac, cucumber garnished with diced tomatoes, lettuce
COOKED DISHES:
Rice ring No. 234 D with peas No. 119 and mushrooms and mushroom sauce No. 311
Beans No. 119
Castle potatoes No. 217

DESSERT:
Viennese pears No. 348

Everyday Menus	*Festive Menus for Special Occasions*

FRUIT
RAW SALAD:
  carrots, peppers, lettuce
COOKED DISHES:
  Tomato soup No. 80 D
  Carrots Nos. 111 D–113
  Bread dumpling No. 277

FRUIT
RAW SALAD:
  celeriac or beetroot, spinach, lettuce
COOKED DISHES:
  Cream soup Nos. 65 D, 66 D
  Fennel Nos. 108 D, 109, garnished with carrots Nos. 111 D–113
  Lyons potatoes No. 214

FRUIT
RAW SALAD:
  fennel, tomatoes, lettuce
COOKED DISHES:
  Endives as a vegetable No. 102 D
  Cheese patties No. 285

FRUIT
RAW SALAD:
  radishes or carrots, lettuce
COOKED DISHES:
  Clear soup No. 51 D with pancake strips No. 55
  Cauliflower au gratin No. 173
  Caraway potatoes No. 194 D

FRUIT
RAW SALAD:
  cauliflower, cress, lettuce
COOKED DISHES:
  Bean soup No. 93
  Squash No. 137
  Tomato Rice No. 227 D

Festive Menus for Special Occasions column:

FRUIT
RAW SALAD:
  tomatoes stuffed with Russian salad and grated or chopped celery or celeriac, lettuce
COOKED DISHES:
  Squash Nos. 136 D, 137
  Risotto, No. 224
DESSERT:
  Apricot tartlets as in No. 392

FRUIT
RAW SALAD:
  tomatoes, endives, radishes
COOKED DISHES:
  Ravioli No. 262
  Cauliflower No. 153 and filbert potatoes No. 216
DESSERT:
  Apple porcupines with vanilla sauce No. 349

Everyday Menus	*Festive Menus for Special Occasions*

FRUIT
RAW SALAD:
  carrots, squash, endives
COOKED DISHES:
  Peppers with tomatoes
    Nos. 142–144
  Millotto No. 247

FRUIT	FRUIT
RAW SALAD:	RAW SALAD:
radishes, cucumber, white cabbage, lettuce	squash, cress, white cabbage
COOKED DISHES:	COOKED DISHES:
Broth No. 51 D with dumplings No. 52	Cheese turnovers No. 408
Lettuce as a vegetable No. 101 D	Carrots and peas No. 114 D, garnished with potatoes cooked in vegetable stock No. 195 D
Spaghetti à la Napolitaine No. 254	DESSERT:
	Stuffed melon No. 335 D

OCTOBER

Everyday Menus	*Economical Menus*
FRUIT	FRUIT
RAW SALAD:	RAW SALAD:
beetroot, squash, cress	celery, lettuce
COOKED DISHES:	COOKED DISHES:
Pea soup No. 94	Browned wholewheat soup No. 78
Celeriac as a vegetable No. 121	Potatoes with tomatoes No. 199 D
Filbert potatoes No. 216	
FRUIT	FRUIT
RAW SALAD:	RAW SALAD:
cauliflower, lettuce, cabbage	carrots, red peppers, lettuce
COOKED DISHES:	COOKED DISHES:
Beans No. 119	Tomatoes as a vegetable No. 129 D
Risotto No. 224	Spaghetti No. 254
DESSERT:	
Apple tart No. 390	

Everyday Menus

FRUIT
RAW SALAD:
 radishes or carrots, spin-
 ach, lettuce
COOKED DISHES:
 Broth No. 51 D with pan-
 cake strips No. 55
 Stuffed potatoes No. 222
 Chopped cabbage No. 157

FRUIT
RAW SALAD:
 carrots, fennel or chicory,
 lettuce
COOKED DISHES:
 Tomato soup No. 80 D
 Red cabbage with apples
 No. 162
 Spaetzle No. 263

FRUIT
RAW SALAD:
 celery or celeriac, spinach,
 lettuce
COOKED DISHES:
 Fennel Nos. 108 D, 109 or
 chicory No. 103 D gar-
 nished with carrots Nos.
 111 D–113
 Potato balls No. 202 D
DESSERT:
 Lemon soufflé No. 383

FRUIT
RAW SALAD:
 carrots, sauerkraut or
 white cabbage, cress
COOKED DISHES:
 Browned wholewheat soup
 No. 78
 Tomatoes as a vegetable
 No. 129 D
 Millotto No. 247 D

Economical Menus

FRUIT
RAW SALAD:
 fennel or cauliflower, en-
 dives
COOKED DISHES:
 Lettuce as a vegetable No.
 101 D
 Mashed potatoes No. 201 D

FRUIT
RAW SALAD:
 tomatoes, lettuce
COOKED DISHES:
 Farmer's omelette No. 271

FRUIT
RAW SALAD:
 black radishes or celery,
 lettuce
COOKED DISHES:
 Chestnuts in their shells
 with butter No. 175 D
DESSERT:
 Apple purée No. 337 D

FRUIT
RAW SALAD:
 beetroot, lettuce
COOKED DISHES:
 Farina gnocchi No. 239

Everyday Menus	*Festive Menus for Special Occasions*

FRUIT
RAW SALAD:
  beetroot, lettuce, cabbage
COOKED DISHES:
  Tapioca soup No. 60 D
  Peperonata No. 144 D
  Spaghetti No. 254

FRUIT
RAW SALAD:
  salsify, cucumber, lettuce
COOKED DISHES:
  Stuffed rolls No. 295
  Lettuce as a vegetable No.
    101 D
  Fruit jelly No. 336

FRUIT
RAW SALAD:
  peppers, carrots, cress
COOKED DISHES:
  Turkish rice No. 233
  Beans No. 119 and potato
    snow No. 200 D
DESSERT:
  Lemon whip Nos. 357–
    358

FRUIT
RAW SALAD:
  cauliflower, squash, let-
    tuce
COOKED DISHES:
  Vegetable and rice soup
    No. 63 D
  Vegetable fritters: celery
    or celeriac, cauliflower,
    salsify No. 174 with
    Remoulade sauce No.
    320
  Potatoes cooked in vegeta-
    ble stock No. 195 D

FRUIT
RAW SALAD:
  radishes, or carrots, en-
    dives, lettuce
COOKED DISHES:
  Cream of oatmeal soup
    No. 69 D
  Eggplant au gratin No.
    146
  Mashed potatoes No. 201 D

FRUIT
RAW SALAD:
  black radishes or carrots,
    squash, lettuce
COOKED DISHES:
  Celeric slices with sauce
    Hollandaise No. 123
  Caraway potatoes No.
    194 D
DESSERT:
  Grape tart No. 391

Everyday Menus	*Festive Menus for Special Occasions*

FRUIT

RAW SALAD:
  beetroot, sauerkraut or white cabbage, lettuce

COOKED DISHES:
  Spinach Nos. 97–100 D
  Cheese patties No. 285

DESSERT:
  Banana sweet No. 364

FRUIT

RAW SALAD:
  tomatoes, cress, lettuce

COOKED DISHES:
  Chervil soup No. 85 D
  Carrots Nos. 111 D–113
  Risotto No. 224

FRUIT

RAW SALAD:
  cauliflower, fennel or chicory, lettuce

COOKED DISHES:
  Barley soup No. 72
  Onions as a vegetable in sauce No. 167
  Caraway potatoes No. 194 D

FRUIT

RAW SALAD:
  carrots, chicory, lettuce

COOKED DISHES:
  Cauliflower au gratin No. 173
  Lyons potatoes No. 214

DESSERT:
  Chestnut purée and cream No. 365

FRUIT

RAW SALAD:
  celery or celeriac, lettuce

FRUIT

RAW SALAD:
  celery or celeriac, cucumber, lettuce

COOKED DISHES:
  Pizza napolitana No. 298
  Brussels sprouts No. 155
  Potato snow No. 200 D

DESSERT:
  Apple whip and biscuits No. 354

FRUIT

RAW SALAD:
  beetroot, sauerkraut or white cabbage, lettuce

Everyday Menus	*Festive Menus for Special Occasions*

COOKED DISHES:
  Barley soup No. 72 D
  Chicory No. 103 D
  Farina gnocchi No. 239
	COOKED DISHES:
	  Vegetable cutlets No. 276
	  Lettuce as a vegetable No. 101 D
	  Potatoes cooked in vegetable stock No. 195 D
	DESSERT:
	  Almond pudding No. 377 with raspberry syrup

NOVEMBER

Everyday Menus	*Economical Menus*

FRUIT
RAW SALAD:
  beetroot, sauerkraut or white cabbage, lettuce
COOKED DISHES:
  Potato soup No. 89 D
  Spinach Nos. 97–100 D
  Bread and egg dish No. 278
	FRUIT
	RAW SALAD:
	  black radishes or celery, lettuce
	COOKED DISHES:
	  Rice pudding No. 375 with apple purée No. 337 D

FRUIT
RAW SALAD:
  carrots, leeks, spinach, lettuce
COOKED DISHES:
  Chicory No. 103 D
  Tomato rice No. 227 D
DESSERT:
  Apple pudding No. 380
	FRUIT
	RAW SALAD:
	  fennel or cauliflower, tomatoes, lettuce
	COOKED DISHES:
	  Chicory No. 103 D
	  Cheese soufflé No. 283

FRUIT
RAW SALAD:
  celery or celeriac, tomatoes, lettuce
COOKED DISHES:
  Minestra No. 95
  Lentils No. 170
  Potato salad Nos. 181, 182
	FRUIT
	RAW SALAD:
	  celery, savoy
	COOKED DISHES:
	  Baked tomatoes No. 130 D
	  Risotto No. 224

Everyday Menus

FRUIT
RAW SALAD:
  black radishes or carrots,
  cress, lettuce
COOKED DISHES:
  Rice soup Nos. 61 D–64 D
  Cauliflower au gratin No.
  173
  French fried potatoes No.
  218

FRUIT
RAW SALAD:
  beetroot, fennel or chic-
  ory, lettuce
COOKED DISHES:
  Carrots Nos. 111 D–113
  Spinach spaetzle No. 263
DESSERT:
  Almond pudding with rasp-
  berry syrup No. 377

FRUIT
RAW SALAD:
  cauliflower, chicory, let-
  tuce
COOKED DISHES:
  Broth No. 51 D with
  golden cubes No. 59
  Stuffed cabbage leaves No.
  159
  Potato balls No. 202 D

FRUIT
RAW SALAD:
  salsify, tomatoes, lettuce
COOKED DISHES:
  Leek soup No. 87
  Red cabbage with apple
  No. 162
  Farina gnocchi No. 239

Economical Menus

FRUIT
RAW SALAD:
  carrots, lettuce
COOKED DISHES:
  Spinach Nos. 97–100 D
  Potatoes with cottage
  cheese No. 193 D.

FRUIT
RAW SALAD:
  chicory, tomatoes
COOKED DISHES:
  Red peppers stuffed with
  rice No. 142

FRUIT
RAW SALAD:
  beetroot, sauerkraut or
  white cabbage, lettuce
COOKED DISHES:
  Vaudois farina soup No.
  75
DESSERT:
  Apple tart No. 390

Everyday Menus

FRUIT
RAW SALAD:
   celery or celeriac, sauer-
   kraut or white cabbage,
   lettuce
COOKED DISHES:
   Mixed vegetable platter
   (carrots, tomatoes, Brus-
   sels sprouts, cauli-
   flower). See individual
   recipes.
   Wheat cakes and cran-
   berries No. 280
DESSERT:
   Lemon whip and biscuits
   Nos. 357, 358
FRUIT
RAW SALAD:
   beetroot, chicory, lettuce
COOKED DISHES:
   Tapioca soup No. 60 D
   Brussels sprouts No. 155
   Noodles with tomato sauce
   No. 254
FRUIT
RAW SALAD:
   black radishes or carrots,
   tomatoes, lettuce
COOKED DISHES:
   Farina soup with egg No.
   74
   Spinach beet stalks au
   gratin No. 173
   Caraway potatoes No.
   194 D
FRUIT
RAW SALAD:
   carrots, white cabbage, let-
   tuce
COOKED DISHES:
   Fennel Nos. 108 D, 109 or
   chicory No. 103 D
   Castle potatoes No. 217
DESSERT:
   Apple tart No. 390

Festive Menus for Special Occasions

FRUIT
RAW SALAD:
   Vegetable Aspic No. 189 D,
   garnished with grated
   beetroots, cress and
   canapés No. 190
COOKED DISHES:
   Brussels sprouts No. 155
   Filbert potatoes No. 216
DESSERT:
   Savarin No. 405 with
   chaudeau No. 362

FRUIT
RAW SALAD:
   carrots, fennel or chicory,
   lettuce
COOKED DISHES:
   Vegetable turnovers No.
   290
   Salsify à la polonaise No.
   125
   French fried potatoes No.
   218
DESSERT:
   Orange jelly No. 336 D

Everyday Menus	*Festive Menus for Special Occasions*

FRUIT
RAW SALAD:
  black radishes or carrots,
  squash, lettuce
COOKED DISHES:
  Oat groat soup No. 71 D
  Celeriac slices with sauce
  Hollandaise No. 123
  Millotto No. 247

FRUIT
RAW SALAD:
  tomaoes, celery, lettuce
COOKED DISHES:
  Cheese soup No. 77
  Carrots Nos. 111 D–113
  Spinach pudding No. 274
    with caper sauce No.
    302

FRUIT
RAW SALAD:
  salsify, cress, lettuce
COOKED DISHES:
  Lettuce as a vegetable No.
    101 D
  Stuffed peppers with noo-
    dles No. 143
DESSERT:
  Black currant jelly with
    biscuits No. 336 D

FRUIT
RAW SALAD:
  tomatoes, cauliflower, en-
  dives
COOKED DISHES:
  Broth No. 51 D with diced
    egg No. 57
  Salsify in sauce No. 124 D
  Rice cakes No. 235

FRUIT
RAW SALAD:
  cauliflower with pine ker-
    nels, radishes and let-
    tuce
COOKED DISHES:
  Farina gnocchi No. 239
  Chicory No. 103 D
  Duchess potatoes No. 206
DESSERT:
  Oranges and cream No.
    344

FRUIT
RAW SALAD:
  chicory, tomatoes, lettuce
COOKED DISHES:
  Vegetable served in shells
    No. 175 D
  Fennel Nos. 108 D, 109 or
    celery hearts No. 107 D,
    garnished with potatoes
    cooked in vegetable
    stock No. 195 D
DESSERT:
  Almond slices with apri-
    cot sauce No. 385

DECEMBER

Everyday Menus	*Economical Menus*

FRUIT
RAW SALAD:
    Stuffed tomatoes with
    celery or celeriac No.
    39, lettuce or watercress
COOKED DISHES:
    Barley soup No. 72 D
    Dried beans No. 120
    Potato salad Nos. 181, 182

FRUIT
RAW SALAD:
    salsify, cress, lettuce or
    watercress
COOKED DISHES:
    Cauliflower au gratin No.
    173
    French fried potatoes No.
    218
DESSERT:
    Chestnut cream cake No.
    412

FRUIT
RAW SALAD:
    carrots, cauliflower, let-
    tuce or watercress
COOKED DISHES:
    Vegetable soup No. 96
    Fennel Nos. 108 D, 109 or
    celery hearts No. 107 D
    Millotto No. 247

FRUIT
RAW SALAD:
    beetroot, chicory, lettuce or
    watercress
COOKED DISHES:
    Cauliflower soup No. 84
    Tomatoes as a vegetable
    No. 129 D
    Macaroni soufflé No. 256

FRUIT
RAW SALAD:
    carrots, lettuce or water-
    cress
COOKED DISHES:
    Millotto with diced toma-
    toes as in No. 248 D
DESSERT:
    Apple pudding No. 380

FRUIT
RAW SALAD:
    red peppers with cauli-
    flower
COOKED DISHES:
    Potato soup No. 89 D
    Cream cheese on Ryvita or
    wholewheat rolls with
    lettuce or watercress

FRUIT
RAW SALAD:
    beetroot, lettuce or water-
    cress
COOKED DISHES:
    Cheese soup No. 77
DESSERT:
    Fruit salad and cream No.
    334 D

FRUIT
RAW SALAD:
    lettuce or watercress, to-
    matoes, carrots
COOKED DISHES:
    Potato pudding No. 204

Everyday Menus

FRUIT
RAW SALAD:
  carrots, sauerkraut or
    white cabbage, lettuce or
    watercress
COOKED DISHES:
  Chicory No. 103 D
  Cream patties No. 284
DESSERT:
  Stuffed apples No. 346

FRUIT
RAW SALAD:
  black radishes or carrots,
    savoy, lettuce or water-
    cress
COOKED DISHES:
  Broth No. 51 D with fried
    bread
  Boiled potatoes No. 191 D
  Various cheeses

Everyday Menus

FRUIT
RAW SALAD:
  celery or celeriac,
    black radishes, carrots,
    spinach or watercress
COOKED DISHES:
  Tomato soup No. 79
  Lettuce No. 101 D
  Sweet corn cakes Nos. 245,
    246

FRUIT
RAW SALAD:
  cauliflower, chicory, let-
    tuce or watercress
COOKED DISHES:
  Brussels sprouts No. 155
  Vegetable turnovers No.
    290
DESSERT:
  Orange whip Nos. 359, 360

Economical Menus

FRUIT
RAW SALAD:
  celeriac or celery, sauer-
    kraut or white cabbage
COOKED DISH:
  Spaghetti à la napolitaine
    No. 254

FRUIT
RAW SALAD:
  black radishes or chicory,
    lettuce or watercress
COOKED DISH:
  Rice with spinach No.
    231 D

Festive Menus for Special Occasions

FRUIT
RAW SALAD:
  cauliflower, tomatoes
COOKED DISHES:
  Cream patties and lettuce
    No. 284
  Spinach Nos. 97–100 D
  Browned potatoes No.
    211 D
DESSERT:
  Lemon whip, uncooked,
    No. 358

Everyday Menus

FRUIT
RAW SALAD:
  beetroot, savoy, lettuce or
    watercress
COOKED DISHES:
  Oat groats soup No. 71 D
  Carrots Nos. 111 D–113
  Mashed potatoes No. 201 D

FRUIT
RAW SALAD:
  carrots, fennel or chicory,
    endives
COOKED DISHES:
  Tapioca soup No. 60 D
  Stuffed tomatoes Nos. 132,
    133
  Noodles No. 254

FRUIT
RAW SALAD:
  salsify, red cabbage, let-
    tuce or watercress
COOKED DISHES:
  Celeriac slices with sauce
    Hollandaise No. 123
  Japanese rice No. 223 D
DESSERT:
  Filbert whip No. 351

FRUIT
RAW SALAD:
  radishes or carrots, Brus-
    sels sprouts, lettuce or
    watercress
COOKED DISHES:
  Potato and leek soup No.
    90
  Chinese artichokes in
    sauce No. 173
  Millotto with vegetables
    No. 248 D

Festive Menus for Special Occasions

FRUIT
RAW SALAD:
  carrots, chicory
  Choux puffs No. 297 or
    fleurons No. 292 for
    vegetables with lettuce
COOKED DISHES:
  Brussels sprouts No. 155
  Duchess potatoes No. 206
DESSERT:
  Halved apples with jelly
    No. 340 D and vanilla
    sauce No. 366

Everyday Menus

FRUIT
RAW SALAD:
celeriac, tomatoes, lettuce
or watercress
COOKED DISHES:
Cheese soup No. 77
Cauliflower au gratin No.
173
Swiss potatoes roesti No.
213

FRUIT
RAW SALAD:
beetroot, spinach, lettuce
or watercress
COOKED DISHES:
Leeks as a vegetable No.
166
Rice with saffron No. 225
DESSERT:
Almond pudding with rasp-
berry syrup No. 377

FRUIT
RAW SALAD:
carrots, sauerkraut or
white cabbage, corn-
salad
COOKED DISHES:
Barley soup No. 72 D
Beetroot as a vegetable
No. 126 D
Caraway potatoes No.
194 D

Festive Menus for Special Occasions

FRUIT
RAW SALAD:
black radishes, savoy,
lettuce
COOKED DISHES:
Pea purée with diced to-
matoes No. 169
Endives as a vegetable No.
102 D
Browned potatoes No.
211 D
DESSERT:
Splits No. 406

FRUIT
RAW SALAD:
salsify, fennel or chicory,
lettuce
COOKED DISHES:
Stuffed rolls No. 295
Chinese artichokes with
sauce No. 173
French fried potatoes No.
218
DESSERT:
Rice pudding with pine-
apple No. 374

5. KITCHEN AND MODERN COOKING UTENSILS

WARNING ABOUT UNSUITABLE EATING AND COOKING UTENSILS

Some metals may be corroded by foodstuffs, and this may in certain circumstances lead to slight upsets in health. This applies particularly to copper, zinc, tin, iron and silver plating, but also to certain glazes used on pottery, earthenware and china containers.

Care must, therefore, be taken that fruit and vegetables containing acid are not left to stand in such containers after cooking, since the acid may dissolve the metals. The juice of berries soon deteriorates in a zinc vessel, because the acids of the fruit dissolve the zinc and combine to form zinc salts which spoil the flavor of the juice. Similarly, soluble copper salts, which damage the gastro-intestinal tract and destroy Vitamin C, may easily form from the use of a copper utensil. Iron saucepans are also unsuitable for the cooking and storage of acid foodstuffs. Furthermore, acid foods may dissolve the poisonous lead in the glaze of cooking and eating utensils that have been badly fired and perhaps contain this metal.

Nickel spoons may be corroded by acid apple, rhubarb and sauerkraut dishes, etc. It is, therefore, advisable to use caution with such implements. The same applies to the so-called German silver, which consists of an alloy of nickel, zinc and copper. Aluminum utensils must not be cleaned with hydrochloric acid or soda solutions, nor is it desirable to keep acid foods in them for days at a time. With this reserve, such utensils may be used for eating, drinking, and cooking purposes.

MODERN COOKING UTENSILS

The following utensils are advisable for use in the preparation of Bircher Muesli, fruit dishes, raw vegetables and cooked dishes:

1. *In small households*

Stainless steel knives, potato-peeler, chopping knife, tomato knife, etc. Chromium-plated or stainless steel Bircher or two-way grater, chromium-plated egg whisk, small hand-driven shredder (Mouli grater). Juice extractor or electric blender, garlic juice extractor, etc.

2. *In large households*

Stainless steel knives as above. Small and large chromium-plated Bircher or two-way grater, electric grater with attachment for juice extracting, electric blender or mixer with motor with attachments for juice extractor, etc.

Hydraulic juice extractors are too expensive for any but the very large household. They extract a maximum quantity (about 90 per cent).

If possible, saucepans should be of stainless steel. Most aluminum alloy pans are also recommended; although care must be taken that no food containing acids are cooked in them. They are best used for cereals and are not really suitable for cooking or straining fruit and vegetables.

Enamel saucepans are very good except for baking and roasting, when the glaze may easily crack unless the very best makes are used.

Glazed steel or iron pans with heavy bottoms for electric cookers are excellent for fruit and vegetable cooking.

Pyrex, now available for many cooking purposes, is most useful. It does not enter into any chemical combination with acids or any other substance, is non-porous, thus preserving the value of aroma substances of the food. After cleaning it does not retain flavors.

Utensils for Modern Methods

PRESSURE COOKERS

Cooking in a pressure cooker has some advantages:

1. The food is cooked in steam at over 212° F., so that cooking time may be considerably reduced. For example, in the usual saucepan carrots may need 40 minutes; in a pressure cooker 3 minutes.

2. Cooking may be done without—or with only a very little —water, which is specially valuable in the case of fruit and vegetables. Moreover, the cooker is completely sealed and so practically no oxygen from the air can enter. Thus the danger of loss of values from food is reduced to a minimum and also the aromatic substances are retained to a large degree. Oxidation processes are decreased and Vitamin C better retained despite the greater heat. Contact with oxygen causes this vitamin to be destroyed fairly rapidly by an enzyme contained in the fresh vegetables themselves; but this oxidation requires time and is most active at a temperature of 113° F., decreases at higher temperatures and stops completely at a temperature of 194° F. If food containing vitamins is heated slowly

to boiling point, the Vitamin C runs great risk of being destroyed. The risk is much smaller during the far shorter period of heating in a pressure cooker.

If, however, sufficient care is not taken, the shorter cooking times also increase the danger of over-cooking. Cooking time should be strictly adhered to, if necessary with the aid of an automatic timer.

At temperatures above 212° F., protein and carbohydrates may enter into a combination (Maillard reaction) which impedes the utilization of protein by the organism. Whether and to what degree this reaction must be taken into account when cooking with a pressure cooker has not yet been sufficiently investigated and requires further research.

PART III

SPECIAL DIET SUGGESTIONS

---

1. GENERAL GUIDE TO THE FEEDING
OF CHILDREN

We have a few words to say on the nutrition of the healthy child, giving mothers a brief outline of how the growing child is most healthily fed, from early childhood to the end of adolescence. Children's invalid diets and measures to be taken in cases of illness cannot be discussed here, since this is a matter for the physician, nor can we touch on the wider subject of infant feeding. We shall limit ourselves to giving suggestions for the diet of healthy children from the age when they are able to chew. For more details we refer the reader to *Children's Diet* by Dr. Bircher-Benner (C. W. Daniel and Co., Ltd., Rochford, Essex).

The mother should know the best way to choose and combine a diet to ensure well-balanced nutrition containing all the important factors, so that her child grows up strong and healthy, free of deficiencies and resistant to disease. One can take it for granted that today every mother knows, either instinctively or from personal study, all that has been written and taught in recent years on the subject and what important responsibilities she undertakes with the planning of a diet—important not only for the child's future, but also, it is not too much to say, for the healthy development and economic welfare of the race. The years of growth are a time of increased needs and more rapid renewal of tissues and exchange of food into energy. A nutrition of high biological value has a more rapid and powerful effect on the health of children and adolescents than is the case with adults; the damage caused by deficient and incorrect diet is more deep-seated and less easily corrected.

Dr. Bircher-Benner says 'the laws of nutrition apply fundamentally to children in the same way as they do to adults, save that the effects of their violation are graver and more significant for later life during the years of growth.'

In his book, *Children's Diet,* Dr. Bircher-Benner deals exhaustively with the whole question and gives much useful advice and a number of recipes from his long and varied experience, in order to bring children's diet into line with up-to-date results of work on nutrition. 'Three conditions,' says Dr. Bircher-Benner in his foreword, 'determine the constitution, health and later lives of our children: heredity, mental and emotional experience in childhood and diet,' and further on in the same book (p. 26): 'out of respect for the whole food—and what is of ultimate importance—in order to achieve in our diet a harmonious accord of the different factors, we need to fulfill the following requirements':

1. *Plant organisms which can be eaten fresh and raw should, preferably, be eaten in this form.* These are: fruit of all kinds, berries, many roots, tubers, bulbs, leaf vegetables, vegetable fruits, filberts and almonds.

2. *Shortening cooking times, moderate heating, use of cooking water.* Cooked food should be a mere supplement to a plentiful supply of raw food. Any heat, particularly sterilizing and blanching, weakens and destroys nutritional value and many important constituents of food are transferred to the water and therefore lost if the latter is thrown away. Sterilized and blanched preserves should only be used in times of need. The natural wholeness of vegetables is best retained by stewing them—finely cut up—in fat and their own juices. Potatoes especially (whose protective and active principles lie immediately beneath the peel) should be eaten when possible steamed or baked in their skins. (See Recipe No. 194 D, p. 121, for Caraway Potatoes.)

3. *Our diet should contain the whole cereal grain, with its germ and inner husk.* Therefore, only wholewheat bread should be used, never white bread. Rolls and biscuits made with white flour should be reduced to a minimum. White flour and refined sugar are irritating and also a burden to a child's digestive organs and metabolism. They lead to over-acidity, rob the system of the vitamins of the B complex, which are of supreme importance for the processes of digestion and absorption, and alter the bacterial flora of the cavity of the mouth (saliva and teeth) and that of the whole digestive tract down as far as the large intestine.

Whole cereals are a major factor in children's diet from the moment when the child can chew and should be provided in the form of wholewheat bread, germinated wheat, crushed whole cereal dishes and flakes, and with the Bircher Muesli instead of or in combination with oatflakes or oatmeal. A dish made with whole cereal groats should often be given for supper, alone or as a supplement to Muesli; also wholewheat soup, whole unpolished rice, barley, etc. Anyone who has ever become accustomed to the appetizing and varied whole-cereal and brown-sugar dishes, cakes, cookies, etc., will not want to do without them, nor desire to replace them in their children's diet with cookies and cakes made with white flour. (The dish made with various kinds of whole cereals on Kollath's system is given on p. 142, Recipe No. 251.)

4. *Refined sugar, sweets and cookies should be reduced to a minimum in children's diet.* The craving for sweet things is best satisfied exclusively with fresh and dried fruit, fruit concentrates, honey, carrots, etc., all of which contain natural sugar. A large consumption of refined sugar results in a disturbance of the balance of nutrition, which may have grave consequences.

5. *The protein part of the child's diet must not be disproportionately increased by the arbitrary addition of protein-rich food such as meat, eggs and cheese.* A continual protein surplus leads to severe disturbances in health. Nuts, green vegetables, whole cereals and mild, soft cheese, as well as milk (especially yogurt) should be employed as the chief source of protein.

It is, unfortunately, still too little known that the whole cereal grain, green leaves and milk contain the complete sum of all protein components, and that the protein of the whole cereal grain, supplemented by the comparatively limited yet essential protein contained in green vegetables and potatoes, provides a supply of complete protein of ideal quality, not surpassed even by milk protein. For this reason also children should be given wholewheat bread and whole-cereal dishes as their main daily food. Among the various kinds of plant proteins, that in soya beans, sesame seeds and nuts is of particularly high value; and from animal sources that of milk: T.T. milk, sour milk, yogurt, buttermilk, cream cheese and mild kinds of cheese; as well as raw eggs (twice weekly at most).

As regards meat, the remarks made in the introduction to this book are doubly valid when dealing with children. Meat should have no place in the young child's diet.

6. *The consumption of fat should also be moderate, since a continual surplus of fat disturbs the balance of nutrition,* with harmful consequences to health. Vegetable fats that have not been hardened (hydrogenated), cold-pressed sunflower and olive oil and good quality butter (from correctly fed, healthy cows) are preferable to all other fats. Vegetable fats (nut butter) and sunflower and olive oil should be used for cooking. Butter and cream should, if at all possible, be eaten without

previous heating.

7. *Salt should never be used on raw salads and only in very moderate quantities, as an addition to cooked foods, and then preferably sea salt.* In districts where goiter is common, the use of iodized salt is recommended.

8. *Alcoholic beverages of every kind must be excluded from children's diet.* Their damaging effects are far greater than in the case of adults—often irreparable.

9. *Stimulants such as coffee, tea and cocoa, to which refined sugar is usually added, are in no way beneficial to the growing child.* They all have an unhealthy exciting action on the nervous system and on the most delicate blood vessels, but above all, they distort the natural instinct for food and thus upset the nutritive balance which is normally controlled by the sense of taste.

10. *Milk.* From a child's second year of life onwards, milk has fulfilled its task, since the childish body has now developed the tools—i.e. the teeth—for dealing with solid food, and thus the needs of the organism have gradually changed. The iron reserve supplied to the newly born baby for the breast-feeding period has now been used up. Milk, which contains no iron, is now inadequate also in this respect. Cow's milk has sometimes wrongly been recommended as the perfect nourishment for children. A two-year-old would waste away if given milk as the only form of nourishment. Neither the toddler nor the older child should be allowed more than 2½ cups daily. It should be drunk unboiled, and should be a hygienically obtained, high-quality and tuberculin-tested milk, with low bacterial content, coming from healthy, grass-fed cows. Unpasteurized milk should only be consumed if obtained from T.T. attested herds. The effects of heat, which vary according to the length of time during which milk is exposed to it, cause fundamental changes in the substance and nutritive quality of the milk. The change in the quality of fat is easily recognizable by the fact that no more cream can be skimmed off, the lecithin in the milk is destroyed by the splitting off of the phosphorous salts, the casein alters its reaction upon acid and rennet, the sugar of milk becomes caramelized, the citric acid destroyed, the soluble lime salts become insoluble and the oxygen content is decreased. Above all, the enzymes, vitamins and the antibiotic properties of the milk are all destroyed.

All this means that boiled milk can no longer be considered a valuable supplementary nourishment for children but only as an addition to the cooked part of the diet.

On the other hand, yogurt, buttermilk and sour milk are of unique importance among milk products as a whole.

Yogurt. The drawback of the brief warming process is off-set by the advantage of its excellent action on the intestinal flora by means of the lactic acid bacillus. Delicate children, or those with deficient or delayed development of digestive functions, may thrive better if given additional yogurt, especially with a low fat content, as when made with skimmed milk. Constipation, flatulence and chronic dyspepsia respond very favorably to yogurt, particularly during the summer. The full benefit is, however, only obtained if the yogurt is pure and given after or between meals. Mixing it with other foods leads rapidly to satiety and cancels out most of its beneficial effects. Yogurt should not be used regularly as a salad dressing. Salads should always remain exclusively raw food to children.

Sour milk. This is a valuable food, particularly in summer, when milk can be rapidly soured. Its special advantage is that it is made with fresh milk; it has an effect, similar to yogurt, of increasing beneficial lactic acid bacteria, thus having a cleansing action on the intestines. T.T. milk must, however, be used for making it (see Recipe No. 48, p. 63).

Buttermilk is particularly valuable on account of its lack of fat (a property specially needed by children with liver and pancreas complaints), for its abundance of vital substances of the auxon* group and of mineral substances and amino acids, which are important for building up teeth, bones, intestinal health and powers of resistance. Buttermilk quenches thirst in summer and, together with fruit and vegetable juices, is a valuable aid in the treatment of acute diarrhea.

11. *Quantities of food required.* Long experience, as well as the investigations of the American nutritionists Chittenden and Benedict (and more recently those of Clive McCay), have made it very clear that we thrive best and acquire a higher degree of efficiency throughout our lives, on an economical supply of food, just sufficient for our needs.

This economical supply will, however, only be adequate if the diet is well balanced and the food is properly chewed and absorbed. Children often experience cravings, for even the richest and most varied diet is not satisfying, if the food is devitalized and not well balanced. It may, therefore, lead to excessive and too-frequent eating between meals as long as the digestive organs can still manage this sufficiently well. If they are weak, or finally break down after being continually strained, a poor appetite is the result. Insatiable appetite at a certain age is often regarded as a good sign—proof that the child's growth demands this nourishment—and a lack of appetite as a reason for forcing the child to eat more.

* See chapter on Vitamins (Vitamin B), pp. 25–7.

Thus more children today are given something to eat five and more times daily, with chocolate in between meals. Few people realize how detrimental to health is this too frequent and excessive eating. Provided the child's constitution is good and the digestive organs sufficiently robust, the organism may perhaps be stimulated by such over-feeding to premature and powerful development. This method often begets the biggest and most splendid-looking young people, who appear strong and highly efficient. Premature aging and early disease may, however, already be inherent in them and both these possibilities are still further accelerated by this early habit of eating too much and too frequently. Their premature maturity is achieved by over-exciting the nervous system, overburdening the organs and uneconomical metabolic processes, which—seen as a whole—will reduce their total achievements.

To sum up, the foundation for a long, productive life, is laid in childhood with a well-balanced, not too lavish, diet. Every sort of between-meal snack, specially all sweets and similar foods, should ideally be avoided. Mid-morning snacks should be omitted and the mid-afternoon one be limited to fruit and one piece of wholewheat bread with butter, always provided that the suggestions of the 50 per cent uncooked part of the diet (one or two Muesli; one raw salad per day, and fresh fruit before each meal) are closely followed.

Editor's Comment

In these few words on the nutrition of the healthy child, the staff of the B-B. Clinic has tried to lay down some ideal basic principles desirable for creating wholesome feeding habits and the building up of healthy, happy and bright children.

The Editor—in her work with children—has experienced the results of this teaching in healthy and gravely ill children and cannot stress enough the surprising effects which can be achieved.

There is no doubt that the habits in the child's surroundings—of parents, school meals and, above all, the likes, dislikes and habits of his school friends—may make it difficult always to keep to these apparently somewhat restricted lines. Psychological problems arising from being 'different' from other children may cause situations necessitating compromise.

However, if these basic principles are adhered to with the small child before he gets too much involved with other children's feeding habits, the child's likes and dislikes will already have been formed and a sound physical foundation laid which may later prove to be of inestimable value.

SUGGESTIONS FOR A DAY'S MENUS
FOR CHILDREN

For Children 1–2 years

Breakfast (between 7 and 8 a.m.)

1 ripe fruit, cut up, or Muesli of apples or ripe berries, passed through a sieve or prepared in mixer or electric blender, with addition of various kinds of flakes.

1 cup unboiled T.T. (tuberculin tested) milk, slightly warmed if desired, or 1 cup yogurt.

Crust (later on slice) of wholewheat bread.

Lunch (between 12 and 1 p.m.)

Raw vegetables, very finely chopped or grated, or raw vegetable juice.

Vegetable stew, crushed with a fork or left whole, made of various steamed or stewed vegetables with potatoes, rice and a little fresh butter.

For Children over 2 years

1 portion of Muesli, or 1–2 ripe fruits, or stone fruit or berries.

T.T. (tuberculin tested) milk, yogurt or herb tea.

1–2 slices of wholewheat bread with butter or nut butter, possibly honey, rose hip jam, soft cheese, *or*

crushed wheat or other whole cereal, with fruit, milk or cream.

A little raw fruit. 2–3 kinds of salad and raw vegetables, cereals or vegetable soup.

If desired, 1 cooked, steamed or stewed vegetable, potatoes or wholewheat noodles, rice, farina, millet, etc.

Once or twice weekly, dessert preferably made of fruit sweetened with brown sugar, or dish made with eggs.

Occasionally, stewed fruit with brown sugar, or honey, or fresh fruit.

Afternoon snack (between 3 and 4 p.m.)

Mashed banana or fruit juice, Nut Cream or Almond Cream (made into fruit milk) or yogurt, No. 45 D

Bread crust

Fruit, fruit juice or buttermilk.

If necessary, one slice wholewheat bread with cream cheese, butter, soft cheese *or* honey, or wholewheat biscuits or wholewheat fruit cake.

Supper (between 5 and 6 p.m.)

Cut-up fruit or fruit juice.

Cereal dish of wholewheat, groats or other cereals, barley flour, oatmeal, corn, barley, millet, crushed oats, etc., or flakes, should be cooked in half water, half milk *or*

Muesli (Familia for babies over 6 mos.)

Muesli, usual kind with whole nuts, or fresh fruit.

Small hot dish (soup or potatoes in their skins or wholewheat dish) *or*

Wholewheat bread and cream cheese, *or*

1 cup T.T. (tuberculin tested) milk or yogurt, according to season and requirements.

Keep individual menus simple. The above suggestions should be understood as being capable of variation. They should not all be given daily.

2. GUIDE TO THE COMPILING OF DIET MENUS

Medical instructions or prescriptions cannot, of course, be given here. However, if the housewife or cook has to look after a sick member of the family suffering from a disorder which necessitates special feeding under the physician's direction (such as problems of digestion and circulation or liver complaints) or if particular attention has to be paid after treatment to definite organic weaknesses or susceptibilities (as in tendency to obesity, diabetes and allergy, especially of skin diseases), it is usually necessary to restrict or avoid certain foodstuffs and methods of preparation. Thus the task of compiling and preparing attractive menus is a difficult one, even for expert cooks; yet with sufficient experience and some imagination, it is quite possible.

The following suggestions, based on our own experience, may prove helpful as a general guide to the compiling of such menus.

Raw food must always be eaten before cooked food

If raw food is properly prepared and adapted to individual requirements, every type of human organism can tolerate and derive great benefit from it. Our sixty years of experience have confirmed that raw food, in a form correctly adapted to the digestive powers (e.g. juices) is always tolerated. How often do we hear at the beginning of dietetic treatment such remarks as 'fresh fruit and salads do not agree with me, therefore I haven't eaten any raw food for many years'! If, however, fruit and raw vegetables are given *before* the meal, if necessary in the forms mentioned below, they can always be tolerated, and indeed usually taken with pleasure. It goes without saying that all uncooked food must be thoroughly masticated.

No discomfort will be felt from eating salads made of raw vegetables if prepared without vinegar and salt, and if neither egg nor mustard be added. Instead, a dressing should be used of unrefined oil, e.g. sunflower oil, lemon juice and some herbs, or a yogurt dressing. The salad must be finely chopped, or made into a purée in a blender; in exceptional cases it should be given in the form of juices with cream of cereals (gruel) or cream, or be made into jellies with Agar-Agar. In this way the impoverished body, having suffered deficiencies by inability to deal with whole uncooked fruit and vegetables, is once again revitalized.

To summarize: fresh food should always come first. Its selection and combination, and the degree of fineness of grating and smoothness of texture (of purées and juices) should be adapted to the individual case. For fuller details, see the chapters on fresh fruit, raw vegetables and juices, pp. 55, 57–9, and examples of raw food and juice days, pp. 296–9.

The importance of thorough mastication

The most valuable components of food are wasted if it is not thoroughly chewed; starch is not changed into sugar and pieces of food are swallowed which are too large for the stomach and intestines to digest, thus causing an apparent intolerance to certain foods. 'I can't do with cold food: I must heat everything or else I get bilious, colic or gastric attacks' is a common complaint. This may be because the food has been bolted without being sufficiently chewed, thus missing the contact with the pre-digestive saliva. This also prevents the food's adaptation to the body's temperature in the mouth.

Man's inherently delicate sense of taste and instinctive healthy choice of food can only be developed as a result of thorough mastication. Quiet, relaxed eating with sufficient time for taking one's food in leisure are essential for the diet patient.

Avoid over-stimulation and irritating substances

Invalid diet demands—even more than the normal diet—the avoidance of all highly seasoned ingredients which overpower the natural flavors. No mustard, pepper or curry should be taken, nor any coffee, tea or nicotine. In addition to any toxic and possible cancerogenic effects these may have, they also blunt the sense of taste.

3. PRACTICAL SUGGESTIONS FOR DIET COOKERY

FATS

Details of various types of fat will be found on pp. 18, 40. Fat is a reserve and storage substance. As protein and carbohydrates can also be converted into fat in the body, the intake of fat can to a large extent be replaced, if it is not available, either during times of shortage due to war and famine or to economic reasons, or if it cannot be tolerated.

Fat also replenishes reserves; it can be given in more abundant quantities for short periods to help gain weight and strength after prolonged illness and during periods of an expenditure of excessive physical energy, such as sports and mountain-climbing, etc. In such cases only a fat of high biological value should be used, unrefined and in as natural and fresh a condition as possible, such as nut butters made from nuts, butter, cream, sesame, etc. It must, however, be remembered that prolonged periods on a diet with a high fat intake *without sufficient exercise* are dangerous for liver, pancreas, stomach and intestines, and may be followed by chronic damage to these organs. Epidemic jaundice attacks such overburdened organs more severely. Diabetes is more common and takes a more serious course than is the case with more austere diets containing less fat, as has been proved in times of war.

The daily total intake of fat should not exceed 1¾–2½ oz. (50–70 gm.). All fat is prohibited in cases of acute liver disease. Fat should also be greatly reduced during a slimming diet. It should not be forgotten that the moderate amount of fat supplied by the germs in whole cereals—which is, however, of exceptionally high quality—is normally quite sufficient to meet all requirements for fat-soluble vitamins, if used together with raw vegetables. This economical supply of fat is also helpful for maintaining a slim figure.

Only vegetable oils and fats of a low melting point, carefully extracted with respect to their biological value, that is with regard to their balance of essential fatty acids, should be used for cooking. Best of all are cold-pressed olive and sunflower oils on account of their great nutritive value and easy digestibility. All hardened (hydrogenated) fats should be avoided. These oils and fresh butter are the most easily-digested and are therefore the first fats to be allowed after liver disorders. One disadvantage of butter, however, is that it is rich in cholesterol, a substance which is mentioned in connection with factors causing thrombosis. If animal fat is permitted at all, fresh liquid, pasteurized cream is a fat of high value to be added to juices, binding and improving their flavor. Fats which are browned and heated to a high temperature, in short, everything deep-fried, must be omitted. The blue smoke arising from hot fats should never be seen in the diet kitchen! Special note should be taken of the cooking methods recommended in our recipes and menus; these tend to prevent the formation of the wrong kind of fatty acids that irritate the mucous membrane linings of the alimentary tract, and protect the liver from being overburdened. The fat should either be warmed only or added as fresh fat or butter to the dishes before they are served.

Sauces are not easily digested by liver patients owing to their usually high content of heated butter or fat, milk, eggs and cream—a combination of over-rich ingredients. They are also unsuitable for people suffering from kidney diseases and disorders of the metabolism owing to their salt and high protein content, and also because of the increase in fluids they entail. Those with cardiac and blood pressure disturbances should refrain from eating much protein and salt. This means avoiding sauces which, as a rule, are highly seasoned. There are, however, exceptions in the simple and yet attractive sauces made of tomatoes and herbs, etc., which can be found in the recipes Nos. 301 and 304.

PROTEIN

Protein is the substance which supplies the material to build up the body tissue, and many important enzymes effective in the body in minute quantities, as well as providing repair of their wear and tear. It is, therefore, essential and should—from our point of view and clinical experience—be supplied in regular but nevertheless moderate amounts. Excessive protein creates over-acid residues, burdening liver, blood vessels, kidneys and skin. Additional protein in the diet may be useful after severe loss of tissue in convalescence. It should then be given in the form of easily digestible protein, if possible plant protein (see Part I). We do not give any protein in diseases of the kidneys and certain heart complaints, not even foods rich in vegetable protein; and we do not suggest any animal protein (eggs, meat, milk and cheese) in allergic and skin complaints and in cases of high blood pressure. Supply of the most complete protein of high biological value is possible by combining whole-grain cereals with green vegetables or milk protein. Soya beans, nuts, cereal germs and germinated pulses are rich in equally valuable vegetable proteins. The following practical suggestions are made with regard to the foods rich in protein: cheese, eggs, dairy products and meat.

Cheese. The hard, strong-flavored cheese should be avoided altogether in diet menus, or only be used grated and in very small quantities. Soft cheeses (for example, cream cheese, Gervais, etc.) and other kinds which are not too rich are far more easily digested than hard cheeses and contain protein in its most readily assimilated form.

Eggs. If permissible at all, they must be absolutely fresh. They are most easily digested raw, lightly beaten and mixed with fruit juice and a little brown sugar. Raw egg yolk is sometimes prescribed to stimulate bile in cases of an inactive gall bladder. The white of eggs is rich in amino acids but promotes decomposition in the intestines and should therefore be given in moderation. Egg yolk is rich in calories, minerals and vitamins (B complex). It is, however, also rich in cholesterol and is thus unsuitable in cases of obesity, poor thyroid activity, arteriosclerosis, high blood pressure, rheumatism and gout. Since eggs, in particular egg yolk, put a great strain on the liver, they should be avoided in cases of liver disorder or, at the most, used very sparingly, to bind other ingredients in cooked dishes, for which purpose they can be replaced by soya. Eggs are absolutely forbidden in cases of jaundice.

The cooking of eggs not only renders them less easily digestible but alters them and reduces their nutritional value, robbing them of their enzymes and a number of their vitamins. In Switzerland, many hard-boiled eggs are eaten over Easter and the health of many children and adults is subjected to a severe strain at this time, a number of serious cases of dyspepsia (fermentative) and liver disease result. On the other hand, a raw egg twice a week may be of dietetic value to children and convalescent adults.

Milk. If milk is to be used unboiled it should be tuberculin-tested. In special light diets milk plays the part of a liquid protein-fat-sugar-salt mixture, with a high mineral, in particular calcium, content. Its binding properties make it valuable from a cookery point of view as an enriching, creaming agent for cereal mixtures, puddings, junkets, etc., and condensed in Muesli. It is not suitable as an addition to fruit juices because of its tendency to curdle. It is important to realize that the majority of patients suffering from liver trouble cannot tolerate milk, either boiled or unboiled, and react with severe flatulence, discomfort, nausea and irritation of the mucous membranes. In such cases milk must first be soured and given as yogurt and, if necessary, also skimmed and given as buttermilk and yogurt made of skimmed milk. As such it becomes a valuable addition to the menu.

Varieties of milk which can be used in diets

(a) *Sour milk*. Tuberculin-tested sour milk, yogurt made of skimmed or unskimmed milk, buttermilk or milk beaten up with citric acid tablets or lemon juice. Excellent in cases of acute gastro-intestinal trouble. Used in India for every type of dyspepsia.

(b) *Skimmed milk*, if fat is not allowed. Skimmed at home or bought already skimmed; buttermilk or semi-skimmed milk powder, skimmed milk powder (free of salt and fat), which can also be made into yogurt.

(c) *Milk treated with rennet*. Junket (diet protective for the stomach).

(d) *Salt-free milk*. For diets in which animal protein is allowed and salt forbidden. For dehydration and weight reduction.

(e) *Plant milk*. When animal protein is not allowed: Soya milk, almond milk.

See recipes Nos. 45–8 for the preparation of various kinds of milk.

Editor's Notes

The 'ready to use' soya milk, Soyamel,* is an easily digestible milk of plant origin, supplemented with essential vitamins and minerals to be as near as possible to the proportion of nutrients in mother's or cow's milk. Soyamel looks like dried milk and when reconstituted with water, as directed on the box, it can be used instead of fresh and cooked milk.

It is valuable for infants and children who have to avoid milk proteins and for cases of allergy.

Meat. We serve no meat at all in our invalid diets, since our sixty years' experience has shown that the protein in meat is

* Available at health food stores.

a greater burden to the digestive and filtering organs than the protein from plants and dairy products. The latter, moreover, contains all the essential proteins (amino acids).*

Meat is not necessary or even helpful when recovering from illness and is better left to the diet of the healthy, when, in our opinion, it can be taken once or twice weekly. See Preface for further details.

CARBOHYDRATES OR STARCHES
(FLOUR PRODUCTS AND SUGARS)

All foods of the cereal group are rich in carbohydrates, and so are many kinds of fruit and vegetables (potatoes, carrots, beetroot, turnips, Jerusalem artichokes, etc.). Wholemeal cereals have, in addition, an adequate content of protein and fat with trace elements. This group of foods is of essential value in human nutrition and can play the chief part in invalid diets, provided the right kind of carbohydrates are used.

Cereals. Whole-grain cereals are an excellent aid to the treatment of digestive ailments; they regulate the working of the intestinal tract in cases of constipation, etc. However, if the digestive organs of the patient are weak, the cereals should be opened up by a brief heating or soaking process (see Recipes Nos. 249, 250, 251) and Ryvita is another example. Whole or coarsely ground cereals (or coarse wholewheat bread), or finely crushed to finely ground whole cereals, can be used according to the patient's condition. The form of preparation easiest to digest, however, is gruel made with whole rice, barley, oats, etc., when all fibrous particles are strained off. Care must be taken that whole-grain cereals are always used for all of these variations of texture. Diets based exclusively on white flour for the purpose of avoiding discomfort in affected digestive organs, subsequently produce more or less severe deficiency diseases (e.g. European beri-beri) according to the duration of the diet. This type of diet belongs, we now hope, to the errors of the past, although there are unfortunately still too many chronic gastric patients who live on white bread and milk, white fish and white toast. Modern methods of preparing whole cereals make this unnecessary. Strained gruel, whole cereal cream, milk and finer or coarser cereal dishes, or raw cereals may be used, according to the physician's prescription. Coarsely ground wholewheat bread should be the normal bread of the healthy. The Bircher wholewheat bread (see recipe on

---

* It may happen that protein deficiency conditions develop, in spite of an adequate or even abundant, quantity of meat, in cases where the digestive organs cannot digest it. Such conditions can often be cured by vegetable proteins which can be more easily absorbed.

p. 210), made of coarsely crushed cereal, fulfills these requirements. Our clinical experience has proved that, if well chewed, it is digested without any difficulty whatever, even by patients with weakened digestion. For this reason it is also used with success in the gastric wards of many hospitals on the Continent.

Special conditions, like peptic ulcers and their consequences, can be met by the use of much more finely ground wholewheat flour, complete with all its values, than recommended above for the healthy, or the use of specially prepared breads like wholewheat rusks, Ryvita, Vita-Weat and pumpernickel. White bread, and rusks made of white flour, should be given only as an exception and never regularly in the daily diet, the same applying to white cereal and milk dishes, puddings, etc., which should be considered only as an occasional possible variation.

Wheat. The chief bread cereal, used with yeast to make wholewheat bread; also used uncooked as germinated fresh wheat, No. 40 D; as uncooked or cooked crushed wheat (Kollath breakfast), see recipe No. 252; as farina, wheatflakes, and flour, milled to various degrees of fineness.*

Rice. A soothing, anti-diarrheal, dehydrating effect (e.g. Kempner's rice diet in cases of dropsy: salt-free rice three times daily, if necessary sweetened, together with fruit); can also be used as cream* (gruel), whole rice and rice pudding.*

Sweet Corn: used as fresh corn-on-the-cob, farina, and flour.* In the case of gastro-intestinal conditions whole kernels and corn farina may cause difficulties. Cornstarch can be used instead of oatflakes or oatmeal, as a fine binding substance in Mueslis for toddlers. Cornflakes can be used for puddings.

*Barley:** a demulcent, soothing effect on the intestines as cream* (gruel) added to freshly expressed juices, and to soups; as groats, flour, flakes, whole grains (not good coarsely ground or crushed, in which form it is too mucigenous).

Rye: used as whole grains, flakes,* groats, flour; made into whole-grain bread with or without the addition of wheat.

Millet: used as grains, flakes,* groats, flour, coarsely ground; particularly rich in minerals (silicon, for growth of hair and nails); used in the same way as wheat and rye.

*Buckwheat:** used as grains, groats, flour; specially good as groats with cream or sour milk (see recipe No. 249).

Oats: a very nourishing cereal, stimulates circulation and peristalsis; used as flakes (rolled), as cream* (gruel) and groats.* Can cause irritation if eaten in large quantities for

* Available at health food stores.

too long; excellent in small quantities, for instance, in Bircher Muesli.

Potatoes: the most concentrated source of starch and in contrast with cereals an alkaline-forming food, and as such equal in value to other vegetables, salad and fruit, but also valuable as a concentrated, high-calorie food. Potatoes are easily digested, rich in mineral substances, dehydrating and of great dietetic value, enriching, soothing and uniting certain foods not otherwise comfortably combined. For light diets they are best served whole in their skins (steamed or baked), as potato snow or purée, or with other vegetables (see diet recipes). Raw potato salad (made with one potato) taken before each meal is valuable for preventing gastric spasms and gastritis.

SWEETS

In the invalid diet menu sweets should be restricted to dried and fresh fruit, fresh vegetables containing sugar (carrots, onions, Jerusalem artichokes), fruit concentrates (pulp) and honey. Cooked sweets should be given even less often than in the ordinary diet; if given at all, they should be made of pure and whole natural products. Refined white sugar is irritating to the gastro-intestinal tract, has an excessive acid-forming effect, robs the body of mineral substances (especially calcium) and vitamins of the important B complex, and fundamentally disturbs the bacterial flora in the gastro-intestinal tract by causing constant fermentation. If additional sweetening is required, honey, brown sugar or fruit concentrates should be used instead—and sparingly!

Chocolate contains fat and cocoa as well as much refined sugar, and therefore imposes a heavy burden on the gall bladder, slows up digestion and nearly always causes relapse in liver conditions. Patients with bad skin, spots and boils should not eat chocolate or any other sweets.

Dessert can be selected from the following: stewed fruit, moderately sweetened as suggested above, wholewheat biscuits, rusks and fruit tarts made of wholewheat flour, honey and brown sugar, deep-frozen fruit, fruit juice jellies, fresh fruit whips and cold fruit dishes.

Dried Fruit is valuable but concentrated and should only be taken in small quantities, especially dates (which should be obtained in their natural form, untreated by chemicals), dried bananas and grapes, also apricots and raisins, provided they are hygienically dried. Otherwise quantities of bacteria may collect on their sticky surface. Dried figs, pears, and prunes or a mixture of all three, are extremely useful for constipation. Figs or other fruit with seeds should not be given to patients with chronically delicate, gastro-intestinal tracts, with tendency to ulcers. Many conditions of weakness or near collapse, caused by a fall in the blood sugar, may be checked by a few sultanas, instead of by devitalized substances such as glucose or drugs like coramine. Honey is hematogenic, that is improving the hemoglobin, disinfectant and also strengthens the action of the liver. It is rich in Vitamin C and helps to restore the intestinal flora to normal. It must, however, be the genuine unadulterated and unheated variety.

VEGETABLES AND THEIR DIETETIC VALUE

Whenever possible, vegetables should be given in their uncooked form. The method of their preparation, the mechanical means of achieving any degree of fineness, that is, whether whole, chopped, grated, puréed or as juice—can be adapted to each individual case. It is important that the vegetables are fresh and, if possible, compost-grown. Like fruit, raw vegetables must precede the cooked courses and, if offered daily, ensure a regular supply of mineral trace elements and also of vitamins (see chapters on raw vegetables, pp. 49–55, and examples of diet days with raw foods, p. 294, and juices, pp. 296–9). Cooked vegetables, properly prepared, are also an indispensable addition to the diet because of the endless possibility of their variety, to enrich the menu and stimulate the palate. Dietetically speaking, they are a food rich in minerals, vitamins and vegetable protein of high quality; they nourish without supplying too many calories and do not demand too much effort on the part of the digestive organs. They are particularly valuable for diabetics (vegetable days) and for anyone wishing to retain a slim figure.

Certain vegetables of the cabbage group, and also garlic, onions and leeks, should be temporarily avoided by sufferers from intestinal disorders. Garlic and onions, however, can soon be resumed in juice mixtures, where they have a very valuable therapeutic effect on the circulation and the intestinal tract. The high content of fibrous material in cabbage easily produces flatulence, especially (as is usually the case) if the cabbages are forced with artificial fertilizers or liquid manure. Compost-grown cabbage is the most easily digested. The nutritive substances of cabbage and other vegetables are not properly utilized if the necessary enzymes are not available in the intestines. Patients with colitis are specially sensitive in this respect. Once a therapeutic diet has improved conditions in the intestines, cabbage can gradually be reintroduced. It should be given either raw (finely chopped) or steamed or sautéed in its own juice. Cabbage has a pronounced curative action on an inflamed lining (mucous membrane) of the stomach (Vitamins K and V) and is therefore given raw in the form of juices in gastric and intestinal conditions, in which form it is always readily digested, as it then contains no roughage. Raw cabbage is more easily digested than cooked.

Sauerkraut requires special mention, since it is easily digested in its uncooked state. It cleanses the intestines, has a stimulating effect on the digestive juices and on the action of the gall bladder.

Asparagus should not be eaten too frequently on account of the sulphur compounds it contains, which have a mildly irritating effect on the tissues of the kidneys. Furthermore, asparagus is poor in the usual therapeutic factors commonly contained in vegetables.

Globe artichokes, on the other hand, are to be recommended, particularly in liver conditions, on account of their mildly stimulating effect on the gall bladder. If possible, they should be given as raw juice. The same applies to chicory and small quantities of horseradish, which contain enzymes and stimulate the liver.

Spinach should not be given in the case of diarrhea unless it is compost-grown. It has a slightly purgative action. It is valuable as a blood-builder (improving the hemoglobin) because of the iron, folic acid and chlorophyll it contains. Small quantities may be given to patients with weak digestive organs as an addition to raw food, and later in the form of salad or as a vegetable dish. If special care in preparation is taken and the recipes (Nos. 99 D, 100 D) followed, it is liked even by most children.

Legumes (haricot beans, ripe peas, lentils, and soya beans) are rich in minerals and vegetable protein. They should be avoided if the supply of protein has to be kept to a minimum and they are also acid-forming foods. They are not easily digested by gastro-intestinal patients. They are more valuable and more easily digestible if germinated.

The vegetables most easily digested are carrots, beetroot, celery or celeriac (rich in iron), fennel, Jerusalem artichokes, Chinese artichokes, tomatoes, zucchini, chicory and salsify or scorzonera.

4. MENUS FOR LIGHT DIETS

EASILY DIGESTIBLE, PROTECTIVE FOR STOMACH, INTESTINES AND LIVER.

Note:

1. All recipes in this book which have a D against their numbers are suitable for a diet menu; some become diet recipes if suggested alterations are followed.

2. For Raw Salad recipes see Nos. 8–39.

FRUIT
RAW SALAD—radishes (long), white cabbage, endives.
Tomatoes as a vegetable No. 129 D.
Rice No. 223 D.

FRUIT
RAW SALAD—carrots, chicory, lettuce.
Cauliflower soup No. 84.
Beetroot as a vegetable No. 126 D.
Potatoes with cream cheese No. 193 D.

FRUIT
RAW SALAD—celery, or celeriac, savoy, lettuce.
Carrots No. 111 D.
Millet No. 247 D.
Mashed bananas, cold.

FRUIT
RAW SALAD—fennel, tomatoes, lettuce.
Spring soup No. 86 D.
Celery hearts or celeriac Nos. 107 D. 121.
Baked potatoes No. 192 D.

FRUIT
RAW SALAD—salsify, tomatoes, lettuce.
Clear vegetable broth, No. 51 D.
Apple slices.
Farina shape No. 371 D.

FRUIT
RAW SALAD—carrots, cauliflower, endives.
Salsify without sauce No. 124 D.
Tomatoes and potatoes No. 199 D.

FRUIT
RAW SALAD—beetroot, white cabbage or sauerkraut, lettuce.
Tomato soup No. 80 D.
Spinach No. 100 D.
Potatoes cooked in vegetable stock No. 195 D.

FRUIT
RAW SALAD—tomatoes stuffed with chopped celery or celeriac,
   lettuce.
Barley soup No. 72 D.
Carrots No. 111 D.
Spinach noodles No. 258.

FRUIT
RAW SALAD—celery or celeriac, tomatoes, lettuce.
Endives as a vegetable No. 102 D.
Spaghetti No. 254 D.

FRUIT
RAW SALAD—radishes (long), red cabbage, lettuce.
Minestra No. 95 D.
Spinach No. 100 D.
Tomatoes with noodles Nos. 304 and 254.

FRUIT
RAW SALAD—carrots, radishes (long), lettuce.
Spinach soup No. 82 D.
Chinese artichokes, see No. 173.
Rice No. 223 D.

FRUIT
RAW SALAD—beetroot, cress, lettuce.
Chicory No. 103 D.
Mashed potatoes No. 201 D.

FRUIT
RAW SALAD—cauliflower, endives, lettuce.
Baked tomatoes No. 130 D.
Noodles No. 259 D.

5. RAW FOOD DIET

RAW FOOD DAY
RAW FOOD DAY WITH ADDITIONS
TRANSITIONAL DAY
FULL B-B. DIET

These diets are examples of the classical Bircher-Benner
diets, as they have always been prescribed and served at the
Bircher-Benner private clinic in Zurich. They are prescribed
for different lengths of time, there are various degrees of
mechanical breaking down of the fruit and vegetables, and
different methods of preparation, according to the case in
question. Based on sixty years' experience, they provide diets

of first-class quality with curative and protective properties of the highest order. Fuller details of these diets will be found in Dr. Bircher-Benner's book, *Fruit Dishes and Raw Vegetables* (C. W. Daniel and Co., Ltd., Rochford, Essex).

A WEEKLY DIET PLAN

AS AN EXAMPLE OF THREE RAW FOOD DAYS WITH SUBSEQUENT TRANSITION TO B-B. FULL DIET.

For convalescence after severe illnesses (epidemics, feverish disorders). Given after acute attacks of rheumatism.

This diet plan, with perhaps only 1–2 Raw Food Days weekly and one week of Raw Food Days every spring and autumn, is an ideal preventive measure in cases of constitutional predisposition to high blood pressure, cardiac and kidney conditions, disturbances of the liver, migraine, chronic constipation and gastro-intestinal inertia. It is also valuable as a general preventive measure and for providing increased resistance to infection as well as for chronic rheumatic conditions.

THREE-DAY RAW FOOD DIET

Breakfast: (the same on all three days)

Bircher Muesli* with addition of germinated wheat or wheat germ Nos. 1 D–6 D.

Nuts, fruit or dried fruit.

Herb tea if desired.

Lunch:

Fruit, nuts.

Raw salad: 1st day: celery or celeriac, tomatoes, lettuce.*

2nd day: beetroot, cucumber, white cabbage.†

3rd day: carrots, kohlrabi, cress.*

Evening Meal:

The same as breakfast (the same on all three days).

4th Day: Raw Food Day with additions:

---

* Raw vegetables fat-free: without oil, only lemon or buttermilk or skimmed yogurt.

† Raw vegetables fat-free: without oil, only lemon or buttermilk or skimmed yogurt.

Breakfast:

Same as for Raw Food Day with addition of one slice of wholewheat bread, Ryvita or pumpernickel.

About 1 level teaspoon butter.

Herb tea.

Lunch:

Fruit.

Raw salad—radishes (long or large ones), tomatoes, lettuce.

Vegetable broth No. 51 D.

Baked potatoes No. 192 D.

Evening Meal:

The same as for breakfast. If preferred, germinated wheat can be taken instead of wholewheat bread with the addition of some dried fruit.

5th Day: Transitional Day

Breakfast:

Bircher Muesli with milled nuts.

2 slices wholewheat bread.

About 1 tablespoon butter.

Fruit.

Herb tea or milk or yogurt.

Lunch:

Fruit.

Raw salad—cauliflower, spinach, lettuce.

Potato soup No. 89 D.

Baked tomatoes No. 130 D.

Whole rice with fresh butter only, without cheese and with very little salt. No. 223 D.

Evening Meal:

The same as for breakfast. If desired, rose hip jam, honey or helva purée can be spread on the bread.

6th Day: Full B-B. Diet

Breakfast:

The same as for Transitional Day.

Lunch:

Fruit.

Raw salad—zucchini, beetroot, lettuce.

Oat groats soup No. 71 D.

Spinach No. 100 D.

Potatoes with cream cheese No. 193 D.

Evening Meal:

> The same as for breakfast, with the addition of cream cheese No. 48 *a* D, or some other soft cheese such as Gervais.

7th Day: Full B-B Diet

Breakfast:

> The same as on the 6th day.

Lunch:

> Fruit.
>
> Raw salad—finely chopped celery or grated celeriac, cress, lettuce.
>
> Cooked dishes—zucchini No. 137 D, mashed potatoes No. 201 D.
>
> Fruit juice jelly with cream No. 336 D.

Evening Meal:

> Bircher Muesli.
>
> Minestra No. 95 D.
>
> Wholewheat bread No. 420.
>
> Butter mixed with herbs (Herb Butter) or soya sandwich filling.
>
> Herb Tea.

6. FASTING ON JUICES AND FRUITS

JUICE DAY WITH PROTEIN · · · · · · · · · · STRICT JUICE DAY

FASTING ON FRUIT

The essence of this diet is that it is liquid food and is, therefore, the most easily assimilated nourishment for all severe illnesses and feverish conditions, especially for acute cases of gastro-intestinal disorders and disturbances of the liver and pancreas, as well as for peptic ulcers. It is free of fiber and cellulose and therefore does not tax the digestive organs, yet it is rich in first-class quality vitamins and minerals.

The physician can adapt the juice diet by different methods of preparation and in various combinations, according to the prevailing conditions and requirements of the patient. Such a diet can be continued for days and even weeks.

Chronic conditions such as cardiac and circulatory disorders, rheumatism and particularly obesity, also respond extremely well to a juice diet taken a day at a time, owing to its relieving, 'detoxicating' and dehydrating effect. Such Juice Days are best followed by a Raw Food Day, then by a Raw Food Day with Additions and a Transitional Day. Juice Days may be prescribed in different forms, varying from strict juice days—which means 'fasting on juices'—to juice days with additional liquid protein, an adequate form of nourishment even over long periods.

JUICE DAYS WITH PROTEIN

A nutrition of high value, relatively satisfying. This may be continued for one week or more. If strenuous physical and mental exertion is avoided, it may even be continued for weeks with the addition of cereals in the form of cream* (gruel).

Juice with protein periods are prescribed at the beginning of any change of diet treatment, for dehydrating and reducing diets and also in cases of vitamin and mineral deficiency, such as may happen in chronic digestive conditions in which a 'protective diet' without fresh uncooked foods, as often used by the old schools of thought, has been carried out for any length of time. In such cases, one-third of the fruit juice should be replaced by linseed, cream of barley or cream of rice (gruel—Recipe No. 44) or by Agar-Agar jellies (Recipes Nos. 336 D and 361 D). During dehydrating cures, urine and weight must be regularly checked and a diuretic tisane (such as solidago or rose hip, p. 220) given if necessary.

DAILY MENU FOR A 'JUICE WITH PROTEIN' DAY

Breakfast: 1 glass freshly extracted mixed fruit juice (Recipe No. 42 D).

¾ glass Almond Milk or soya milk or yogurt (Recipe Nos. 45, 47, 48 D).

1 cup rose hip or solidago tea (p. 220) with brown sugar if desired.

Lunch: 1 glass freshly extracted mixed fruit juice.

¾ glass Almond Milk No. 45 D *or* Sesame Milk No. 46 D *or* yogurt No. 48 D.

¾ glass any freshly extracted vegetable juice or 2–3 kinds mixed (Recipe No. 43 D).

1 cup solidago tea with brown sugar if desired.

Evening Meal: 1 glass mixed freshly extracted fruit juice.

¾ glass Almond Milk or yogurt.

1 cup solidago or lemon peel tea (p. 220) if desired.

If the diet must be kept entirely fat-free, the milk part may be given in the form of buttermilk, yogurt made with skimmed milk, or skimmed salt-free milk (made into yogurt if desired).

* See p. 59.

STRICT JUICE DAYS
(TO BE TAKEN WHILE RESTING IN BED)

If more intensive action with regard to fasting, general 'detoxication', dehydration and rejuvenation is desired, a stricter fruit juice day may be suggested before the Juice with Protein period. It may also be carried out once a week in a normal diet. This day must, however, only be undertaken if absolute rest is possible, mental as well as physical, best of all in bed. Without such rest, the full effect of the treatment is not achieved. Weariness and hunger prevent relaxation and relief from tension, consequently the desired spectacular discharge of urine does not result.

The patient should not be disheartened by reactions such as headache, nausea or sensations of weakness (especially in the afternoon). These are signs that the fasting is causing the organism to start the work of detoxication, and that such days really achieve their purpose. These observations should, nevertheless, be reported to the doctor.

DAILY MENU FOR A STRICT JUICE DAY

(a) 3 *glasses juice* (*severe*)

8 a.m.   1 glass freshly extracted, unsweetened fruit juice No. 42 D: grapefruit, orange, tangerine, berry, peach, melon, etc.

12.30 p.m.   1 glass fruit juice as above, *or*
                    1 glass fresh vegetable juice No. 43 D, with a few drops lemon juice; for instance, carrot, tomato, spinach, beetroot, plain or mixed.

6 p.m.   1 glass fruit juice as at 8 a.m.

Note: Absolute rest in bed is necessary. Weight and urine check during the 24 hours is advisable. Not more than 1–3 days should be carried out in succession unless under a doctor's supervision.

This type of day is advisable before Raw Food treatment and before Juice Days with Protein and once per week regularly (see above).

If the patient suffers badly from thirst, or there is insufficient discharge of urine (less than 24 oz. in 24 hours), 1–3 small cups of solidago or rose hip tea may be given in addition, between the juice meals.

(*b*) 4 *glasses juice* (*less severe*)

8 a.m.	1 glass freshly extracted fruit juice.
Midday	1 glass freshly extracted plain or mixed vegetable juice.
4 p.m.	1 glass freshly extracted fruit juice of different kinds.
8 p.m.	¾–1 glass carrot or tomato juice, *or* ¾ glass plain orange juice at 4 p.m. and 1 glass at 8 p.m.

The duration and application is the same as for the stricter form (*a*).

FASTING ON FRUIT

This may replace the Strict Juice Day, i.e. the strict form of the Fasting on Juice day if, for instance, a change in the metabolism and stimulation of the intestines with fiber or cellulose is required instead of a protective diet, free of fiber or cellulose. The sense of satisfaction is stronger, for which reason single days of Fasting on Fruit are possible without absolute rest, and such a diet may be continued for a longer period. However, the effect of Fasting on Juice—that is Strict Juice Days—is more intense.

Fasting on Fruit is indicated in cardiac conditions, chronic weakness of the liver, intestinal inertia; an apple day is effective in cases of acute diarrhea, a strawberry day is more effective in cases of sprue. They can be taken with all precautions about rest for 1–5 days, longer only if prescribed by the physician.

DAILY MENU

3 times daily:
> About ½ lb. washed, fresh, ripe, unsweetened fruit, for instance, berries, citrus fruits (oranges, grapefruit, tangerines), grapes, figs, melon.

DAYS OF FASTING ON INDIVIDUAL FRUITS

Apple day (5–6 times daily):
> 1 large apple, finely grated, in cases of acute gastrointestinal inflammation with diarrhea.

Strawberry day (3–4 times daily):
> About ½ lb. very ripe strawberries, unsweetened, in cases of sprue (chronic diarrhea in the tropics), Vitamin C deficiency.

Blueberry day (3 times daily):
About ½ lb. Mildly constipating, disinfectant.

Blackberry day (3 times daily):
About ½ lb. Particularly rich in natural sugar and Vitamin C, easily digestible and nourishing.

Currant day (3 times daily):
About ½ lb. two-thirds red and white, one-third black. Rich in Vitamin C, especially refreshing and thirst-quenching for liver patients.

Grape day (4–5 times daily):
Grape cure of old repute: total amount of about 1–2 lb. grapes divided into 4–5 portions. Whole fruit to be eaten, well washed and freed of residues of poison spraying Poor in vitamins but specially nourishing owing to its high content of fruit sugar, which is so easily assimilated. Protects the liver. Seeds stimulate intestines. Can be carried out for 1–2 weeks, or up to 6 weeks if prescribed by a physician.

Fig day (3 times daily):
About ½ lb. Stimulates bowels, nourishing. Not for more than one day.

7. DIET DURING PREGNANCY AND BREAST-FEEDING

Although pregnancy is in itself a healthy condition, there are special dietetic requirements which the expectant mother has to consider.

(*a*) Dietetic measures to be taken to ensure that mother and child are supplied with all the substances necessary for the development of the child, and for the special task of the mother's organism, without overtaxing or depleting her strength.

(*b*) Suitable nutrition to combat the transitional symptoms, particularly of the early months, such as nausea and vomiting, also abnormal cravings and aversions.

We cannot give detailed instructions in this book but a few general directions for diet during pregnancy and breast-feeding are suggested.

1. The healthy woman should follow her natural instinct, which is often an excellent guide to the choice of correct foodstuffs.

2. It is not necessary to 'eat for two' since the mother's organism selects and utilizes efficiently and economically everything it receives.

3. The same general rules as in the Bircher-Benner Full Diet for the healthy are applicable but stricter adherence to its principles are necessary, i.e. fresh food as a start to every meal, two or three raw vegetables daily, as many green leaf salads as possible, only whole-grain cereals of every type, no devitalized food (canned goods, white flour, refined sugar, etc.), meat as a rare addition, if at all, no stimulants such as coffee, tea, alcohol and nicotine. Only a little salt; mild seasonings such as herbs should be used.

If, during the early months, the expectant mother suffers from nausea, heartburn, unnatural cravings, various digestive disturbances and abnormal flow of saliva, she should base her diet strictly on the following rules:

1. Whole food, in its natural state.
2. Low fat diet. The following fats are most easily assimilated: sunflower oil, fresh butter and nut butter. No fatty cheeses or chocolate are pemitted.
3. Dry, plain food, requiring long and thorough chewing, thus making good use of the saliva and gastric juices secreted in excessive quantities.
4. Little ordinary unskimmed milk should be taken; instead 2–2½ cups daily of sour milk, yogurt, buttermilk, cream cheese and Gervais or other soft cheeses.
5. Raw vegetables without dressing. Once or twice daily whole leaves, tomatoes, long radishes, carrots, cucumbers, etc. Green leaves as juice, raw or cooked.
6. Germinated whole cereal grains, coarsely ground, or dry flakes (rich in vegetable protein, Vitamin B complex and Vitamin E) twice or three times daily. Acts as an intestinal stimulant. Recipe No. 40 D.
7. Raw Food Days (see p. 293) with nuts and dried fruit once or twice weekly, or one whole week per month.
8. Coffee, tea, alcohol, nicotine and refined sugar are harmful (causing heartburn) and should be strictly avoided.
9. Meat should not be eaten during any period of vomiting.
10. Little fluid should be taken; thirst should be quenched with fruit.

Specimen Menu if nausea (morning sickness) is troublesome

If the expectant mother feels nausea on waking, a few raisins, pine kernels, mint or peppermint leaves can be chewed (p. 217).

Breakfast: Fruit, dried fruit, 3–5 nuts (to be well chewed); yogurt, wholewheat bread, dry or with cream cheese.

10 a.m. Fruit juice if thirsty. Bitter Tea (see p. 219) for nausea.

Midday: Plate of fruit without sugar; ½ cup spinach juice, 1 whole tomato, 1 whole carrot, 1–2 cabbage leaves (whole and well washed); whole rice or potatoes in their skins with cream cheese, Gervais or other soft cheese; real fruit jellies (see Recipe No. 336 D, p. 175) with brown sugar.

4 p.m. Fruit juice or small cup Bitter Tea; one slice Ryvita or pumpernickel or similar bread if desired.

Evening: Bircher Muesli or fruit; flakes cereal grains (coarsely ground) with a little honey and dried fruit; if desired one potato in its skin, or a cereal soup; buttermilk or yogurt.

1 apple to be left by the bed so that small pieces can be chewed if feelings of nausea should occur during the night.

Note: If the vomiting is severe, consult a doctor as soon as possible.

If the bowels are not working regularly, 1 tablespoon psyllium seeds should be taken twice daily.

A fortnight before the birth is expected, raw food should be eaten almost exclusively, with fresh whole grains, yogurt and potatoes in their skins. Such a diet keeps the metabolism and all the bodily functions in the best condition and prevents the retention of fluids, causing swelling of the tissues in mother and child.

Foods which stimulate milk secretion: Almonds, Almond Cream and Milk, soya and sesame cream, germinated wheat, coarsely ground whole cereals, wheat germ, oats, grapes, grape juice, honey, all fresh fruit, T.T. (tuberculin tested) milk, yogurt, cream cheese and other soft cheeses.

In addition, exposure of the breasts to sunshine or ultra-violet light, exercises and hydrotherapy improve the circulation in the breasts.

Excessive drinking should be avoided. It is harmful to the metabolism of the mother and the quality of her milk.

8. DIET FOR REDUCING AND FOR RETAINING A SLIM FIGURE

One important fact should be stressed at the outset: overweight or obesity is the result of disturbed health, a disorder resulting in exaggerated growth of fatty tissue and therefore a disturbance of metabolism. Glandular trouble is often, but not always, the cause. Abnormal overweight is never caused *solely* by over-eating, otherwise everyone with a good appetite would be fat. Unbalanced nutrition and over-eating are factors leading to disease, but there are both fat and thin gluttons who fall ill. *Weight reduction of the obese must, above all, mean recovery of good health,* and once a slim figure has been achieved, only good health will retain it. Fashions in reducing diets, many of them short-lived but very popular, forcing a weight reduction within a definite period of time, do not belong to our work nor to the ideas on which this book is based.

Forced reduction of weight *within a brief period* may occasionally be justified for the purpose of special film or stage parts, or particular types of sport (light athletics). However, it is dangerous to extend or repeat this period as the metabolic balance and general health will be disturbed. Nicotine and drugs to check the appetite have no place in a healthy reducing diet.

In all slimming diets reducing must proceed at a rate to suit each individual organism until the ideal weight has been reached.

We give below a few brief and practical suggestions as to how this can be achieved without damage to the metabolic and eliminative organs and, what is more, how it may be combined with an increase in vitality and improved health altogether. Behind this brief summary are the sixty years of clinical experience of the Bircher-Benner school.

Basic Principles for Reducing Weight

1. The total consumption of cooked food should be decreased to achieve a higher proportion of fresh uncooked food for the purpose of retaining as many of the active principles as possible.

2. To allow a more economical utilization of this raw food, it should always be eaten at the beginning of the meal.

3. *Fat* should be strictly reduced and limited to the unrefined types containing the highest proportion of unsaturated fatty acids, see pp. 19–20 and 283.

4. *Starch and sugars*—except for natural fruit sugar—should also be strictly reduced or temporarily omitted.

5. *Protein* (animal and vegetable). Animal protein should be taken only in the form of low-fat milk products. Vegetable proteins such as are contained in raw vegetables and whole cereals only should be taken.

In the case of hypofunction of the thyroid, confirmed by a physician, a more abundant, but still relatively moderate quantity of milk protein (buttermilk, yogurt made of skimmed milk, salt-free milk, soft cheese with low fat content, cream cheese, etc.) is advisable.

We would like to warn against unbalanced, excessive high protein diets for the purpose of reducing. According to our experience they are based on a fallacy, achieve only a short-lived success, followed by a relapse and damage to the organism, due to over-burdening it with protein (injury to the liver, inflammation of the large intestine, rheumatic disorders, etc.).

6. *Cooking salt,* hot spices and stimulating substances, such as coffee, and nicotine, should be restricted.

Diet Treatment for Reducing

1–2 Strict Juice Days (see chapter on 'Fasting on Juices', pp. 296–7).

2–3 Juice Days with Protein, fat-free (see chapter on 'Fasting on Juices', p. 296–7).

2–3 Raw Food Days, fat-free (see chapter on 'Raw Food Days', p. 294).

Subsequently, 'Diet for Retaining a Slim Figure' (weekly plan below) with inclusion of one Strict Juice Day or Fruit Fasting, or one Juice Day with Protein per week, fat-free.

Stricter reducing diets must be carried out under a doctor's supervision.

The weekly Strict Juice Day, p. 298, particularly if adhered to for some time, requires rest in bed and a weight check. A rapid reduction in weight is most pronounced at the beginning (dehydration), though some of the loss will be made up again in the course of the week. However, as time advances and general weight reduction increases, such fluctuations become slighter and the weight curve more dependable and permanently low. The improvement in general health will be considerable.

The Fruit Juice or Fruit Fasting Day should be carried out at longer intervals, for instance, once per month if possible. It may, however, be replaced by a buttermilk day (the same quantity, up to 2 good pints daily) or a salt-free milk day, provided the patient can tolerate milk.

WEEKLY PLAN FOR A DIET FOR RETAINING A SLIM FIGURE

These menus are intended to help all those who have completed a reducing diet treatment under the supervision of a doctor, and whose problem now is to maintain the weight reduction they have achieved. This plan offers a frugal but adequate diet, even for working days.

At the same time we should like to point out how important it is to see that bowel action is regular and spontaneous without the aid of medicines, and that sufficient urine is discharged (over 2 pints every 24 hours). The latter may be encouraged by rose hip tea; should this prove insufficient, 1–2 cups of solidago tea must be drunk daily (see chapter on Herb Teas, p. 211). Nothing should be eaten between meals.

Day preceding the Weekly Diet Plan: Strict Juice Day or Fruit Fasting Day (see pp. 298 and 299).

1st day: Breakfast:

About 5 oz. Bircher Muesli (see No. 3D) with yogurt made of skimmed milk and some honey.

1 level tablespoon milled nuts.

1 slice wholewheat bread with cream cheese No. 48 *a* made of skimmed milk.

1 cup rose hip, lime blossom or solidago tea, unsweetened (p. 211).

Lunch:

FRUIT (equivalent of 1 apple).

RAW SALAD

2–3 heaping tablespoons raw vegetables with low-fat (e.g. sunflower oil) dressing.

COOKED DISHES:

1 cup vegetable broth, No. 51 D, if desired with fat-free garnish (small quantity noodles, etc.).

Steamed celery No. 107 D or celeriac, No. 121 (fat-free or only a little fat).

1 large or 2 small potatoes with curd made of skimmed milk, No. 193 D.

Evening Meal:

About 5 oz. Bircher Muesli or ½ grapefruit, or about 5 oz. yogurt Muesli made of skimmed milk (see No. 3 D).

1 slice wholewheat bread.

About 1 level teaspoon butter, nut butter or curd, or about 5 oz. crushed whole wheat or other whole cereals with milk, or buttermilk, and a brown sugar.

2nd day: Breakfast
Same as above.

Lunch:
FRUIT (as 1st day)

RAW SALAD:
2–3 heaping tablespoons raw vegetables, with low-fat
dressing.

COOKED DISHES:
Steamed endives (without fat), No. 102 D.
Stuffed tomatoes (with cheese slices). See No. 133.

DESSERT:
Jelly made of fresh fruit juice with a little sugar,
No. 336 D.

Evening Meal:
About 5 oz. Bircher Muesli or ½ grapefruit.
Mixed salads, Salad Niçoise if desired, No. 185 D.
1 cup vegetable stock, No. 51 D.

3rd day: Breakfast:
Same as above.

Lunch:
FRUIT (as above)

RAW SALAD:
2–3 heaping tablespoons raw vegetables, with low-fat
dressing.

COOKED DISHES:
Dish of mixed vegetables (cauliflower, beans, carrots,
1 potato cooked in vegetable stock). Very small
portions of each.

DESSERT:
1 tablespoon blueberries or any other soft fruit.

Evening Meal:
About 5 oz. fruit salad.
About ¼ cup yogurt or buttermilk.
1 slice wholewheat bread.
About 1 teaspoon nut butter or curd.
3 walnuts.

4th day: Breakfast:
Same as above.

Lunch:
FRUIT (as above).

RAW SALAD:
2–3 heaping tablespoons raw vegetables, with low-fat
dressing.

COOKED DISHES:

1 small portion carrot soup, No. 81 D.

Tomatoes with rice, lettuce, Nos. 132–3.

Evening Meal:

¾ cup freshly extracted fruit juice, p. 58.

2 open sandwiches or canapés (one of tomato and one of curd or other cheese), No. 190.

1 cup Herb Tea, p. 219.

5th day: Breakfast:

Same as above.

Lunch:

FRUIT (as above).

RAW SALAD:

2 raw stuffed tomatoes (celery, celeriac or carrot, white cabbage), No. 39.

1 spinach omelette with a little fat, No. 272.

DESSERT:

Apple purée, No. 337 D.

Evening Meal:

About 5 oz. Bircher Muesli.

COOKED DISH:

1 soup plate minestra without noodles, No. 95 D.

6th day: Breakfast:

Same as above.

Lunch:

½ grapefruit.

1 glass freshly extracted carrot and tomato juice.

Millotto with vegetables, No. 248 D, and corn-salad (lamb's lettuce).

Evening Meal:

About 5 oz. Bircher Muesli.

2–3 caraway potatoes No. 194 D.

1 small portion soft cheese (Gervais) or curd made with skimmed milk, No. 48 a.

1 portion lettuce.

7th day: Breakfast:

FRUIT (as above).

About 5 oz. crushed whole cereal.

½ cup yogurt or buttermilk.

Lunch:

FRUIT (as above).

RAW SALAD:

2–3 heaping tablespoons raw vegetables, with low-fat dressing.

COOKED DISHES:
2–3 potato cakes with spinach, No. 203.
DESSERT:
Orange Whip No. 359, Version 2, or fruit jelly No. 336 D, with a little beaten egg white instead of whipped cream.

Evening Meal:
About 5 oz. Bircher Muesli.
About 1 tablespoon ground or whole almonds.
1 slice wholewheat bread.
1 tablespoon curd made of skimmed milk, mixed with a little milk, chives, Marmite or other yeast extract, or soya spread, No. 48 *a*.

9. LOW-FAT DIET

FOR GASTRIC, INTESTINAL, LIVER, GALL BLADDER AND PANCREATIC CONDITIONS, AND OBESITY

Since the digestion of fat puts a special burden on the liver, care must be taken that the diet for liver and gall-bladder conditions contains little or even no fat. These diets may have to be prescribed for short or long periods under the supervision of a physician.

A low-fat diet must be prepared with great skill so that it may be of high quality and, at the same time, tasty and stimulating to the appetite, despite the restrictions necessary. Since the stomach, intestines and pancreas take part in the digestion of fat, and as, in the cases of liver disorder, the stomach and intestines are nearly always in an irritated and weak condition, a low-fat diet must also be easily digestible. Thus a low-fat protective liver diet must be combined with a gastro-intestinal protective diet. In chronic cases it must be possible to continue this diet also over long periods without any deficiencies resulting.

A weekly plan with menus for a low-fat diet which is tasty and varied and, at the same time, of full value, is suggested below.

If an entirely fat-free diet has been prescribed, the fat must be omitted altogether from the low-fat menus. Thus: no nuts or nut butter; also no butter should be used. Only yogurt made of skimmed milk or buttermilk is allowed. Salads should be dressed with lemon juice or, for instance, buttermilk instead of oil. Bircher Muesli must be made only with yogurt of skimmed milk or buttermilk. Curd must be made only of skimmed milk. Vegetable stock should not contain any fat, nor must butter be added to any vegetables and other cooked dishes before serving. Junket can also be made with skimmed milk.

The recipes in this book marked D are intended for use in such low-fat protective diets.

WEEKLY PLAN FOR A LOW-FAT PROTECTIVE DIET

1st day: Breakfast:

Bircher Muesli, small portion (about 3½ oz.), perhaps with yogurt made with skimmed milk (see No. 3 D).

1 teaspoon milled nuts, pine kernels if desired.

Wholewheat bread with a teaspoonful of butter, a little nut butter and honey or with curd made with skimmed milk, No. 48 *a*.

A herb or rose hip tea, sweetened with brown sugar, p. 220.

Lunch:

FRUIT

RAW VEGETABLES:

Beetroot, zucchini with lemon juice and a little yogurt, lettuce with French dressing.

COOKED DISH:

Tomato soup without cream, No. 80 D.

Steamed fennel with a little fresh butter, No. 108 D.

Caraway potatoes, No. 194 D.

Evening Meal:

Bircher Muesli.

Wholewheat bread with nut butter.

COOKED DISHES:

Oatmeal gruel soup without cream, No. 70 D.

Fruit.

2nd day: Breakfast:

As above.

Lunch:

FRUIT

RAW VEGETABLES:

Celery or celeriac, tomatoes, lettuce, with lemon juice and a little oil or yogurt.

COOKED DISHES:

Steamed lettuce, No. 101 D.

Whole rice, No. 223 D, with tomato sauce, No. 304.

DESSERT:

Apple purée, No. 337 D.

Evening Meal:

During the berry season, berries with yogurt or junket made with skimmed milk, and brown sugar: otherwise Bircher Muesli.

Potatoes in their skins, No. 192 D, with curd (dressed with milk, chives, a little salt or caraway seeds), No. 48 b.

Lettuce with a little French dressing and chives.

3rd day: Breakfast:

As above.

Instead of wholewheat bread, perhaps a crushed cereal dish with milk or yogurt and brown sugar.

Lunch:

FRUIT

RAW VEGETABLES:

Carrots (with yogurt, lemon juice and herbs), spinach and lettuce with a little olive oil, lemon juice, onion and mint.

COOKED DISHES:

Farina soup without cream, No. 74 D.

Cooked celery or celeriac with a little fresh butter added before serving, No. 107 D.

Potato snow, No. 200 D.

Evening Meal:

Bircher Muesli, milled nuts if desired.

Wholewheat bread with nut butter and rose hip jam.

Fruit and a little dried fruit if desired.

Herb Tea.

4th day: Breakfast:

See above.

Lunch:

FRUIT

RAW VEGETABLES:

Long or large round radishes, cress and lettuce with French dressing (little oil).

COOKED DISHES:

Steamed or stewed zucchini, Nos. 136 D and 137 D.

Noodles without cheese and with a little fresh butter, No. 258 D.

DESSERT:

Fruit jelly made from freshly expressed fruit juice, No. 336 D.

Evening Meal:

Bircher Muesli.

Wholewheat bread.

COOKED DISH:

Thick minestra, if necessary without cheese, No. 95 D.

5th day: *Breakfast:*
As above.
Lunch:
FRUIT
RAW VEGETABLES:
Cauliflower with yogurt, lemon juice and herbs, cucumber and lettuce with French dressing.
COOKED DISHES:
Tomato soup, No. 80 D.
Steamed or stewed stalks of spinach beet, No. 105 D.
Potatoes cooked in vegetable stock, with a little fresh butter, No. 195 D.
Evening Meal:
Bircher Muesli or ½ grapefruit.
COOKED DISHES:
Baked potatoes and a little soft cheese, No. 192 D.
Salad.
Wholewheat bread.

6th day: *Breakfast:*
As above.
Lunch:
FRUIT
RAW VEGETABLES:
Kohlrabi with yogurt, lemon juice and herbs, spinach and lettuce with French dressing (little oil).
COOKED DISHES:
Vegetable stock with tapioca, No. 51 D.
Steamed carrots, No. 111 D.
Millotto with a little fresh butter, No. 247 D.
Evening Meal:
Bircher Muesli or fruit.
Open sandwiches or rolls with curd, tomatoes, radishes, cress.
Rose hip tea.

7th day: *Breakfast:*
As above.
Lunch:
FRUIT
RAW VEGETABLES:
Fennel and lettuce with French dressing (little oil), cauliflower with yogurt, lemon juice and herbs.
COOKED DISHES:
Steamed or stewed chicory, No. 103 D.
Tomatoes and potatoes, No. 199 D.
Red fruit shape, No. 378.

Evening Meal:
Bircher Muesli with a little banana.
Wholewheat noodles with very little fresh butter, No.
258 D, served with lettuce if liked.
Cup of vegetable broth, No. 51 D.

10. SALT-FREE DIET

This diet is often prescribed by a physician in cases of edema (abnormally large amounts of fluid in the tissues), cardiac and circulatory disease, and for certain kidney disorders. In these menus not only is no salt used but furthermore only those vegetables and fruits are included whose sodium content is low. Since many vegetables, especially tubers, contain sodium, the menus are, consequently, of limited variety. However, as the diet usually has only to be followed for a short time, the patient will not find it difficult to carry out.

The following basic principles should be carefully noted:

1. Do not use any common salt at all.
2. Use only salt-free butter for all cooking and eating.
3. For seasoning, use a salt-free yeast extract such as Marmite (unsalted).
4. Use salt-free milk powder for all recipes requiring milk (p. 286).
5. Use soya flour instead of eggs.
6. Adapt the dressings used for raw salads as follows:
    (*a*) cream sauce without cream cheese;
    (*b*) mayonnaise with soya flour or sesame purée, as suggested in the recipes (No. 10 D).
7. The breakfast menu is the same for each day.

Not all the items listed in the Weekly Plan need be included. A choice can be made to suit the appetite of the individual patient.

Vegetables rich in sodium, and therefore to be avoided, are: beetroot, dandelion, celeriac, corn-salad (lamb's lettuce), tomatoes, carrots and kohlrabi. All other vegetables may be freely used.

The outer husk of natural rice grains contains sodium, so if a strict sodium-free diet has been prescribed, whole brown rice cannot be used. If a partly polished variety is available, this is advisable, otherwise white rice must be used.

As a rule, however, the sodium contained in vegetables need not be avoided to the same extent as if taken with a mixed diet, since the former contain far more potassium, which offsets the sodium.

The same applies to culinary herbs which, though they contain sodium, are used in such small quantities that this does not matter. Herbs are excellent for seasoning salt-free diets if used in moderation.

When small quantities of salt are once again allowed in the cooking, sea salt should be used instead of cooking salt.

Salt substitutes should not be taken without the physician's permission. They vary considerably as to content and suitability and may disturb the balance of the mineral metabolism of the body.

WEEKLY PLAN FOR A SALT-FREE DIET WITH LOW SODIUM CONTENT

1st day: Breakfast:
>
> Almond Muesli.
> Salt-free wholewheat bread.
> Unsalted butter.
> FRUIT:
> Selected from the following: oranges, pears, apples, cherries, plums, damsons, watermelons, cantaloupes, tangerines, currants (red and black), bananas, dried figs, raisins or sultanas.
> Nuts: almonds, filberts, Brazil nuts, walnuts.
> Tea: Herb Tea with brown sugar if desired.
>
> *Lunch:*
> FRUIT (as above).
> RAW VEGETABLES:
> Cauliflower, lettuce.
> COOKED DISHES:
> Green beans, No. 119, fried potatoes, No. 213.
> DESSERT:
> Banana whip as in No. 354, with salt-free milk* and a little cream and brown sugar, or Rice and Lemon Pudding, No. 373 D.
>
> *Evening Meal:*
> The same as breakfast, with the addition of Oatmeal Soup, No. 69 D.

2nd day: Breakfast:
>
> See above.
>
> *Lunch:*
> FRUIT
> RAW VEGETABLES:
> Long or round large radishes, lettuce.

* See p. 286.

COOKED DISHES:

Vegetable broth (of onions, leeks, curly kale, potato peel, sorrel), No. 51 D.

Cauliflower, No. 153.

Parsley potatoes, No. 196 D.

Evening Meal:

The same as breakfast, with the addition of a whole cereal dish with raisins.

3rd day: Breakfast:

See above.

Lunch:

FRUIT

RAW VEGETABLES:

Parsnips, lettuce.

COOKED DISHES:

Steamed or stewed peas, No. 116 D, in rice ring, No. 234 D.

DESSERT:

Fruit jelly: from fresh fruit juice prepared with Agar-Agar, No. 336 D.

Evening Meal:

The same as breakfast with the addition of thick potato soup, No. 89 D.

4th day: Breakfast:

See above.

Lunch:

FRUIT

RAW VEGETABLES:

Cauliflower, cress.

COOKED DISHES:

Barley soup, No. 72 D, steamed or stewed parsnips, mashed potato, No. 201 D, prepared with salt-free milk.

Evening Meal:

Fruit and nuts.

Rice pudding with salt-free milk, No. 374.

Stewed plums.

5th day: Breakfast:

See above.

Lunch:

FRUIT

RAW VEGETABLES:

Chicory, spring cabbage or curly kale.

COOKED DISHES:

Steamed lettuce, No. 101 D, wheat cakes with soya (instead of eggs), No. 280.

DESSERT:

Stuffed apples (with raisins and nuts), No. 346 D.

Evening Meal:

The same as breakfast, with salt-free milk instead of tea.

6th day: *Breakfast:*

See above.

Lunch:

FRUIT

RAW VEGETABLES:

Parsnips, Brussels sprouts.

COOKED DISHES:

Browned wholewheat soup, No. 78, broccoli (steamed or stewed) as No. 154, but omit sauce. French fried potatoes, No. 218.

Evening Meal:

See above.

7th day: *Breakfast:*

See above.

Lunch:

FRUIT

RAW VEGETABLES:

Chicory, lettuce.

COOKED DISHES:

Steamed or stewed Brussels sprouts, No. 155, but omit sauce, Japanese rice, No. 223 D.

DESSERT:

Cold fruit dish with bananas.

Evening Meal:

The same as breakfast, with the addition of sodium-free cheese (soft cheese, cheese made of cream).

11. ALLERGY DIET

EXCLUSIVELY PLANT DIET

This is a diet for cases of hypersensitiveness, or allergic reaction, to certain outside influences which manifests itself in skin disorders, asthma, hay fever, rheumatic disease, digestive conditions of allergic origin, etc.

It is a simple matter to keep to purely plant nutrition, containing no animal substances whatsoever, with the aid of the Bircher diet. This can be extremely valuable in allergic conditions, above all in cases where experience has shown that hypersensitiveness toward animal substances (protein and fat) is present. It appears that an exclusively vegetable diet is even able to reduce an allergic tendency altogether. Such a diet may, for instance, be tried out in cases of disorders of suspected allergic origin such as those of the gastro-intestinal tract and of the joints, in cases of chronic nettle rash (urticaria), of bronchial asthma and specially of eczema.

If an exclusively plant nutrition proves to be the only way to achieve permanent freedom from these unpleasant symptoms, the food must be selected with special care, so as to avoid any deficiency. The body of the patient in question requires in addition sufficient natural sunlight or ultra-violet rays, to ensure that adequate quantities of the essential Vitamin D (otherwise contained only in animal food, milk and milk products) are formed in the skin.

The calcium content of the diet, normally well provided by milk and milk products, must also be replaced in a plant diet by the special addition of vegetables containing calcium (see chapter on Mineral Substances). Such a long-term diet may be carried out only under the supervision of an experienced physician.

WEEKLY PLAN FOR ALLERGIC CONDITIONS

Exclusively plant diet, free of animal protein and other animal products. Soyamel can be used as a milk substitute (see p. 286). Low salt content.

For cases of hypersensitiveness (allergy) towards animal protein and fat. Also for skin diseases and allergic phenomena such as certain intestinal symptoms, and asthma, hay fever, etc., high blood pressure, kidney disease, acute feverish conditions and certain forms of general gastro-intestinal disturbances which have to be diagnosed by the physician.

1st day: Breakfast:

    Bircher Muesli (for preparation see Recipe No. 2), with Almond Cream or Nut Cream and honey.

    Wholewheat bread with nut butter.

    Milled or whole nuts of all kinds.

    Herb Tea sweetened with brown sugar (p. 219).

    Fruit if desired.

    Lunch:

    FRUIT of all kinds.

    RAW VEGETABLES:

Carrots (with Nut Cream, Almond Cream or French dressing), cucumber and lettuce (with French dressing).

Note: All dressings for raw vegetables must be made without cream, curd, yogurt or mayonnaise.

COOKED DISHES:
Minestra No. 95 D.
Zucchini, steamed or stewed, with nut butter, No. 137 D.
Rice with nut butter, without cheese, No. 223 D.
Evening Meal:
Bircher Muesli (prepared as for breakfast).
Wholewheat bread with nut butter and rose hip purée.
Milled or whole nuts.
Fruit or dried fruit.
Herb or rose hip tea.

2nd day: Breakfast:
This always remains the same. See above.
Lunch:
FRUIT
RAW VEGETABLES:
Beetroot, white cabbage, lettuce (dressings as suggested for the first day).
COOKED DISHES:
Steamed lettuce with nut butter, No. 101 D.
Filbert potatoes with nut butter, No. 216.
DESSERT:
Stuffed apples (raisins, nuts and brown sugar), No. 346 D.
Evening Meal:
Bircher Muesli, No. 2, or fruit.
Wholewheat bread with nut butter.
Nuts.
COOKED DISHES:
Potato soup with nut butter, No. 89 D, or farina, No. 74 D, or barley soup, No. 72 D.
An herb tea.

3rd day: Breakfast:
See above.
Lunch:
FRUIT
RAW VEGETABLES:
Salsify, red cabbage, lettuce.

COOKED DISHES:

Cream of leek soup with nut butter, No.87.

Tomatoes as a vegetable with nut butter, No. 130 D.

Soya spaetzle (soya replaces egg), No. 264 D.

Evening Meal:

Bircher Muesli, No. 2, or fruit.

Nuts.

Wholewheat bread with nut butter.

COOKED DISHES:

Potatoes cooked in vegetable stock (sprinkled with a few herbs such as chives and rosemary), No. 195 D.

Lettuce.

4th day: Breakfast:

See above.

Lunch:

FRUIT

RAW VEGETABLES:

Cauliflower (with Nut Cream, Almond Cream or French dressing), chicory mixed with tomatoes, lettuce.

COOKED DISHES:

Steamed or stewed carrots with nut butter, No. 101 D.

French fried potatoes fried in nut butter, No. 218.

DESSERT:

Chestnut purée, No. 365, or vermicelli without milk; a little apple purée, No. 337 D can be added if too dry.

Evening Meal:

Bircher Muesli, No. 2, or ½ grapefruit with brown sugar.

Wholewheat bread or soya noodles with fresh nut butter.

Tomato salad.

An herb tea.

5th day: Breakfast:

See above.

Lunch:

FRUIT

RAW VEGETABLES:

Celery or celeriac (with Nut Cream, Almond Cream or French dressing), spinach, lettuce.

COOKED DISHES:

Vegetable stock, No. 51 D, with bread cubes fried in nut butter.

Steamed or stewed fennel with nut butter, No. 108 D.

Millet, cooked with diced carrots and nut butter, as in No. 248 D.

Evening Meal:

Bircher Muesli, No. 2, with nuts or fruit.

Wholewheat bread.

COOKED DISHES:

Boiled potatoes with herb-nut butter.

Radishes and lettuce.

Instead of a herb tea, apple juice or a mineral water, such as Perrier, may be served.

6th day: *Breakfast:*

See above.

Lunch:

FRUIT

RAW VEGETABLES:

Long or round large radishes (with Nut Cream, Almond Cream or French dressing).

Zucchini, lettuce.

COOKED DISHES:

Chopped spinach with nut butter (recipe as for light diets without cheese), No. 97 D.

Swiss fried potatoes with nut butter, No. 213.

DESSERT:

Black-currant jelly as No. 336 D.

Evening Meal:

Bircher Muesli, No. 2, with nuts or fruit.

Wholewheat bread.

COOKED DISHES:

Minestra with rice and nut butter, No. 95 D.

An herb tea.

7th day: *Breakfast:*

See above.

Lunch:

FRUIT

RAW VEGETABLES:

Carrots, cress, lettuce.

COOKED DISHES:

Browned wholewheat soup with nut butter, No. 78.

Brussels sprouts with nut butter, No. 155.

Rice shape, No. 234 D, with tomato sauce, No. 304, without cream.

Evening Meal:
Bircher Muesli, No. 2, and nuts.
Wholewheat bread with nut butter and rose hip jam,
   or honey.
Fruit, dried fruit.

12. DIABETIC DIET WITH WEEKLY PLAN

The best permanent type of diet for the diabetic should be
of a somewhat frugal nature, with particular emphasis on raw
plant food (i.e. raw vegetables, specially green ones, and fresh
fruit). Every diabetic must replace white bread by the more
beneficial, satisfying and more easily tolerated wholewheat
bread and crushed whole cereal dishes. Double the quantity
of wholewheat bread may be eaten and yet the number of carbohydrates remains the same. The carbohydrates in green
vegetables and fresh fruit are better utilized than those in
cereal dishes, particularly those which are made from white
bread and refined sugar.

There are many cases of diabetes in which reduction of
protein intake leads to a permanent marked improvement in
metabolism. It is just such cases which will derive the greater
benefit from the Bircher diet. Individual Raw Food Days, periods of Raw Food Days, or a permanet diet containing abundant quantities of raw food and vegetables, may produce
excellent results in diabetic conditions, with improved carbohydrate tolerance and a reduction in the quantity of insulin
required—if indeed any insulin at all is still needed in severe
cases.

Simultaneously, the development of arteriosclerosis and
high blood pressure is checked, a condition which is often encouraged by diabetic metabolism and the usual diabetic diet,
which is often so rich in animal fats. On the other hand, the
carbohydrate content of friut and vegetables need be considered only in severe cases, or if large quantities are eaten.
Legumes and root vegetables (i.e. celery or celeriac, large and
small radishes, salsify) should only be eaten in moderate
quantities, and carrots, beetroot, and kohlrabi only as an occasional exception. Small quantities of Jerusalem and Chinese
artichokes (stachys) are permitted, and little or no sweet
fruit, according to the individual case (sweet pears, cherries,
plums, greengages, grapes, fresh figs, bananas, chestnuts and
peanuts). Best of all are tart apples, berries and especially
citrus fruits (oranges and grapefruit), whose high alkali
content (sodium citrate and sodium salts) greatly promotes

the increase of alkaline reserve in the blood and, as experience has shown us, also checks diabetic coma.

As a general rule—applicable to all diabetics—keep the diet frugal. In times of war and famine there are considerably fewer cases of diabetes.

We do not recommend the use of saccharin: being a substance foreign to the body, it may lead to disturbances.

WEEKLY PLAN FOR A DIET FOR MILD CASES OF DIABETES

In moderately severe and severe cases, every item of diet must be prescribed by the physician.

1st day: Breakfast:

The same every day.

Bircher Muesli, made of tart apples or grapefruit. Cream, Nut Cream, Almond Cream or yogurt should be used instead of condensed milk (the latter can be used if unsweetened), see Recipe No. 4.

Small quantity of rolled oats can be left out if not permitted. Avoid fruit such as bananas, grapes, peaches, sweet apples, tangerines, sweet berries.

1 slice wholewheat bread or Ryvita with butter.

Walnuts, almonds and filberts as desired.

An herb tea without sugar (p. 219).

Lunch:

FRUIT:

Oranges, grapefruit, currants, blueberries (without sugar), apricots, damsons, plums, tart apples, nuts.

RAW VEGETABLES (Large portions):

Cauliflower with cream, lemon juice and herbs, tomatoes and lettuce with French dressing (see Recipe No. 8).

COOKED DISHES:

Vegetable soup, No. 86 D.

Lettuce and zucchini, No. 137 D, sautéed or stewed, No. 138, with cream, one potato in its skin if allowed, or Jerusalem artichoke, No. 128 D.

If the patient is thirsty, 1 glass alkaline mineral water, or apple juice.

Evening Meal:

Bircher Muesli with Nut Cream, Almond Cream or cream, without honey or sugar.

Lettuce.
Salsify (raw) with cream, lemon juice and herbs.
1 slice wholewheat bread, if permitted.
Nuts.
Butter.
Cheese.
An unsweetened herb tea or vegetable broth, No.
51 D.

2nd day: Breakfast:
See above.
Lunch:
FRUIT:
Non-sweet or tart fruit, nuts.
RAW VEGETABLES (large portions):
Long or round large radishes (with cream, lemon
juice and chives), zucchini, with mayonnaise and
herbs, lettuce (with French dressing).
COOKED DISHES:
Tomato soup, perhaps a small quantity of potatoes
for thickening instead of flour, No. 80 D.
Spinach, Nos. 97 D–100 D.
Steamed cauliflower with butter and cream, No. 153.
Small portion whole rice with cheese, No. 224.
Evening Meal:
Same as above, with other raw salads (no carrots or
beetroot).
Cheese.

3rd. day: Breakfast and Evening Meal:
See above.
Lunch:
Tart fruit and nuts.
RAW VEGETABLES:
Celery or celeriac with cream dressing, cucumber
with mayonnaise, lettuce with French dressing.
COOKED DISHES:
Steamed cabbage, N. 156.
Stalks of spinach beet with cheese, No. 105 D.
1–2 baked potatoes, No. 192 D.
DESSERT:
Whipped cream with tart fruit without sugar.

4th day: Breakfast and Evening Meal:
See above.

322

Lunch:
Tart fruit and nuts.
RAW VEGETABLES (large portions):
Fennel with cream dressing, tomatoes, lettuce, endive or corn-salad (lamb's lettuce), all with French dressing.
COOKED DISHES:
Artichokes with vinaigrette, No. 148 D.
Steamed or stewed Brussels sprouts, No. 155.
Some potato snow, No. 200 D.

5*th day: Breakfast* and *Evening Meal:*
See above.
Lunch:
Tart fruit and nuts.
RAW VEGETABLES:
Salsify with cream dressing, lettuce with mayonnaise, corn-salad (lamb's lettuce) or cress with French dressing.
COOKED DISHES:
Vegetable broth, No. 51 D, with diced egg custard, No. 57.
Steamed or stewed kohlrabi, No. 163.
Tomatoes, No. 129 D.
Small quantity of soya noodles with butter and cheese, No. 258 D, using soya instead of eggs.

6*th day: Breakfast* and *Evening Meal:*
See above.
Lunch:
FRUIT:
Tart fruit.
RAW VEGETABLES (large portions):
Tomatoes with French dressing, spinach with mayonnaise, lettuce with French dressing.
COOKED DISHES:
Lentils, No. 170.
Steamed or stewed lettuce, No. 101 D.
A little potato purée, No. 201 D.

7*th day: Breakfast* and *Evening Meal:*
See above.
Lunch:
FRUIT
Tart fruit and nuts.
RAW VEGETABLES (large portions):

Celery or celeriac with cream dressing, cucumbers with mayonnaise, cress with French dressing.

COOKED DISHES:

Steamed or stewed chicory, No. 103 D.

Halved tomatoes with onions and parsley, No. 135 D.

Soya spaetzle, No. 264 D.

DESSERT:

Apricots and cream without sugar, prepared together in electric blender if available.

REFERENCES

1. Sir Robert McCarrison, *Studies of Deficiency Diseases*, London, 1922, Cantor Lectures, 1936; G. T. Wrench, *The Wheel of Health*, London, 1938; R. Bircher, *Hunsa, das Volk, das keine Krankheit kennt*, Bern, 1954; *Les Hounzas—un peuple qui ignore la maladie*, Paris, 1954.

2. Karl Hintze, *Geographie u. Geschichte der Ernaehrung*, Leipzig, 1936; S. Bommer, *Die Ernaehrung der Griechen und Roemer*, Muenchen, 1943; Dr. med. Karl Kassowitz, *Ernährung der Römer*, Oberst Georg Veit, *Heeresverpflegung der Römer*, Lexikon f. Ernährungskünde, Wien, 1926.

3. R. Bircher, *Wirtschaft u. Lebenshaltung im schweiz. Hirtenland am Ende des 18 Jhs.*, Thesis, University Zurich, 1938, and 'Beitraege zur Ernaehrungsgeschichte der Schweiz,' *Wendepunkt*, 1934; 'Geographie und Geschichte der Ernährung im Dienste der Ernährungsphysiologie,' *Hippokrates*, 1957, pp. 9, 14, 16.

4. Karl Eimer, *Zeitschrift f. Ernaehrung*, July 1933; M. Hindhede, *Gesundheit durch richtige und einfache Ernaehrung*, Leipzig, 1935; W. H. Adolph, 'Nutrition Research in China,' *J. Am. Dietet. Assoc.*, November 1946; A. G. u. Postmus S. van Veen, 'Vitamin A Deficiencies in the Netherland East Indies,' *J. Amer. Dietet. Assoc.*, August 1947; R. S. Harris, 'The Nutrition Problem of Mexico,' *J. Amer. Dietet. Assoc.*, November 1946; G. Stolzenberg, *Die Ernährung des Sportlers*, Baden-Baden, 1959.

5. Dr. G. C. M. McGonigle, Report on Stockton-on-Tees in G. T. Wrench, *The Wheel of Health*, London, 1938.

6. Kaunitz, 'Transmineralisation u. vegetar. Kost,' *Erg. d. Inn. Med. u. Kinderheilkunde*, 51, 1936; H. Eppinger, 'Ueber Rohkostbehandlung,' *Wiener Klin. Wschr.*, 1.7.38; M. Paul, 'Erfahrungen im Allgemeinkrankenhaus mit d. neuzeitlichen Ernaehrung,' *Hippokrates*, 9/38 (1938); M. Bircher-Benner, *Grundzuege der Ernaehrungstherapie auf Grund der Energetik*, Berlin, 1903; *The Nature and Organization of Food Energy*, London, 1938; 'Vegetabile Heilkost, Klin. Fortbildung,' *Neue Deutsche Klinik, Ergbd.*, I, 1933; Sir Robert McCarrison and H. M. Sinclair, *Nutrition and Health*, London, 1953; Jorian Jenks, *The Stuff Man's Made Of*, London, 1959.

7. M. Richard, *Die Heilkunst* (Muenchen), Maerz, 1952.

8. W. Kollath, *Die Ordnung unserer Nahrung*, Stuttgart, 1955.

9. W. Kollath, *Die Ordnung unserer Nahrung*, Stuttgart; A. Kouchakoff, 'Nouvelles Lois de l'Alimentation Humaine basées sur la leucocytose digestive,' *Mem. Soc. Vaudoise des Sciences naturelles*, 1937/5; A. Fleisch, *Volksernaehrung in Mangelzeiten*, Basel, 1947.

10. Kuratsune Mansanore (Klinik Mizushima), Kyushu, 'Experiment on Low Nutrition with Raw Vegetables,' *Kyushu Memoirs of Medical Sciences*, 2/1–2 June, 1951.

11. Mueller-Hesters, *Die Heilkunst*, Muenchen, Maerz, 1952.

12. A. Fleisch, *Volksernaehrung in Mangelzeiten*, Basel, 1947.

13. V.p. Dole *et. al.*, *Amer. J. Clin. Nutr.*, 1954, 2, 381.

14. C. M. McCay (Cornell), 'Chemical Aspects of Ageing and the Effects of Restricted Feeding upon Ageing and Chronic Diseases in Rats and Dogs, *Amer. J. of Public Health*, 27/5, May, 1947. For similar experiments with cattle, we note the work done by Dr. Artur Hansson, Director of the Institute for Domestic Animal Improvement at Wiad. See their *Feeding Experiments in Identical Twins*, Stockholm, 1956. More applicable results with elderly persons appears in *Zeitschrift f. Alternsforschung*, Dresden, 1968, in the article "Ernährungsverhältnisse während d. Kindheit b. langlebigen Personen," pp. 159–164, by Dr. S. Hejda of the J. Mašeks Institute for Nutritional Research of the Univ. of Prague.

15. R. Bircher, 'Perspektiven zur Eiweissfrage,' Eine Sammlung weniger beachteter Ergebnisse, *Hippokrates*, 1956/1, Jan.; W. Abelin, 'Schweiz. Med. Wschr.,' 21.3.1942—Reynolds and Beyer (Wisconsin), *J. Am. Diet. Assn.*, August, 1950; M. Kuratsune, 'Experiments on Low Nutrition with Raw Vegetables,' *Kyushu Memoirs of Medical Science*, 2/1–2 June, 1951; H. A. Schweigart, 'Der Biologische Grundeffekt von Nahrungs-proteinen,' *Diaita* 1/3, 1955; W. Schuphan, *Gemuesebau auf ernaehrungswiss. Grundlage*, Hamburg, 1939; C. M. McCay, 'Diet and Ageing,' *Vitamins and Hormones*, VII, 1939; 'Chemical Aspects of Ageing and the Effects of Restricted Feeding upon Ageing and Chronic Diseases in Rats and Dogs,' *Amer. J. of Public Health*, 27/5, May, 1947; E. S. Schmid, 'Leistungsfaehigkeit b. eiweissknapper Ernaehrung, Mitt. Lebensmitteluntersuchung u. Hygiene,' *Eidg. Gesundheitsamt Bern*, VXXIV (1933), 1/2, S.195–225; H. C. Sherman, *The Nutritional Improvement of Life*, New York, 1950; A Fleisch, *Volksernaehrung in Mangelzeiten*, Basel, 1947.

16. H. A. Schweigart and G. Quellmalz, *Diaita* 1/3, 1955.

17. C. Sherman (Cornell), *Nutritional Improvement of Life*, New York, 1950.

18. D. M. Hegsted (Harvard), *Journal of the Amer. Dietet. Association*, March, 1957, pp. 225–232.

19. Report of the Annual Congress of the American Society of Experimental Biology, 1952. Paper by Dr. Ernest Geiger (Pharmacology), University of Southern California.

20. Professor Staub, 'Einfluss der spezifisch-dynamischen Wirkung auf die Leber,' *Helvetica Medica Acta*, 17 (1950; 378).

21. Dr. med. C. D. de Langen, University of Utrecht, 'Een klinisch panorama van een teveel in de voeding,' *Genees Kundige Bladen mit Klinick en laboratorium voor de praktijk*, 48/III, Haarlem, 1957.

22. Dr. A. G. van Veen and Dr. S. Postmus, Eijkman Institute and Institute for Nutrition Research, Batavia, 'Vitamin A Deficiencies in the Netherlands East Indies,' *J. Amer. Dietet. Assoc.*, August, 1947.

23. W. Heupke and G. Rost, *Was enthalten unsere Nahrungsmittel?* Frankfurt, 1950.

24. W. Schupan, *Gemuesebau auf ernaehrungswissenschaftlicher Grundlauge*, Hamburg, 1948; W. Halden, *Vitamine Therapie u. Praxis*, II, Wien, 1949; A. Fleisch, *Volksernaehrung in Mangelzeiten*, Basel, 1947.

25. B. S. Schweigart, 'Significance of Vitamin B_{12} and Related Factors,' *J. Amer. Diet. Assoc.*, October 1950; R. Bircher, 'Das Fleisch-vitamin (B_{12}),' *Der Wendepunkt*, Maerz, 1951.

26. S. K. Kon and E. H. Mawson (1950), 'Human Milk,' *Med. Res. Coun. Spec. Red. Ser.*, No. 269; R. A. McCance and E. M. Widdowson (1946), 'The Chemical Composition of Foods,' *Med. Res. Coun. Spec. Rep. Ser.*, No. 235; F. Wokes, J. Badenoch and H. M. Sinclair (1957) paper read to Fourth International Congress of Nutrition; F. Wokes and C. Klatzkin (1949), J. Pharm, *Pharmacol*, 1, 903; F. Wokes and M. H. Woollam (1957), J. Pharm., *Pharmacol*, 9, 850.

GENERAL INDEX

INDEX OF RECIPES

The page number (in italics) is followed by the recipe number.

Some other books published by Penguin
are described on the following pages.

MODERN VEGETARIAN COOKERY

Walter and Jenny Fliess

All about modern vegetarian cooking.
From Bortsch to Lemon Soufflé, some five
hundred recipes cover soups, sauces, vegetable dishes of all kinds, uncooked meals,
juices, sandwich spreads, and desserts.
Each recipe is given in step-by-step style
so that even an inexperienced cook can
follow it, and the authors have anticipated
—and answered—the questions most
likely to arise. Their fresh and imaginative
dishes will open up new worlds for the
American cook by showing how attractive
meatless cooking can be. Born in Ger-
many, Walter and Jenny Fliess have
served more than five million meals as the
owners of restaurants on the Continent
and in England.

THE PENGUIN SALAD BOOK

*Compiled by the editors
of Sunset Books and Sunset Magazine*

A complete guide to the art of salad making. Nearly three hundred recipes cover green salads; fruit salads; vegetable salads; meat, poultry, and seafood salads; egg, cheese, rice, and pasta salads; frozen and moulded salads; and salad dressings. A few of the exciting salads you can make with this book: Spanish Salad, Avocado-Popcorn Salad, Cranberry Grape Salad, Frosted Cauliflower Salad, Coconut Crab Salad, Western Patio Salad, and Moulded Peach Salad. With photographs, a glossary, and a full index.

COOK'S QUICK REFERENCE
Essential Information on Cards

Catherine Storr

This supplement to cookbooks gives you the basic information that cooks always need. Produced in the form of cards on a spiral binding, it stands open on the table for easy reference while the cook is working from a recipe book. Topics covered include oven temperatures, roasting times, weights and measures (American, British, and Continental), sauces and roux, pastries, basic batter, and uses for extra egg yolks and whites. With a full glossary of cookbook terms. Catherine Storr is an author and former physician who finds cooking a change from her more sedentary occupations.

THE PENGUIN COOKERY BOOK

Bee Nilson

A complete cookbook containing some 850 basic recipes for all sorts of dishes from soups to desserts. The book is fully indexed and cross-referenced, and the recipes are given both in metric measures and in pounds and ounces. There are also diagrams to assist in buying the different cuts of meat and in preparing fish; a glossary of French terms often used in cooking; and helpful advice on kitchen equipment, food values, cooking time, temperatures, and how much food to buy for how many people. Bee Nilson is a British nutrition expert.